AN ILLUSTRATED ENCYCLOPAEDIA OF
BRITISH POTTERY AND PORCELAIN

Geoffrey A. Godden F.R.S.A.

SECOND EDITION

Barrie & Jenkins
London Melbourne Sydney Auckland Johannesburg

Barrie & Jenkins Ltd

An imprint of the Hutchinson Publishing Group

17–21 Conway Street, London W1P 6JD

Hutchinson Group (Australia) Pty Ltd
30–32 Cremorne Street, Richmond South, Victoria 3121
PO Box 151, Broadway, New South Wales 2007

Hutchinson Group (NZ) Ltd
32–34 View Road, PO Box 40–086, Glenfield, Auckland 10

Hutchinson Group (SA) (Pty) Ltd
PO Box 337, Bergvlei 2012, South Africa

First published in 1966 by Herbert Jenkins Ltd
Reprinted in 1968, 1970 and 1977 by Barrie & Jenkins Ltd
This edition published in 1980
Reprinted in 1982

Printed in Great Britain by
Ebenezer Baylis & Son Ltd
The Trinity Press, Worcester and London
and bound by Wm Brendon & Son Ltd, Tiptree, Essex

ISBN 0 214 20692 0

Contents

This book was planned as a pictorial companion to the *Encyclopaedia of British Pottery and Porcelain Marks*, and the original intention was to confine it to illustrations of key *marked* specimens of English pottery and porcelain from *c.* 1650 to 1900 so that the collector could see the type of wares that bore the marks reproduced in the *Encyclopaedia of Marks*.

As the preparation of the book progressed it appeared advisable to widen its scope to include groups of unmarked wares, the origin of which can be incontestably proved by reference to surviving factory pattern books, and also typical specimens of those classes of pottery which are not found with marks such as tortoiseshell glazes, Jackfield and salt-glazed wares. Illustrations of wasters from factory sites have also been included, together with illustrations from old advertisements, trade cards, etc.

The resulting selection illustrates over two thousand documentary examples of English ceramic art, so that this book, which is virtually an illustrated encyclopaedia of marked specimens, cannot only be used in conjunction with the *Encyclopaedia of British Pottery and Porcelain Marks* but it can be equally useful as a companion to the new revised 15th edition of Chaffer's *Marks and Monograms* . . . or to any other mark book and also to all general ceramic reference books from such nineteenth-century classics as Jewitt's *Ceramic Art of Great Britain* to such modern works as *English Porcelain 1745–1850*, edited by R. J. Charleston (1965). It is also hoped that future authors will be helped by the many illustrations to which they can refer.

In order to assist the beginner characteristics which are usually described in words are here illustrated—pad marks on Derby figures and vases, stilt marks under Chelsea plates and dishes, typical bases of early Chelsea wares with incised triangle marks, workmen's marks on the inside of a Lowestoft foot-rim, etc. The reader is also referred to specialized reference books so that he can delve deeper into the subject of his choice. An outline history of the different types of ware is included in the summary (pages xi–xxvi) and historical details of the major manufacturers is given at the beginning of the relevant sections.

This work foreshadows several new reference books which promise to add much to our knowledge of early nineteenth-century wares. Recent excavations on the site of the Caughley factory in Shropshire have, for instance, shed much light on the later Caughley porcelains and on the early hitherto unidentified Coalport porcelains (Plates 160–2). Plates 403–5 showing drawings from Messrs Mintons early design books (with porcelains matching these pattern books illustrated in Plate 406 and Colour Plate VIII) will surprise many collectors as these wares have hitherto been attributed to Coalport or Coalbrookdale or to one of the other fashionable factories. Early Ridgway porcelain can also be identified from the original pattern book pages reproduced.

Every effort has been made to show prosaic as well as rare specimens; late wares as well as early. It is perhaps difficult to enthuse over some of the objects depicted in the late nineteenth-century advertisements illustrated but my aim has been to show a full range of typical identifiable and datable objects of the 1650–1900 period. Unmarked specimens can be usually identified by referring to these marked key specimens or the designs from factory pattern books.

Numbers given in brackets refer to the mark in the companion *Encyclopaedia of British Pottery and Porcelain Marks* (1964).

Acknowledgements

I am most grateful to the following Antique Dealers, Auctioneers, Librarians, Manufacturers, Museum Curators, and Private Collectors who have permitted examples in their ownership or care to be photographed for inclusion in this book. In the case of objects credited to auctioneers and dealers it must be understood that such a credit is a courtesy one for supplying the photographs and that the objects depicted are now in the possession of new owners:

Messrs Albert Amor Ltd, London
Messrs Ayer & Co (Antiques) Ltd, London
Miss M. A. Beasley
I. M. Booth, Esq.
Mr and Mrs J. F. Breeze
Brighton Museum & Art Gallery
Bristol City Art Gallery
British Museum, London
Cambridge, Fitzwilliam Museum
Cardiff, National Museum of Wales
Chanctonbury Gallery, Washington, Sussex
Messrs Christie, Manson & Woods Ltd, London
Mr and Mrs Coke-Steel
Messrs W. T. Copeland & Sons Ltd, Stoke
Major G. N. Dawnay, Cardiff
Messrs Delomosne & Son Ltd, London
Derby, Museum & Art Gallery
Messrs Doulton & Co Ltd, London
Dublin, National Museum of Ireland
Edinburgh, Royal Scottish Museum
S. W. Fisher, Esq., Bewdley
Fredericton (Canada), The Beaverbrook Art Gallery
Glasgow, Museums & Art Gallery
L. Godden, Esq.
Messrs Godden of Worthing, Suppliers to the Trade only
Messrs W. F. Greenwood & Sons Ltd, York and Harrogate
Mr and Mrs Derek Harper
Hereford, Museum & Art Gallery
Ipswich Museum
Leeds, City Art Gallery & Museums
Messrs E. W. J. Legg, Dorchester

Lincoln, Museum & Art Gallery
Liverpool Museums
Messrs D. M. & P. Manheim, London and New York
Messrs Marshall Field & Company, Chicago
Mrs F. Nagington
Newark (New Jersey) Museum
Newcastle upon Tyne, Laing Art Gallery
Norwich, Castle Museum
Nottingham, Museum & Art Gallery
Messrs R. H. & S. L. Plant Ltd, Longton
Plymouth, Museum & Art Gallery
Rotherham, Museum & Art Gallery
Shoreham (Sussex), Marlipins Museum
Messrs Sotheby & Co, London
Southall Public Libraries
Stoke, City Art Gallery & Museum
W. Ramsey Strachan, Esq.
E. N. Stretton, Esq.
Sunderland, Museum & Art Gallery
Sussex Archaeological Society Museum, Lewes
Swansea, Royal Institution of South Wales
Messrs Tilley & Co (Antiques) Ltd, London
Toronto, Royal Ontario Museum (University of Toronto)
Messrs Trevor-Antiques of Brighton
Ulster Museum, Belfast
Messrs J. & E. D. Vandekar, London
Victoria & Albert Museum, London (Crown Copyright)
Washington (D.C.), Smithsonian Institution
Dr B. Watney
Messrs Josiah Wedgwood & Sons Ltd, Barlaston, Stoke

Messrs Wenger Ltd, Etruria, Stoke   Worthing Museum & Art Gallery
Messrs Worcester Royal Porcelain Co Ltd   Yarmouth Museum

Illustrations from old pattern books, advertisements, trade cards, etc., have either been copied from contemporary magazines or kindly supplied by the following firms and museum authorities:

Bodleian Library, Oxford   Messrs Mintons Ltd, Stoke
Messrs Coalport China Ltd, Stoke   Patent Office Design Registry
Messrs T. G. Green & Co Ltd, Church   Victoria & Albert Museum, London
    Gresley   Messrs Worcester Royal Porcelain Co Ltd

My special thanks are due to C. H. Canning, Esq., of the Photographic Department of the Victoria & Albert Museum for his assistance in photographing the many groups of wares from this source and to Derek Gardiner, A.I.B.P., of Messrs Walter Gardiner of Worthing for his painstaking work in arranging the many complicated selections of services from the stock of Messrs Godden of Worthing and of individual pieces from my own collection. The colour plates are also the work of the above photographers.

Illustrations without acknowledgement depict specimens from my own collection.

Finally, I must acknowledge my indebtedness and offer sincere thanks to Arthur Barker Ltd for permission to quote herein passages from my book *British Pottery and Porcelain, 1780–1850* (published in the United States by A. S. Barnes & Co Inc) to which the reader is referred for more detailed information about the period indicated.

Geoffrey A. Godden, 17–19 Crescent Road,
Worthing, W. Sussex, England

The main pictorial section of this encyclopaedia is arranged in alphabetical sequence to correspond with the arrangement of the companion *Encyclopaedia of British Pottery and Porcelain Marks*, and in order that the productions of any manufacturer may be found on consulting the relevant section without recourse to an index. It therefore follows that the illustrations are not necessarily in date order.

The following notes give a chronological summary of the development of British ceramics and describe the many different bodies or styles of decoration used. This section will also be found to serve as a useful glossary of the terms used in the captions to the illustrations.

This volume deals with the period from 1650 to 1900. Up to the middle of the seventeenth century little or no pottery bore potters' marks. Utilitarian wares were made in several localities by potters using local clays. Decoration, if used at all, was of the simplest and consisted of raised lines, stamped designs, applied motifs, in the same or contrasting colours, patches of coloured glaze, etc. Typical specimens can be seen at the London Museum at Kensington Palace.

"DELFT" WARES *Plates 206–7, 323, 445, 554, 628–9.*

Various methods were employed to make the clay coloured wares more pretentious. One such method was to coat the clay body with opaque or white glaze containing tin, thus giving the outward appearance of a white-bodied article. The technique was an ancient one introduced into Europe from Asia by way of Spain and Italy. English wares of this type are now named after the Dutch pottery centre at Delft, but some early English wares pre-date the Dutch. The word Delft is spelt with a capital "D" when applied to the ware made in Holland, but with a small "d" when it refers to that made in England.

The charm of English delft lies in the vigorous, free, spontaneous style of the painted decoration necessitated by the fact that it had to be applied quickly to the absorbent tin glaze. Blue was the most usual colour, but green, red, brown, yellow, and purple were also used. The main centres of British delft ware manufacture were at Lambeth and Southwark in London, Bristol, Dublin Glasgow, Limerick, Liverpool, and Wincanton. Delft-type tin-glazed pottery very seldom bears a potter's name or mark. Rare documentary specimens are illustrated (see heading) and good dated examples are preserved in the London Museum and at the Victoria & Albert Museum. For the classification of delft wares the reader is referred to *English Delftware* by F. H. Garner (1948).

The nature of the delft-type pottery—a soft clay core coated with a thin opaque tin glaze—makes it extremely susceptible to damage. Edges are normally chipped, exposing the underlying clay body. It was this fragile nature of the ware that led to the decline of the delft potteries in the second half of the eighteenth century when the creamware body (see page xv) which was both new and more stable was introduced.

STONEWARES *Plates 26, 78, 245–51, 295, 331, 375, 446, 448–51, 466, 553.*

The delft wares mentioned previously were low-fired earthenwares which were relatively soft and porous where not protected by glaze.

Various types of clay become vitrified when fired at a very high temperature (about 1300°C.).

The resultant wares, termed Stonewares, are impervious to liquids, strong and resilient. Naturally the process of firing these wares presents its problems, both in the manufacture of the kiln and in the control of the ware at great heats.

A patent was taken out by Thomas Rius and Abraham Cullyn in October 1626 for the "sole making of the Stone Pott, Stone jugg. . . ." In April 1671 John Dwight was granted a patent to make "transparent earthenware . . . as alsoe the misterie of the stoneware, vulgarly called Cologne ware. . . ." This was obviously an attempt to imitate the German stonewares, best known in the form of jugs with mask lips. In a later patent of 1684 John Dwight mentioned "Severall new manufactures of earthenware, called by the names of white gorges, marbled porcellane, vessells, statues and figures, and fine stone gorges and vessells, never before made in England. . . ." Stone-wares made by Dwight at Fulham in London are to be seen in the British Museum and in the Victoria & Albert Museum. The figures include a portrait bust of Lydia Dwight who died in 1673.

In 1693 John Dwight sought to protect his patent rights against those potters who were presum-ably producing stoneware in London, Southampton, Nottingham, and Staffordshire. The reader is referred to the 15th edition of Chaffer's *Marks and Monograms* (1965) for further details of Dwight's career and for several quotations from his, now lost, working records.

An advertisement notice issued by James Morley of Nottingham *c.* 1700 is illustrated in Plate 447. Wares matching the advertisement are shown in Plates 448-9. Other stonewares bearing the place-name Nottingham are illustrated in Plates 450-1. The Nottingham district was one of the main centres of clay coloured stoneware, which was produced well into the middle of the nine-teenth century. Dates in the 1820's and 1830's often occur on specimens which would otherwise be taken for eighteenth-century examples. Several Bristol and London potteries made stonewares, but specimens are seldom marked (see Plates 331, 446) until the second half of the nineteenth century when firms such as Doultons, J. Stiff, and C. J. C. Bailey popularized "Art Stonewares" (see Plates 26, 245-51, 553).

Early in the nineteenth century stoneware was widely used in the manufacture of moulded bottles or flasks, often depicting notable people or events. The Martin Brothers, working in London from 1873 to 1914, produced individual hand-carved and decorated stonewares (see Plates 374-8) and started a tradition of "Studio Pottery" which still gains strength from year to year.

SLIP DECORATED WARES *Plates 30, 274, 318-21, 370, 464, 473, 516-17, 519, 572-3, 577-9.*

A traditional method of decorating pottery was to trail designs in contrasting coloured slip (the name for clay, tinted or not, diluted to the consistency of cream) on to the ware, in the same manner as one would decorate an iced cake. The early slip decorated utilitarian objects were not marked, but in the seventeenth century more ambitious, decorative, or presentation pieces were attempted and these specimens sometimes bear a date, but rarely the initials or name of the maker.

One of the earliest centres for such slip decorated pottery was at Wrotham in Kent. Examples bearing dates from 1621 to 1678 are illustrated in Plates 318-21. These pieces bear initials recurring on several specimens. Mr A. J. B. Kiddell, in a paper in the *Transactions of the English Ceramic Circle*, vol. 3, part 2, has linked many of these initials with Wrotham potters of the period.

Selections of wares attributed to N. Hubble, H. Ifield, T. Ifield, and G. Richardson are illustrated in Plates 318–21, 473.

Although slip decorated pottery was undoubtedly made by most potters, the only documentary signed seventeenth-century specimens originate from Wrotham and the Staffordshire Potteries. In 1686, Dr Plot in his *Natural History of Staffordshire* described slip which would "run out through a quill . . . and is a substance wherewith they paint their wares". As with the Wrotham slip wares, some Staffordshire examples bear initials or names which are attributed to the maker of the object, although these initials or names are prominently displayed on the top or decorative side of the object, rather than underneath where later potters placed their marks.

Staffordshire slip decorated wares by J. Glass, Samuel Malkin, R. Pool, R. Simpson, James Toft, Ralph Toft, and Thomas Toft are illustrated in Plates 274, 370, 464, 516–17, 577–9. Some most effective dishes, etc., have trailed lines of dark slip on a lighter ground, or vice versa, which are "combed" through to give a decorative zigzag effect (see Plate 30).

Slip decorated earthenware has a simple charm of its own and signed and dated examples are keenly sought after and are rarely found in perfect condition. As more pretentious earthenwares came into fashion in the eighteenth century, so the demand for thickly potted slip decorated wares waned. Some country potters, however, continued to use this method and some modern potters still keep up the tradition.

A paper, "Thomas Toft and Associated Slip Ware Potters", by Ronald Cooper, is printed in the *Transactions of the English Ceramic Circle*, vol. 6, part 1.

SGRAFFIATO *Plate 92.*

In the slip decorated wares discussed above the contrasting design was obtained by applying coloured clay in semi-liquid form. With sgraffiato the design is obtained by cutting away part of an overlaying coating to expose a contrasting colour below. While some potters decorated their products with a combination of slip decoration and sgraffiato, others, particularly in the West Country, confined themselves to the sgraffiato technique. A typical specimen of West Country sgraffiato ware is illustrated in Plate 92. Some pieces decorated in this traditional style appear to be earlier than the date found upon them.

RED WARE *Plates 16–17.*

Unglazed red pottery, often with applied relief motifs, is generally known as Elers ware. David and John Elers from Holland settled in London in the 1680's. In 1693 they were cited, with other potters, for infringing John Dwight's patent (see page xii). At this period the two Elers brothers were potting at Vauxhall, on the Surrey side of the Thames, where according to contemporary accounts there was clay for making "all sorts of tea pots". In 1700 the Elers were declared bankrupt and probably soon afterwards left the country.

Prior to the bankruptcy and probably about 1693 a branch factory was established in Staffordshire, but according to Celia Fienners, who sought to visit the works in 1698, the supply of suitable clay had by then run out. Most red wares associated with Elers name are teapots; these were copied from Chinese or Japanese pots of the period and the Eastern seal marks were often imitated.

Josiah Wedgwood, in a letter written in 1777, lists the improvements made by the Elers brothers.

After mentioning salt-glazing and the introduction of ground flint, he continued: "The next improvement introduced by Mr E. was the refining of our common red clay by sifting, and making it into Tea and Coffee ware in imitation of the Chinese Red Porcelaine, by casting it in plaster moulds, and turning it on the outside upon Lathes, and ornamenting it with the Tea branch in relief, in imitation of the Chinese manner of ornamenting this ware".

Apart from the Elers, many other Staffordshire potters made similar red wares, mostly tea and coffee pots, and these constitute the finest ceramic productions of the period. The pots are finely turned, of pleasing proportions and are usually decorated in relief with Chinese or Japanese motifs such as prunus blossom, Chinese figures, etc. The production of red ware was continued up to the second half of the eighteenth century. Some examples were glazed (see Plate 431), but the majority of specimens were unglazed. After the introduction of engine turning, c. 1765, much red ware was decorated by this method (see Plate 17). Very few examples bear a maker's mark. Further information on red ware is given in a paper by R. Rice in the *Transactions of the English Ceramic Circle*, vol. 4, part V.

JACKFIELD WARES   *Plate 324.*

The so-called Jackfield wares are composed of a red clay body entirely covered with a very glossy black glaze. Many specimens were decorated with gilding, but today only traces of this usually remain. Specimens may be decorated with raised motifs like the red ware. Other "Jackfield" objects depend on their graceful form for appeal.

The term "Jackfield" is a generic one. Early ceramic writers suggested that all such wares were made at Jackfield in Shropshire which is on the opposite side of the River Severn to Coalport, but site excavations have shown that several Staffordshire potteries made Jackfield-type black glazed wares and many Staffordshire factory wasters can be seen in the Stoke Museum & Art Gallery.

Several authorities have cited a reference of 1560 to potters "from Jackfield" to show that the pottery industry at the Shropshire Jackfield was of long duration. They have omitted to note, however, that Jackfield is also the name of an estate at Burslem in the heart of the Staffordshire Potteries. So this oft-quoted reference may not therefore refer to the Shropshire Jackfield at all.

Black glazed "Jackfield"-type wares are unmarked and were in the main produced in the 1740 to 1780 period.

SALT-GLAZE WARES   *Plates 245A–51, 375, 508–9.*

Much clay coloured stoneware made in London, Bristol, Nottingham, and other centres was glazed by salt, but the term "salt glazed" is normally reserved for a white or very pale stoneware which was glazed in this manner.

The method of glazing was to fire the unglazed ware in the kiln. When the kiln and its contents reached their maximum heat, salt was thrown in, the heat caused the salt to decompose, forming sodium oxide and hydrochloric acid which settled on the hot ware and, combined with the alumina and silica in the clay, formed a hard glaze, the surface of which is pitted and can be likened to orange-peel in appearance.

The introduction of the standard Staffordshire whitish salt-glazed stoneware body made from Devonshire clay and calcined flints is traditionally ascribed to John Astbury of Shelton who died in 1743. The body quickly became the standard one of the district as it could be moulded into intricate forms, turned to a thin gauge, and was suitable both in price and in appearance for utilitarian objects—teapots, bowls, plates, etc., as well as more pretentious objects, such as figures.

Much utilitarian salt-glaze was sold in the undecorated state, relying for its appeal on its shape or moulded design. Other salt-glaze ware was finely decorated with overglaze enamels. In some instances different coloured clays were mixed together, giving an agate-like effect. A representative selection of eighteenth-century Staffordshire salt-glaze objects is shown in Plates 508–9. Unfortunately Staffordshire salt-glaze pottery does not bear a maker's name, but documents have recently been discovered which promise to shed much light on the makers of salt-glaze stoneware in the Staffordshire Potteries. Staffordshire salt-glaze was mainly produced between 1730 and 1770 when it was superseded by the creamware with its warm tint and smooth surface and glaze. During the transition period some potters made use of their old salt-glaze moulds to make the same objects in the new creamware.

SCRATCH BLUE *Plates 62, 509.*

A variation of the sgraffiato technique is called "Scratch Blue", although it may occasionally occur in colours other than blue. With scratch blue designs, which normally occur on whitish salt-glaze stoneware, the design was incised into the semi-soft unfired clay and blue pigment was then rubbed into the incisions. For simple floral designs this technique was most effective and inexpensive to produce.

As the eighteenth century progressed and salt-glaze wares were superseded by creamwares, the manufacture of scratch blue form of decoration ceased. In the 1870's it was reintroduced on Doulton stonewares, notably in Hannah Barlow's animal studies (see Plate 248). At Doulton the pigment was normally black or brown, but the technique was the same as the seventeenth-century Staffordshire scratch blue wares.

CREAMWARE (QUEENSWARE) *Plates 3–5, 59, 63, 191–2, 238–9, 334–5, 607–8, 634.*

The discovery of creamware or cream-coloured earthenware is generally credited to Thomas Astbury between 1720 and 1740. Light coloured clays imported from Devonshire were used with calcined flints. About 1740 Enoch Booth introduced a fluid glaze, an innovation that did much to establish creamware as the standard earthenware body for the ensuing hundred years. The creamware bowl illustrated in Plate 63 is one of the earliest examples so far discovered; it is inscribed E.B. 1743, the initials probably relating to the above-mentioned potter Enoch Booth.

During the 1740–60 period, the creamware body and its glazes were refined and improved mainly by Josiah Wedgwood who was one of the leading producers of creamware. The Royal patronage that it gained for him did much to increase the popularity of creamware and gave rise to its name "Queensware". In 1767 Wedgwood wrote to his partner Bentley: ". . . The demand for this said cream colour, alias Queensware, alias Ivory still increases. It is really amazing how rapidly the use of it has spread almost over the whole globe, and how universally it is liked. . . ."

The refined lightweight creamware which lent itself to various forms of decoration as well as being highly attractive in its undecorated state, certainly did sweep the markets and caused many Continental potters to either imitate the new English ware or go out of business. Apart from the

Staffordshire potters, creamware was made by most other potters of the period and examples bearing the marks of Birch & Whitehead, Cockpit Hill Works (Derby), Davenports, J. Heath, Hollins, Indeo Pottery (Devon), Lakin & Poole, Leeds Pottery, Neale & Co, Ring & Co (Bristol), Shorthose & Co, Swansea, Turner, J. Warburton (Newcastle upon Tyne), Wedgwood & Co, Josiah Wedgwood, and Enoch Wood are here illustrated.

The better quality creamwares often bear makers' marks, but the majority of the low-priced utilitarian wares are unmarked. The selling price of a hundred-and-eighty-three piece set of "best" Queensware in 1812 was £4 4s., with a blue edge the cost was increased to £5 15s. 6d., and these low prices will indicate the competitive state of the market at this period.

The standard modern reference book is *English Cream-coloured Earthenware* by Donald C. Towner. In the introduction Mr Towner aptly sums up the claims of creamware "with its fine form, thin body, clean and brilliant glaze which formed a perfect background for the ingenious, harmonious and free painting of the earthenware enamellers of that time. It was the prototype of the lead-glazed earthenware that is manufactured today. . . . At its best it did not seek to imitate porcelain either in colour, form or decoration, but remained essentially true to its English earthenware tradition. . . ."

The enamelled decoration on creamware is restrained and often comprises tasteful border designs only. Several firms flourished by printing, or otherwise decorating, creamwares made by other potters. Messrs Sadler & Green of Liverpool printed creamwares for Wedgwood as early as 1771 (see Plate 603). Other outside printed wares are shown in Plates 1, 20, 46, 268.

TORTOISESHELL & WHIELDON WARE *Plates 580–1.*

Much cream-coloured earthenware was enriched with semi-translucent coloured glazes. That known as tortoiseshell is decorated with mottled patterns in blue, green, and brown tints derived from the oxides of cobalt, copper, and manganese. Typical specimens are shown in Plates 580–1. Most commercial earthenware factories of the 1740–80 period produced this type of ware, but examples are normally unmarked. The reason for the name tortoiseshell is self-evident.

Figures and groups decorated with semi-translucent coloured glazes are usually attributed to Thomas Whieldon and the term "Whieldon ware" covers most early or mid-eighteenth-century objects decorated with these pleasing liquid colours. In fact, most of the leading potters produced similar wares which were, in the main, unmarked. These semi-translucent glaze colours were replaced about 1780 by opaque overglaze enamel colours lacking the warm charm of the earlier tints.

AGATE, MARBLED, PORPHYRY, MOCHA, ETC., WARES
Plates 260, 296, 600, 601.

From about 1740 potters intermingled white and coloured clays to form a decorative effect or to emulate natural stones and the early specimens, which might be glazed with either salt- or lead-glaze, were unmarked.

Josiah Wedgwood carried out many experiments to perfect these bodies and the results may bear the Wedgwood mark or that of the Wedgwood & Bentley partnership (1769–80). In letters of 1769 Wedgwood mentions Blue Pebble, Variegated Pebble, Marbled vases (see Plates 600–1), but in March 1774 he wrote to Bentley in London: "The Agate, the Green and other coloured glazes have had their day, and done pretty well. . . ."

Several firms, however, continued to produce earthenware in imitation of agates or marbles, sometimes with the addition of inlaid diced borders. The Leeds factory pattern books show this type of ware.

Mocha decoration is rather similar to marbling except that the tree-like design is formed by the chemical reaction of a dark acid colourant on a pale tinted alkaline slip. Mocha decorated wares are usually utilitarian, mugs and jugs outnumbering all other objects. The style was used by several potters late in the eighteenth century and continued through the nineteenth and into the twentieth century. See Plate 342 for a Leeds pattern book example of c. 1800, and Plates 260, 296 for later specimens. Further details of the Mocha technique are given in *British Pottery and Porcelain 1780–1850* (1963).

PORCELAIN

The distinguishing feature of porcelain is that it is translucent as opposed to earthenware which is opaque, although it is true that vitrified stonewares can be slightly translucent when very thinly potted.

The manufacture of porcelain was not successfully accomplished in England until the mid 1740's. The first essays were made at Bow and Chelsea in London, but within a few years porcelain was being produced at Bristol, Derby, Longton Hall (in Staffordshire), and Worcester and in the 1750's factories were established at Liverpool and Lowestoft. The historic details of these, together with the later porcelain factories, are given in the appropriate places in the main illustrated section. There is one exception to this—the Liverpool factories did not mark their wares and are not therefore included in this volume. For up-to-date information on the several Liverpool potteries the reader is referred to B. Watney's *English Blue and White Porcelain of the 18th century* (1963), or the same author's contribution to *English Porcelain 1745–1850* (1965).

English porcelain is of two main types—hard-paste and soft-paste—and it is absolutely essential that the student of ceramics should be able to differentiate between the two.

Hard-paste porcelain is analogous to that produced in China and in most Continental factories. It is made from a mixture of china clay (kaolin) and china rock (petunse), is resistant to a file and shows a conchoidal or shell-like fracture similar to the surface of a knapped flint. Hard-paste porcelain is glazed with a preparation of petunse and the body and the glaze are fired at a high temperature, usually in one operation.

Expressed in the simplest terms English soft-paste or artificial porcelain was originally ground glass stiffened with white clay to give the mixture stability. It can be marked by a file and when chipped the body is granular. It must be fired in an unglazed state and then re-fired at a lower temperature after glazing. Further firings at successively lower temperatures are necessary to fix the overglaze enamel decoration and gilding. The soft-paste body has been improved from time to time by the addition of other substances, notably soap-rock, bone ash, and feldspar.

Soon after 1790 Spode introduced a refined bone china body that was compact, capable of being thinly turned or moulded and which formed an admirable ground for added decoration. This body soon became standard amongst the leading manufacturers and remains so down to the present day. Plates 77, 393 and Colour Plate I illustrate early nineteenth-century bone china bearing the marks of little known Staffordshire manufacturers. Many other illustrations show typical English bone china made by the better known firms.

About 1820 several potters experimented with the addition of feldspar to their bodies and glazes. John Rose of Coalport was awarded the Society of Arts Gold Medal for a new feldspathic glaze in May 1820, and the fact was recorded in several marks used at the time by this factory (see pages 91, 99 and Plates 167, 168A). At the same period Spode produced a pleasing feldspar porcelain for which a special mark was used. Feldspar was later used as the main constituent of the parian body. It will be observed that the name Feldspar was spelt in various ways on marks—"Feltspar" at Coalport, "Felspar" by Spode.

Of the English porcelains those produced at Plymouth between 1768 and 1770 and at Bristol between 1770 and 1781 are hard-paste and all others are soft-paste. It is true, however, that the New Hall Company did, between 1781 and 1812, make a type of hard-paste but this was fired at a lower temperature than the real hard-paste and for this reason shows none of the flaws associated with the Plymouth and Bristol productions nor has it a conchoidal appearance in fracture. Owing to the much higher temperature at which they were fired it is usual to find in the porcelains of Plymouth and Bristol distortion of the body, slight tears, spiral wreathing (see Plate 88), and slight staining.

Many reproductions of English eighteenth-century soft-paste porcelains were made on the Continent during the nineteenth century, but as these copies are invariably made in hard-paste they are not likely to deceive the experienced collector (see Plates 678-9 and chapter 12 of *British Pottery and Porcelain 1780-1850* (1963)).

BLUE AND WHITE   *Plates 7, 36, 63, 80, 95-9, 129, 190, 243, 357-8, 524, 536, 646.*

The term "blue and white" is used to denote porcelain or other ware decorated in blue under the glaze. The blue pigment which was derived from cobalt was able to stand the high temperature at which the porcelain body was fired. Overglaze enamel colours are applied after glazing and can therefore be fired at a much lower temperature.

The blue decoration was protected from wear by the covering glaze and most blue and white objects are of a useful nature. Purely decorative objects on the other hand were normally decorated with overglaze enamels. Although the ease of manufacture made blue and white popular with the manufacturers, its greatest appeal was probably in its similarity to the fashionable Chinese porcelains of the period and most early blue and white patterns show the influence of Chinese designs (see Plates 80, 96-7, 306, 563, etc.).

With the exception of the sophisticated Chelsea factory (which very rarely produced "blue and white") all eighteenth-century English porcelain factories either painted or printed a large range of utilitarian objects in underglaze blue. Typical marked examples are illustrated, see heading. The reader is referred to B. Watney's excellent and detailed *English Blue and White Porcelain of the 18th century* (1963) for a full appreciation of the charm of "blue and white".

ENAMEL COLOURS

Enamel colours are derived from metallic oxides and are those pigments which are applied to ceramics after they have been glazed and fired. These enamel colours are fired at a lower temperature (about 750–850° C.) than the body and glaze (about 1100° C.), and the range of possible colours is therefore much larger than that of underglaze colours which are fired at a higher temperature.

The porcelain manufacturers quickly mastered the control of enamel colours, and early Bow and Chelsea porcelains of the late 1740's are sometimes attractively enamelled. As the century progressed so did the potters' knowledge and new colours were added to their range.

The earthenware manufacturers did not use enamel colours to the same extent as the larger porcelain manufacturers, but in the eighteenth century specialist enamellers decorated some Staffordshire wares for various potters in the same way that specialist ceramic printers decorated wares sent to them "in the white", and this practice was continued into the early part of the nineteenth century by William Absolon at Yarmouth, by Donovan in Dublin, and by Doe & Rogers of Worcester (see Plates 3–5, 186, 241).

EGYPTIAN BLACK AND BASALT *Plates 19, 32–3, 57–8, 73, 273, 297, 299, 309, 316, 329, 344–5, 392, 435, 530, 590, 593, 599, 601–2, 606, 631, 633, 672.*

A matt surfaced earthenware which was rendered black by the addition of manganese and iron was called Egyptian black. Perhaps mainly due to the ease of manufacture and low cost it was very popular from the middle of the eighteenth century into the late 1820's and is still marketed today by Wedgwood under the name Basalt.

The term Egyptian Black was used in an advertisement in the *New York Gazette* in 1762 when a shipment of "Egyptian black teapots, milk pots, mugs and tea bowls of all sizes" was announced.

Josiah Wedgwood carried out experiments in the 1760's to perfect the colour and texture of black wares. The celebrated vases made in August 1769 to commemorate the first day's production at Wedgwood & Bentley's new factory at Etruria were in this body which was a favourite one with Wedgwood who remarked that it would last for ever. The term "Basaltes" was first used by Wedgwood in his 1773 ornamental ware catalogue to denote his superior version of the standard Egyptian black body. He was later to define basaltes as "a black porcelain biscuit of nearly the same properties with the natural stone, striking fire from steel, receiving a high polish, serving as a touchstone for metals, resisting all acids and bearing without injury a strong fire".

Examples of Egyptian black or basalt bearing the marks of Astbury, Barker, E. J. Birch, Bradley & Co, J. Glass, S. Greenwood, Hackwood, Herculaneum, S. Hollins, Keeling & Toft, Leeds, Mayer, Neale, Spode, Vozey & Hales, Warburton, Wedgwood, and Enoch Wood are illustrated in this book, but very many other potters produced unmarked objects. Examples sold by the London retailers, Messrs Thomas Goode in the 1820's illustrate the ruling prices—"2 Black Teapots 2/–", "1 Black Milk Pot. 8*d*", "1 round Black Sugar Box. 10*d*". It will be observed that most Egyptian Black takes the form of teaware and its popularity probably stems from the fact that the matt black ware showed to advantage the white hands of the hostess. In 1772 Josiah Wedgwood, replying to a letter from his partner Bentley, stated: "Thanks for your discovery in favour of the black teapots. I hope white hands will continue in fashion and then we may continue to make black Teapots."

PRINTING PROCESSES *Plates 1, 11, 31, 36, 39, 46, 153, 213, 238–9, 243, 265, 268, 272, 275–9, 294, 349, 440, 471–2, 503–5, 528, 557, 603, 645.*

The decoration of ceramics by means of transferring the ink from engraved plates to the ware by means of thin tissue-like paper was introduced in the 1750's with the object of reducing the cost of decoration by hand. A pull from an engraved copper plate is shown in Plate 261, and this shows marks which were cut out and applied to the reverse of the object.

Overglaze printed decoration occurs on Bow and Worcester porcelain from the mid-1750's. The most accomplished copperplates were engraved by Robert Hancock and his initials or name occurs on many printed patterns (see Plate 645). Messrs Sadler & Green at Liverpool applied printed decoration to pottery and porcelain for various manufacturers, and their names are found on some specimens (see Plates 294, 505). Printing in underglaze blue on porcelain was much practised at Worcester, Caughley, and at some of the Liverpool factories as well as at Lowestoft (see Plates 97, 362). Later in the eighteenth century and early in the nineteenth century Staffordshire *pottery* was extensively decorated with very fine quality blue prints, often of English or American views or historical events.

Early in the nineteenth century attractive bat printed designs were favoured on both pottery and porcelain (see Plates 382, 534). In this process pliable glue bats replaced the paper transfers and the engraved copper plates were finely stippled, resulting in a very delicate effect. In the late 1840's Messrs F. & R. Pratt of Fenton developed the technique of colour printing by means of separate copperplates, each transferring one primary colour (see Colour Plate X).

JASPER WARE *Plates 8-9, 254, 436, 547, 585, 604-5, 613, 618, 622, 632.*
Jasper is a close-grained stoneware body, hard enough to be polished on a lapidary's wheel, although this was seldom done. The perfection of the coloured jasper body has been called Josiah Wedgwood's most important achievement in ceramics. In the early 1770's the need was felt for a change from the standard black basalt and the contemporary matt white body for the imitation of ancient gems, etc. In December 1772 Wedgwood wrote to his partner Bentley: "You want a finer body for gems . . . I have several times mixed bodies for this purpose but some of these miscarried . . .", but in a further letter dated 6 February 1773 he reported progress—"Some very promising experiments lately upon finer bodies for gems and other things". These experiments were carried on over a long period and it was probably not until 1775 that he was able to market a standard coloured jasper body. Further work on jasper was continued up to at least 1779 before Josiah Wedgwood was satisfied.

In January 1775 he reported to his partner that he had mastered "blue of almost any shade", also "a beautiful sea green and several other colours for grounds to cameos, intaglios, etc.". The coloured jasper body was originally intended for use in the manufacture of small cameos, etc. (see Colour Plate XIV), but other uses which we now associate with the body were a natural development. Wedgwood asked Bentley: "What do you think of vases of our fine blue body, with white festoons, medallions etc.?" Happily Bentley must have thought the idea had merit.

The term "Jasper" was not used until November 1775. The body comprised: flint 10 per cent, barium sulphate 59 per cent, clay 29 per cent, barium carbonate 2 per cent, and this mixture was capable of being stained with various metallic oxides. At first the jasper was stained throughout, but in 1777 it was discovered that a surface layer of tinted jasper saved money for in April 1777 Wedgwood sent Bentley notice of the first "Jasper dipped" plaques—"They are coloured with the Cobalt @ 36/- per lb. which being too dear to mix with the clay of the whole grounds we have washed them over, and I think them by far the finest grounds we have ever made". From November

1785 to 1858 "Jasper dip" was used extensively, but the original solid jasper was reintroduced in 1858.

Wedgwood took great pains to keep the composition of jasper secret, but nevertheless contemporary potters quickly introduced similar bodies to compete with his undoubted success. Marked examples by William Adams, Dudson Bros, Neale & Co, Daniel Steel, John Turner, and Enoch Wood are illustrated. Many other potters made unmarked specimens. The jasper body continued in production throughout the nineteenth century and is still popular today.

PEARL WARE *Plate 620.*

Josiah Wedgwood introduced a whiter version of the standard creamware or Queensware body (see page 340) in 1779. In March 1779 he promised to send samples to London for his partner Bentley to see and on 19 June he wrote: "I thank Her Majesty for the honour she has done to the Pearl White and hope it will have due influence upon all her loyal subjects". Subsequent letters show that the body was introduced to make a change from the creamware which all potters of the period were by now producing, but it was not necessarily considered to be an improvement on the earlier body. Nevertheless other potters copied it and Wedgwoods themselves continued to make it into the nineteenth century. From about 1840 the name "Pearl" was impressed into the body and from *c.* 1868 the initial "P" occurs.

CANE AND BAMBOO WARES *Plates 391, 609.*

Caneware is a tan-coloured and normally unglazed "dry" body much used by Wedgwood in the latter part of the eighteenth century and sometimes slightly enriched with enamels. Often the objects made in this ware were modelled in the form of bamboo shoots, hence the term "Bamboo Ware".

Several authorities have stated that the caneware body was introduced in 1770, but most examples found today would seem to be of the 1785–1810 period and Wedgwood's letters show that experiments in the caneware body were still being carried out as late as 1783.

Many potters other than Wedgwood made caneware. In 1785 Messrs Turner & Abbott, retailers in Fleet Street, London, were advertising "Bamboo, or cane colour teapots, some elegantly mounted with silver spouts and chains, and mugs and jugs with silver rims and covers. . . ." Messrs Turner & Abbott mainly sold wares made by John Turner of Lane End in the Staffordshire Potteries.

TURNER STONEWARE *Plates 6, 10, 24, 425, 459, 582, 627.*

The term "Turner Stoneware" is here used to cover a refined earthenware being a cross between caneware and stoneware. It was much used by John Turner and other potters in the manufacture of decorative jugs, tankards, etc., which were ornamented with hunting or drinking scenes in relief (see Plate 582), and these were often furnished with silver or silver plated mounts. The body was mainly used in the 1785–1810 period and examples can often be dated by the year mark on the contemporary silver mounts.

John Turner was the leading maker of such pieces, hence my descriptive name "Turner Stoneware", but several other potters made similar pieces in this off-white body. Marked specimens by B. Adams, W. Adams, W. Badderley, J. Mist, B. Plant, and Wilson are illustrated in Plates 6, 10, 24, 425, 459, 582, 627. Messrs Davenports also made good examples.

BISQUE *Plates 12, 406, 493.*

The term "bisque" or "biscuit" is used to denote pottery, or more usually porcelain, in its fired but unglazed state. Examples are the fragments from factory sites shown in Plate 161.

During the second half of the eighteenth century the decorative merit of unglazed porcelain was recognized by the French National Sèvres factory and by the Derby factory in England. Graceful, well-modelled figures, groups, and ornamental objects were made in bisque at Derby and these are warm to the touch and often have a pleasing, pale ivory tint. A slight smear glaze is apparent on some specimens. Typical specimens are illustrated in Plates 215–17.

The Derby bisque figures and groups were highly thought of at the period and were more expensive than the decorated examples of the same model. The explanation of this is that only the most faultless specimens could be sold in the white, while, when coloured, any slight blemishes could be hidden by the enamel decoration.

In the early nineteenth century various potters produced bisque figures and groups in a more chalky body than the earlier Derby examples. These can be quite charming (see Plates 406, 493), but are somewhat prone to staining. In the 1840's the newly introduced parian body superseded the earlier bisque (see page xxv).

PRATT WARES *Plates 34, 65, 332, 468–71.*

The name Pratt is given to two entirely different types of pottery. Firstly to jugs and other objects of the 1790–1820 period bearing moulded decoration enriched with underglaze colours—blues, green, browns, yellows, and occasionally black. Some jugs of this type bear the Pratt mark (see Plates 468–9) and these have given the name to the whole class of ware which was in fact made by many other potters in Staffordshire, Yorkshire, and in Scotland. Marked examples by Barker, E. Bourne, and Lakin & Poole are illustrated in Plates 34, 65, 332, 468–71.

The second class of ware to bear the general name "Pratt" is that decorated with multicoloured prints of so-called Pot lid type (see Colour Plate X). Although Messrs F. & R. Pratt of Fenton were the principal producers of objects decorated in this manner, several other contemporary firms also made similar wares, see *Antique China and Glass under £5* (1966).

JAPAN PATTERNS *Plates 107, 158, 160, 200, 223, 283, 384, 479, 551, 663.*

Japan patterns are those bold formal floral designs in underglaze blue with overglaze red and green enamelling and are inspired by the decoration on Japanese Imari wares.

Good quality copies of Japanese Imari patterns had been produced by the Chelsea factory in the 1750's, but in the early 1800's the stylized Japan patterns were used to satisfy the demand for low-priced colourful designs. The manufacturers could produce the patterns at low cost as semi-skilled or child labour could be employed to paint the broad areas of colour and the body itself did not have to be of the finest quality or finish.

The Derby factory is traditionally associated with Japan patterns. It did, of course, produce vast quantities and still does today, but in the 1800–30 period Japan patterns represented one of the standard types of ceramic decoration and were produced by most manufacturers.

The Japan patterns produced by Spode are usually of a very fine quality. Recent excavations at the site of the Caughley factory show that fine Japan patterns were produced there (see Plate 160).

CASTLEFORD-TYPE WARES *Plates 157, 257, 307.*

Teawares in a white stoneware with relief moulded designs, often ornamented with blue enamel line borders, are traditionally attributed to the Castleford Works of David Dunderdale & Co. The teapots often have hinged or sliding covers.

The so-called Castleford stoneware body is translucent and is actually nearer to the later Parian body than to true stoneware. These Castleford-type wares were made by many potters of the 1800–25 period and very few, perhaps not more than one in a hundred examples, will be found to bear the standard "D.D. & Co Castleford Pottery" mark. Most specimens are unmarked except for impressed numerals—often 22 on teapots.

Marked examples of Castleford-type wares are illustrated in Plates 157, 307 and a marked "D.D. & Co. Castleford" teapot is shown in Plate 257. The teapots and related objects are moulded and the relief ornaments indented into the mould and not applied separately as with the Wedgwood jasper reliefs. This moulded method of manufacture is similar to that used on "Egyptian black" (see page xix) teawares of the same period, most of which are unmarked.

TERRA COTTA *Plates 60, 568, 614, 625.*

Although the reddish unglazed earthenware known as Terra Cotta can be of great antiquity it was not until the second half of the eighteenth century that it was reintroduced by Wedgwoods. Vases and other things were made by them in this medium and also in their similar but rather darker Rosso Antico body.

Several other factories also produced similar wares—Dillwyn's Etruscan Ware was made at Swansea from *c.* 1847 to *c.* 1850 and a pottery at Bishop's Waltham made tasteful wares for a brief period from February 1866 to December 1867 (see Plate 60). Later in the nineteenth century several firms, mainly in the West Country, produced decorative Art Terra Cotta.

"STONE CHINA", "NEW STONE", "IRONSTONE", ETC.
Plates 196-7, 384-7, 535, 586-8.

Potters had always sought to produce a refined earthenware body that combined both durability with attractiveness and amongst the first to be successful in this field in England were the Turners, who introduced their "Turner's Patent" earthenware in 1800. Examples bear the red-painted mark "Turner's Patent" (see Plates 586–8). This is a compact body that can on occasions be slightly translucent. The Turners soon ran into financial difficulties (see page 325), and the patent rights were reputedly sold to Josiah Spode.

Spode from *c.* 1805 manufactured this, or a very similar body, under the name "Stone China" or "New Stone", and for many years he produced fine dinner, dessert, and tea services in this strong clean earthenware. The new body quickly won the public's approbation and most pottery manu-facturers of the 1810–30 period made similar wares, using such trade descriptions as "Stone China" or "Semi Porcelain" and these names were often incorporated in their marks.

In July 1813 Charles James Mason patented his famous "Ironstone" china composition and marked the objects made from it "Patent Ironstone China" or "Masons Patent Ironstone China" (see pages 216–220). The name "Ironstone China" was apt as it suggested great strength, coupled with the delicate nature of china. Most manufacturers adopted the name for similar wares that they made throughout the nineteenth century and it is still in current use. The trade description "Granite" was also a popular one from the 1840's onwards.

LUSTRE DECORATION   *Plates 28, 269, 474, 512–13, 555–8, 610, 615, 673.*

Although lustre effects on ceramics were used on both early Near Eastern wares and European maiolica, this shiny metallic decoration, which sought to imitate silver or copper, was not attempted in England until the early 1800's.

"Silver" lustre is made from platinum and "Copper" lustre from gold, but these metallic washes are applied very thinly so that the colour of the underlying body materially affects the colour of the lustre. Copper lustre was usually applied on a dark body, but when the same solution was used on a white ground a pleasant "purple lustre" resulted and this permitted further washes to be added, and these gave great depth of colour and enabled designs such as landscapes to be built up.

Good quality decorative wares were sometimes decorated by the resist process. Parts of an object were painted with wax or some other material that would resist the silver lustre which was then brushed over the whole object so that, after firing and cleaning, the silver lustre adhered only to those parts that had not been treated by the resistant medium. Similar effects were gained by stencilling.

Messrs Wedgwood introduced a decorative type of marbled pink or purple "gold" lustre called "Moonlight Lustre" (c. 1805), and a fine service decorated in this style is shown in Plate 615. A form of "Splash Lustre", formed by splashing drops of oil, etc., on to the copper lustre in a haphazard manner is associated with the Sunderland Potteries (see Plate 558), but it is not confined to them. Articles made in imitation of silver or copper wares and therefore coated with an all-over film of silver or copper lustre are seldom marked and were produced into the second half of the nineteenth century.

The collector must be on his guard against reproductions of "resist lustre" and "Sunderland" type lustre wares. These were made in the latter part of the nineteenth century and are even being produced today. Some of these modern reproductions have the printed mark erased and are then sold by unscrupulous people as old. The removal of the mark, which is usually effected by acids, leaves a dull patch in the glaze.

Old English Lustre Pottery (1951) by W. D. John and Warren Baker is an expensive but most helpful reference book.

COALBROOKDALE   *Plates 169–70, 232–3, 281, 540 and Colour Plates VIII, XI.*

The term "Coalbrookdale" is traditionally associated with a decorative class of ornamental porcelain encrusted with modelled flowers, etc., in relief. This type of porcelain was mainly produced between 1820 and 1840, but some pieces were made either before or after this period.

Some floral encrusted pieces bear the blue painted marks "Coalbrookdale", "C. Dale", "C.D.", or "Coalport", and this is possibly the reason why the name "Coalbrookdale" has been given to all porcelains of this type. Floral encrusted porcelains were very popular and, as a result, were made by many of the leading manufacturers. Marked examples from the Coalport, Derby, Grainger (Worcester), Minton, Rockingham, and Spode factories are illustrated.

Recent research on the pre-1850 Minton wares has shown that much of the floral encrusted porcelain formerly attributed to Coalbrookdale or Coalport was in fact made at Mintons. The factory records include design books in which the floral encrusted objects are drawn (see Plate 404) and the wage books list teams of "Flowerers". Minton floral encrusted porcelains shown in Colour Plate VIII match drawings in the factory design books and show the range of such productions. This recent research suggests in fact that Messrs Minton were the main producers of the so-called "Coalbrookdale" china. Many examples from this factory bear a copy of the Dresden crossed-swords mark in underglaze blue and some of the design book drawings bear titles such as "Dresden Scroll vase, raised flowers" or "Dresden vase R.F.".

REGISTERED DESIGNS   *Plates 41, 61, 74, 154, 176–8, 326–7, 409, 426.*

From 1842 to 1883 designs could be registered at the London Patent Office and thereby be pro-tected against piracy. Such "registered" designs were marked with a diamond-shaped device, from which the date of registration can be discovered, see pages 526–7 of the companion *Encyclopaedia of British Pottery and Porcelain Marks*.

PARIAN   *Plates 15, 40–5, 49, 91, 171, 175, 330, 407, 489, 560.*

The matt white Parian body, originally called "Statuary Porcelain", was introduced in the early 1840's as a refinement of the earlier bisque body (see page xxii). Opinions differ on its date of introduction, but Messrs Copeland & Garrett's "Statuary Porcelain" was reviewed in the January 1845 issue of the *Art Union* magazine—"We have been enabled to examine the material referred to, and can bear testimony to its beauty, as well as very valuable qualities for multiplying the sculptor's work". Messrs Minton were also experimenting with a similar body at the same period.

The original purpose of the body was to facilitate the production in quantity of small-scale copies of antique and modern statuary at a cost low enough to appeal to a large section of the public. The "Art Union of London", a National Art Lottery, did much to popularize and publicize the new productions in "Statuary Porcelain", a name soon superseded by "Parian". The result was that it was not long before Parian figures and groups in vast numbers were being produced by all the leading manufacturers and the foremost of these employed sculptors of international repute to model for them. The names of these sculptors can often be found on the moulded replicas.

Parian figures, groups and busts, were made in quantity from the 1840's to the 1890's. Messrs Robinson & Leadbeater of Stoke were the largest producers in the late nineteenth century (see Plate 489). This versatile body was also used for utilitarian objects—jugs, centre pieces, etc. A full account of the methods of production of Parian and its early history is given in chapter 7 of *Victorian Porcelain* (1961).

MAJOLICA   *Plates 326–7, 414.*

Minton's Art Director, Leon Arnoux, introduced English "Majolica" earthenware in 1850. It was warmly praised at the 1851 Exhibition and remained very popular for the remainder of the nineteenth century.

The earthenware attempted to emulate the early Italian Maiolica in which the basic earthenware was coated with an opaque white glaze or covering slip upon which the design was freely painted. The early Minton "Majolica" wares were painted by leading artists—Thomas Allen, Thomas

Kirkby, and Edouard Rischgitz. Within a few years the name Majolica came to mean earthenwares decorated with deep semi-translucent glazes.

These wares are typically Victorian and large garden ornaments, such as seats, jardinières, etc., were made by the many potters who produced Majolica. These potters included W. Brownfield & Co, Brown-Westhead, Moore & Co, George Jones (& Sons), and Wedgwood. Early Italian Maiolica is spelt with an "i", English Majolica of the Victorian era with a "j".

PÂTE-SUR-PÂTE *Plates 292, 328, 356, 420–2, 427.*

The *pâte-sur-pâte* style of decoration is the most expensive form of ceramic ornamentation. Successive coatings of porcelain slip (diluted to the consistency of cream) are applied to build up a cameo-like design in white semi-translucent porcelain on a tinted Parian ground. The layers of slip are finally carved to accentuate the details and after weeks or even months of work the article is fired and the added ornamentation becomes vitrified and semi-translucent, and only then can it be seen whether or not all the labour has been in vain.

The technique was brought to England from France by Marc Louis Solon, who was engaged by Mintons in 1870 or 1871 and the first Solon *pâte-sur-pâte* entry in the Minton work book is on 23 June 1871. His figure compositions (see Plates 420–1) are eagerly sought after and have always commanded high prices.

Solon trained several artists to work in this technique and one of these, Alboine Birks, worked at Mintons until 1937. Solon's own connection with Mintons was severed in March 1904.

Other firms, W. Brownfield & Sons, George Grainger & Co (of Worcester), George Jones & Sons, Moore Brothers, and the Royal Worcester Company, produced *pâte-sur-pâte* designs which were (with the exception of those of George Jones & Sons) mainly floral in character (see Plates 292, 328, 356, 420–2, 427).

Details of the methods of manufacture are given, with much information, in *Victorian Porcelain* (1961).

INDIVIDUAL POTTERS *Plates 53–6, 209–10, 374–8.*

Most country potters may be regarded as Individual Potters, in that one person or a small team produce by traditional methods wares to meet a local need, and the results show an individuality lacking in mass-produced factory wares. Plates 209–10, 377 show objects of this type.

In the present century numerous "Studio Potters" have carried on the tradition, but most of them enjoy the advantage over their predecessors of having received technical training at art schools or similar institutions.

Late in the nineteenth century several potters created highly individual pottery and may be considered to be the forerunners of today's "Studio Potters". Foremost amongst these nineteenth-century potters were the Martin Brothers (see page 213 and Plates 374–8) and William De Morgan (see Colour Plate VI and Plates 409–10).

N.B. Several references will be found in the captions to BURSLEM, COBRIDGE, FENTON, HANLEY, LONGTON, STOKE and TUNSTALL, these are the towns which collectively make up the STAFFORDSHIRE POTTERIES. See Chapter I, *British Pottery and Porcelain, 1780–1850.*

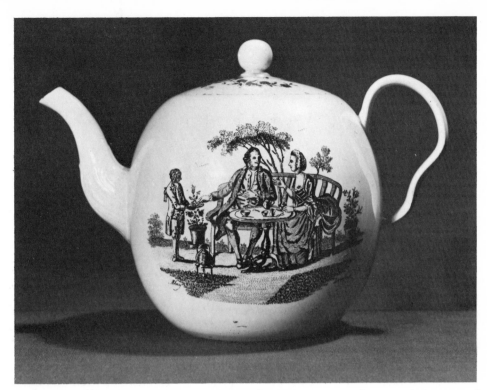

1. *Liverpool creamware teapot, the engraved design signed "Abbey . Liverpool" (c. 1780). 6½ inches high. Abbey was an engraver and printer; he did not produce the wares bearing his signed prints.*

Fitzwilliam Museum, Cambridge

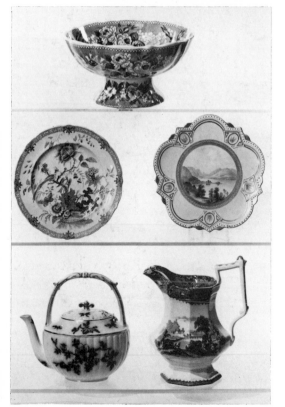

2. *A selection of "A" wares: Blue printed bowl, printed Adams mark (c. 1850–60). Stone china plate, impressed mark "Alcocks" (c. 1840). Porcelain plate hand-painted scenic centre, printed Aynsleys mark (no. 189) (c. 1870). Earthenware teapot with moulded "A Bros" mark of G. L. Ashworth & Bros (pattern registered in 1872). Printed earthenware jug, printed mark "John Alcock" (c. 1853–60). 9 inches high.*

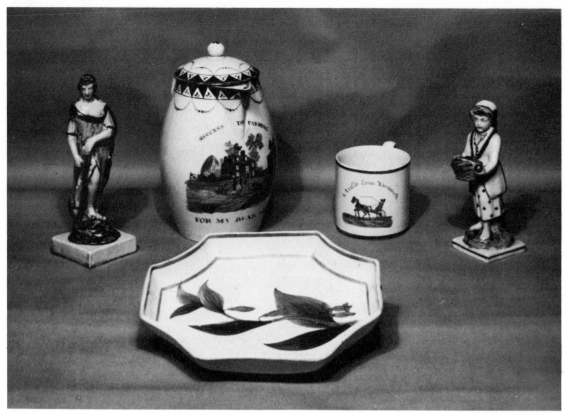

3. *Absolon of Yarmouth decorated English earthenwares, all pieces marked with name marks nos. 6 and 7. Absolon was a decorator not a potter (c. 1784–1814). Covered jug 8¼ inches high.*

Great Yarmouth Museum

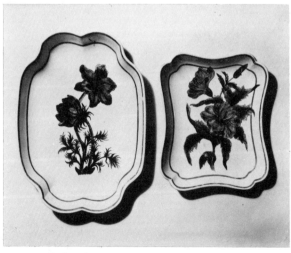

4. *Absolon decorated creamware dishes of Davenport make, signed on reverse (c. 1800–10). He also purchased Worcester porcelains in the 1790's.*

Victoria & Albert Museum

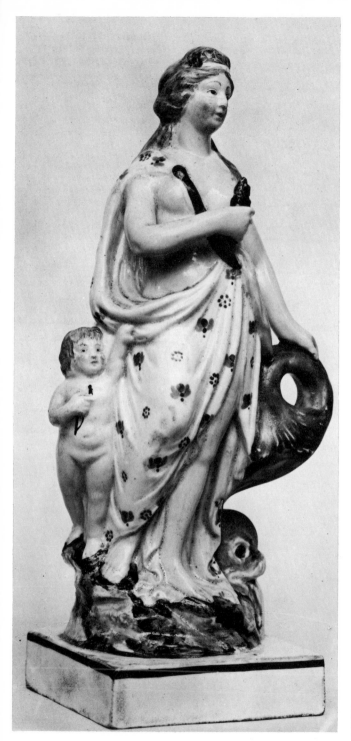

5. *Staffordshire figure decorated and sold by William Absolon. See detail of base for typical painted signature mark (c. 1790–1800). 8 inches high.*

British Museum

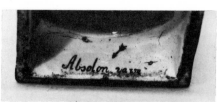

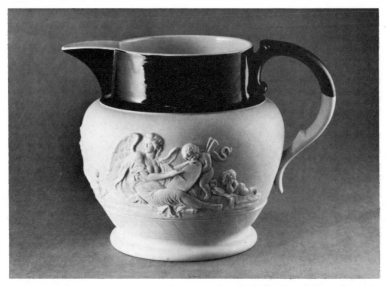

6. *Fine quality stoneware jug, with impressed mark "B Adams" (c. 1800–20).*
6½ inches high.

Godden of Worthing

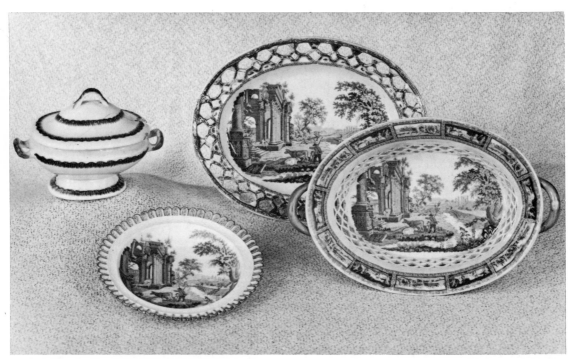

7. *"B Adams" impressed marked, blue printed earthenwares. The covered tureen with simple blue painted borders is of a type made by several potters (c. 1800–20). Tureen. 5½ inches high.*

City Museum & Art Gallery, Stoke-on-Trent

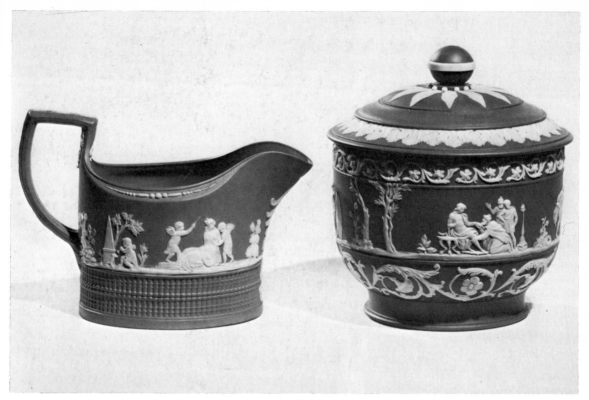

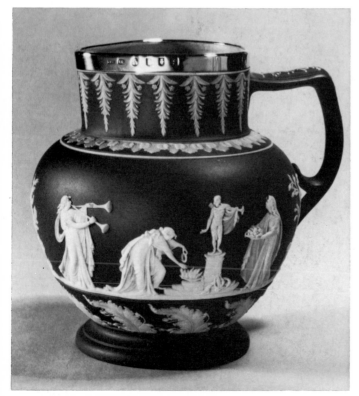

8. *Adams, impressed marked blue jasper (see page xx) wares with white reliefs, in the Wedgwood manner (c. 1800–10). Covered sugar 5¼ inches high.*

Godden of Worthing

9. *Adams, impressed marked blue jasper jug. Contemporary silver rim has year mark for 1821. 6¼ inches high.*

Godden of Worthing

5

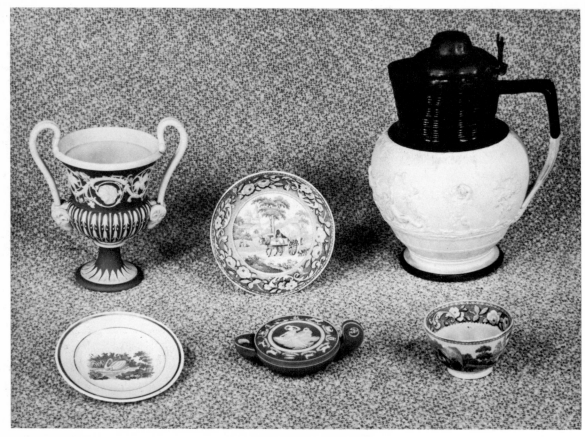

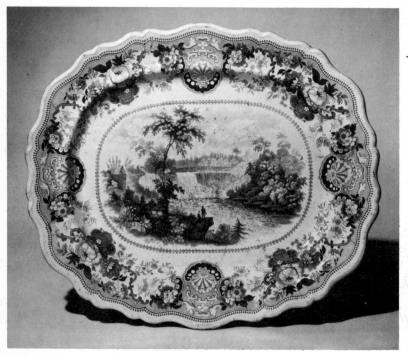

10. *"Adams", impressed marked earthenwares. Blue and white jasper vase and lamp of Wedgwood type (c. 1785–1810). Stoneware jug 10¾ inches high.*

City Museum & Art Gallery, Stoke-on-Trent

11. *Transfer printed earthenware platter, one of several patterns made for the North American market. Marked "W Adams & Sons" (c. 1819–29). 20 inches long.*

Ellouise Baker Larsen Collection, Smithsonian Institution, Washington, D.C.

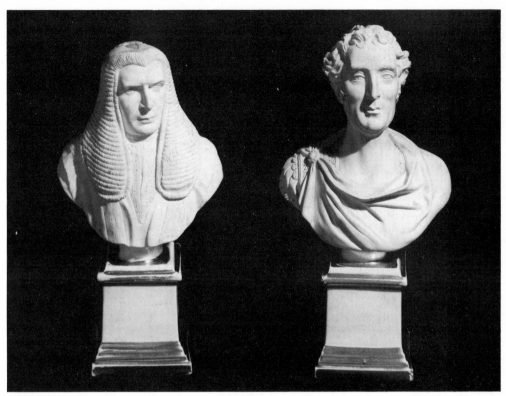

12. *Two early unglazed porcelain busts, marked "Saml Alcock & Co. Cobridge. Staffordshire. Oct 31st 1828". 9 inches high. See G. Godden's* British Pottery and Porcelain, 1780–1850, *page 48.*

D. M. & P. Manheim, London

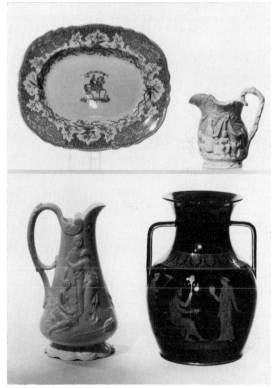

13. *Selection of Samuel Alcock's wares: Blue printed earthenware dish, "SA & Co" mark. Moulded Parian jug in blue and white, printed name mark in full. Moulded Parian jug (c. 1847). Red and black earthenware vase, initial mark with beehive device (c. 1845–50). 10¼ inches high.*

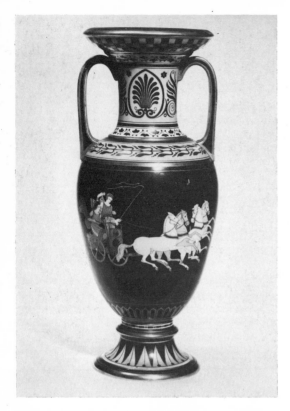

14. *Porcelain vase by Samuel Alcock & Co, initial mark "S A & Co". Many classical subjects were copied by this firm (c. 1840–50). 14¾ inches high.*

Godden of Worthing

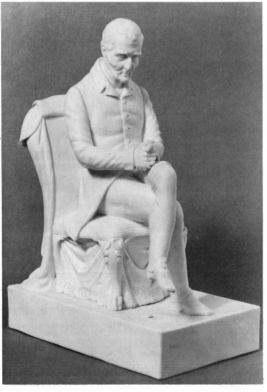

15. *Alcock Parian figure of the Duke of Wellington, modelled by G. Abbott (c. 1852). 11¼ inches high. Many fine Parian articles were issued by this firm.*

For further information see Jewitt's Ceramic Art of Great Britain *(1878 & 1883).* Godden's British Pottery and Porcelain, 1780–1850 *(1963).*

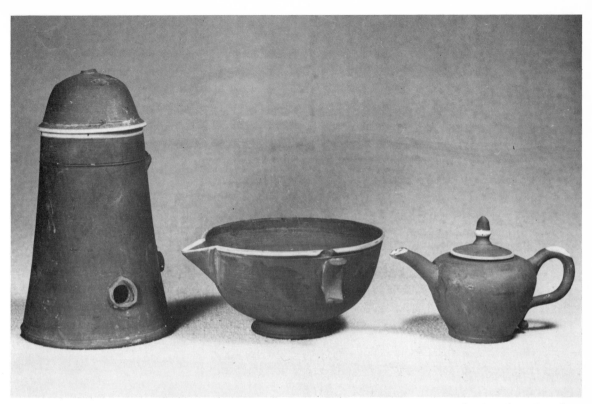

16. *Factory wasters found on the traditional site of John Astbury Works at Shelton. They illustrate the good lines and workmanship of Astbury wares of c. 1740. These wasters are unglazed. When finished the ware would have been brown. Coffee pot 6⅝ inches high.*

Museum & Art Gallery,
Stoke-on-Trent

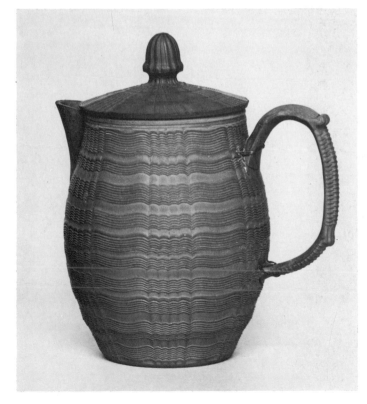

17. *Astbury, impressed marked, unglazed redware jug and cover, decorated with engine-turned pattern (introduced c. 1765). 3¾ inches high.*

Fitzwilliam Museum, Cambridge

Red wares of this type are often attributed to the Elers Brothers, but many potters made similar wares. Marked examples are rare (see page xiii).

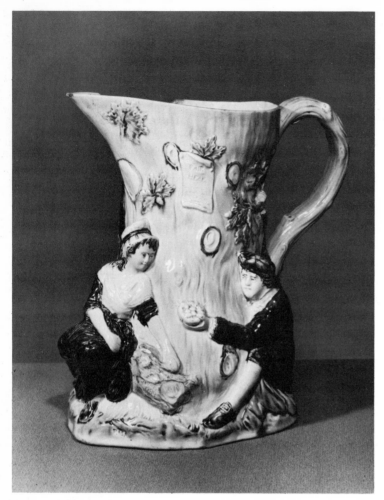

18. *Astbury "Fair Hebe" jug, modelled by J. Voyez (signed and dated 1788). Impressed initial mark R M A on front of base and "Astbury" under the base (c. 1790). 9½ inches high.*

Fitzwilliam Museum, Cambridge

Similar jugs of this basic "Fair Hebe" design were also made by other potters (see page 163).

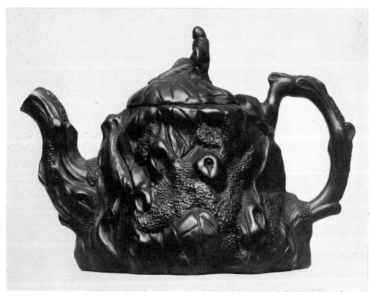

19. *Early basalt (see page xix) teapot, impressed marked "Astbury". Several potters of this name worked in Staffordshire during the eighteenth century. This example is probably by Thomas Astbury, mid eighteenth century. 4⅝ inches high.*

British Museum

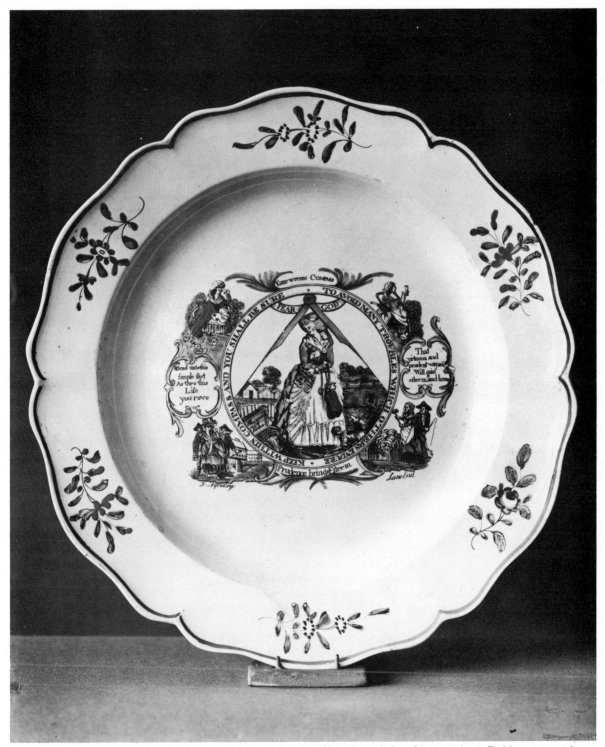

20. *Staffordshire earthenware plate bearing printed pattern engraved by John Aynsley of Lane End, Staffordshire. Many other prints bearing the signature of this engraver in, or near, the main print (c. 1780–1809). 9⅝ inches diameter.*

Victoria & Albert Museum

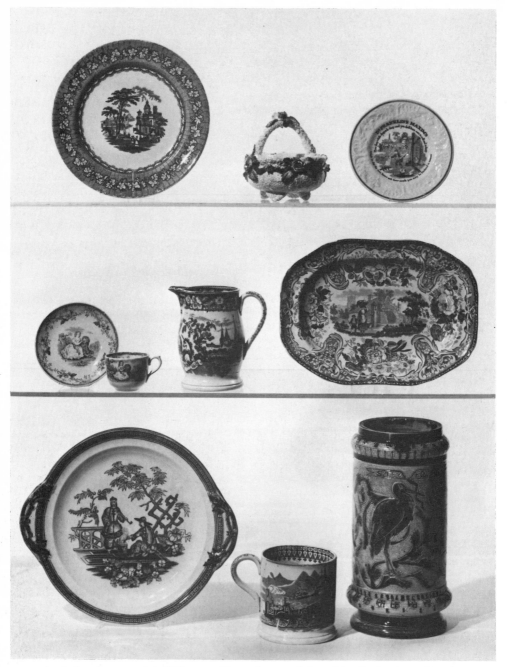

21. *A selection of wares made by "B" potters.* Top to bottom, left to right: *"Baker & Co" earthenware plate (c. 1839); "John Bevington" porcelain basket (c. 1872–92); "B W & Co" (Buckley, Wood & Co) plate (c. 1875); "Beech Hancock & Co" cup and saucer (c. 1851–5); "B & B" (Baggaley & Ball?) jug (c. 1830); "J.D.B." (J. D. Baxter) dish (c. 1823–7); "B & H" (Beech & Hancock) plate "Pekin" pattern (c. 1860–70); "B & T" (Barker & Till) railway mug (c. 1846–50); "C I C Bailey" Fulham stoneware vase (c. 1875).*

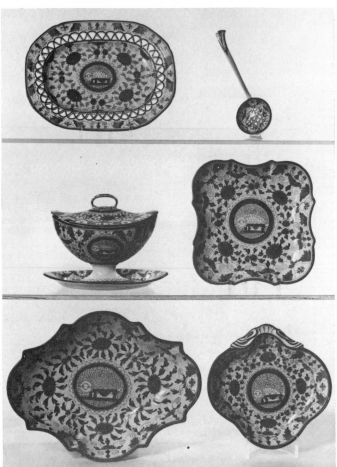

J. AND E. BADDELEY

22. *Part of an earthenware dessert service by John and Edward Baddeley of Shelton, Staffordshire Potteries (c. 1784–1806). Impressed marks I.E.B., I.E.B./W. The plates have the impressed initial B only.*

Godden of Worthing

The shape of these pieces should be noted as other potters used this painted pattern. Minton examples bear the pattern no. 106.

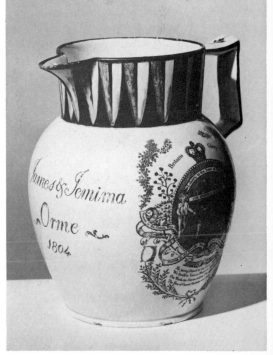

T. BADDELEY

23. *Creamware jug dated 1804. The printed panels depicting spinning machinery and mottoes are signed by the Hanley engraver Thomas Baddeley, mark no. 201. 7 inches high.*

Godden of Worthing

Thomas Baddeley worked from 1800 to 1834; he was an engraver not a potter.

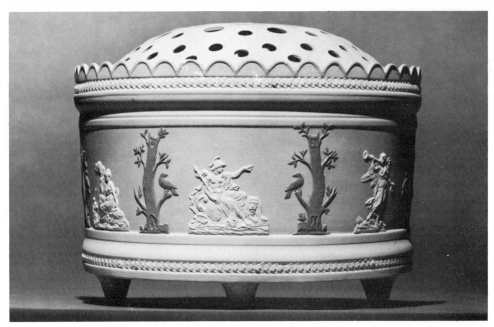

24. *Jasper-type bulb pot with two-colour reliefs. Impressed mark "Eastwood", as used by William Baddeley of Eastwood, Hanley (c. 1802–22). This potter made good quality Wedgwood-type, jasper and basalt wares.* 9¼ *inches long.*   Godden of Worthing

BAGGERLEY AND BALL, LONGTON *c.* 1822–36

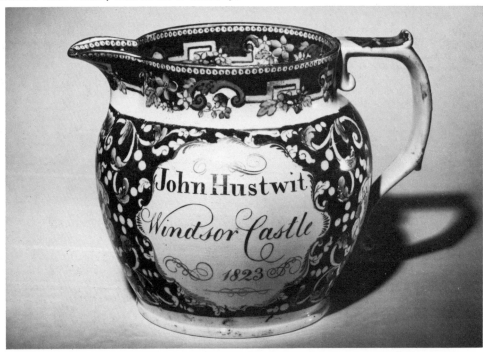

25. *Printed and coloured over earthenware jug dated 1823, by Baggerley & Ball of Longton (c. 1822–36). Printed mark B & B/L (mark no. 207), formerly attributed to other potters in error. 6 inches high. The general form of this jug is typical of the 1820–5 period.*

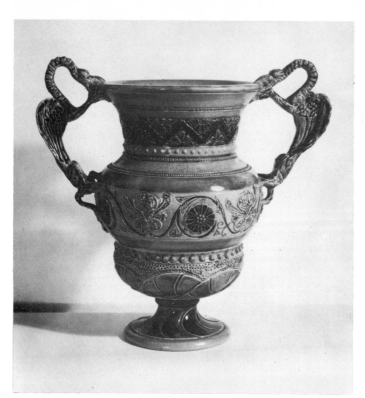

26. *Stoneware vase with typical incised decoration. Incised mark "C J C Bailey. The Pottery Fulham". Working period 1864–89. Doulton-type stonewares were made but are rare.*

Victoria & Albert Museum

27. *A very rare pair of porcelain figures by C. J. C. Bailey. Porcelains were produced at this stoneware factory for a brief period (c. 1873). "C J C B" monogram mark (no. 215) and place-name "Fulham". 6½ inches high.*

Victoria & Albert Museum

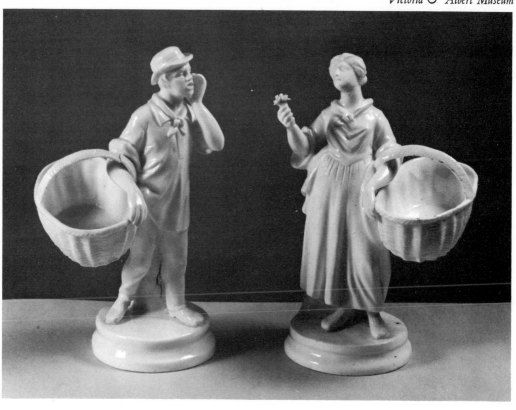

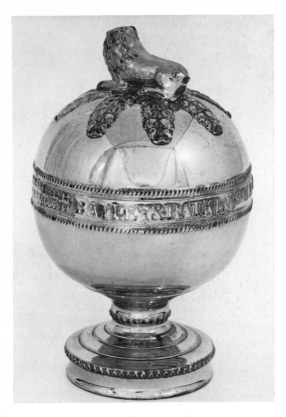

28. *Silver lustre decorated earthenware "perdifume" patented by Bailey & Batkin of Lane End* (c. 1824). *Moulded mark round central band "Bailey & Batkin. sole patentees".* 8½ *inches high.*

Godden of Worthing

Messrs Bailey & Batkin supplied lustre decorated wares to the American market. In 1816 they supplied fifty "lustre edged female figure tea sets" and other lustre decorated wares. Such pieces are normally unmarked.

BAKER, BEVANS AND IRWIN, SWANSEA *c.* 1813–38

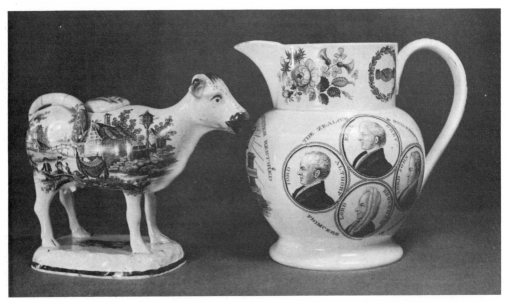

29. *Baker, Bevans & Irwin, Swansea earthenwares bearing printed "B B & I" initial marks* (c. 1813–38). *The Reform jug is of the 1832 period. 6 inches high.*

Willett Collection, Brighton Museum

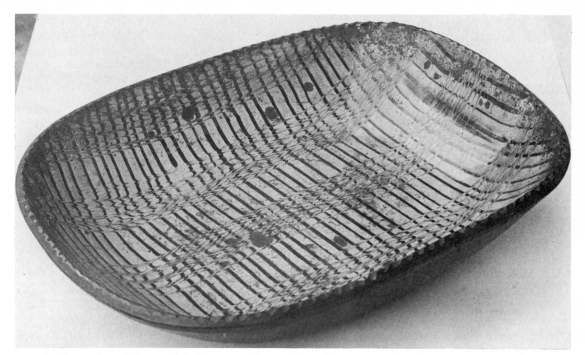

30. *Slip decorated, combed ware dish (see page xii). By W. Balaam. Impressed mark "Rope Lane Pottery. Ipswich".*
17 inches long. Nineteenth century.
Ipswich Museum

Many potters made dishes in this form with this traditional type of decoration. Specimens are very rarely marked.

BALL BROS, SUNDERLAND

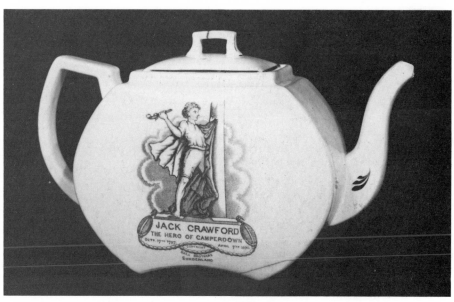

31. *Ball Brothers marked teapot of c. 1890. The Ball Brothers worked the Deptford Pottery at*
Sunderland from 1884 to 1918. This is the only pattern recorded with a mark. 5⅞ inches high.
Sunderland Museum

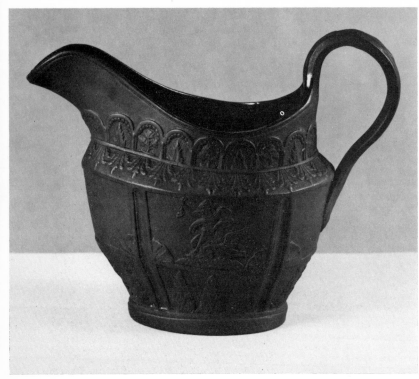

32. *Barker (impressed marked) basalt creamer (see page xix). The form is typical of the 1805 period; note glazed interior. Richard Barker potted at Lane End (c. 1784–1808). Peter Barker worked at the Mexborough Old Pottery, Yorkshire, from c. 1804, and this may be a Yorkshire rather than a Staffordshire example. 4¼ inches high.*

Victoria & Albert Museum

33. *"Barker" impressed marked basalt teapot (c. 1800–10). 6 inches high. See note under Plate 32.*

Godden of Worthing

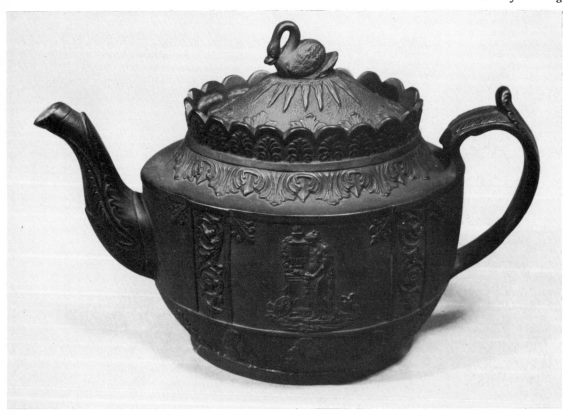

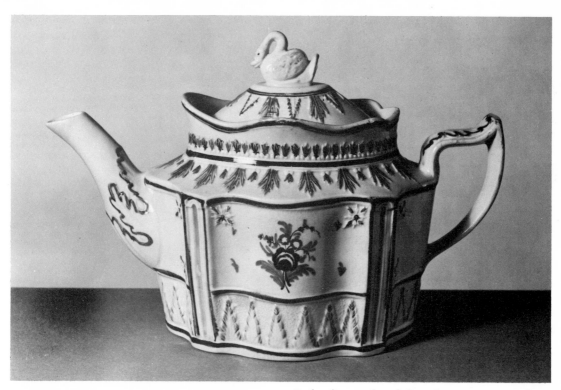

34. *Barker (impressed marked) earthenware teapot, similar in moulded decoration and in colouring to the so-called Pratt wares. Richard Barker was potting at Lane End from 1784 to 1808, but there were many other potters of this name (see Plate 32). 6 inches high.*

Victoria & Albert Museum

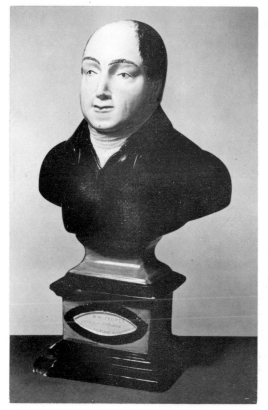

BARKER, SUTTON AND TILL
BURSLEM *c.* 1834–43

35. *Barker, Sutton & Till earthenware bust of the Methodist preacher William Clowes. Rare impressed mark "B S & T/ Burslem". This partnership is of the 1834–43 period. 10¾ inches high.*

Victoria & Albert Museum

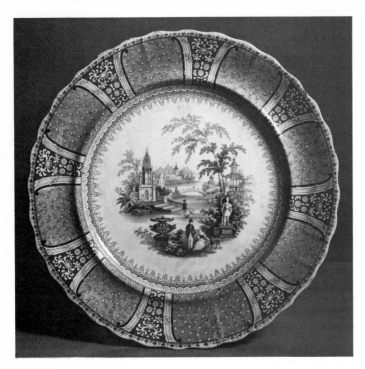

36. *Batkin, Walker & Broadhurst (initial mark) blue printed earthenware plate, showing typical early Victorian scenic pattern. This firm is listed in Lane End, Staffordshire, rate records from 1840 to 1845. 10½ inches diameter.*

Victoria & Albert Museum

BATTAM AND SON

37. *Battam & Son's wares, decorated for the Ceramic and Crystal Palace Art-Union. "B S" and "C & C P Art Union", painted marks (c. 1858–72). Vase 10 inches high. Most Battam wares were made by Copelands; Battams were decorators in London.*

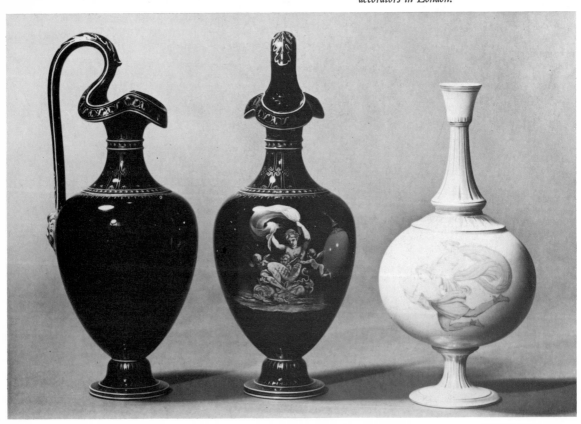

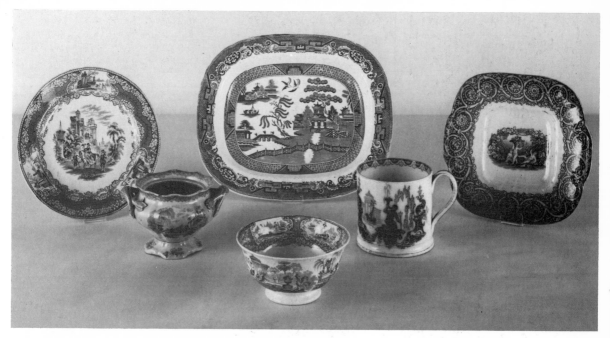

38. *J. & M. P. Bell & Co's transfer printed earthenwares, bearing printed name or initial marks (c. 1842–70). Platter 15 × 12 inches.*

Glasgow Art Gallery & Museum

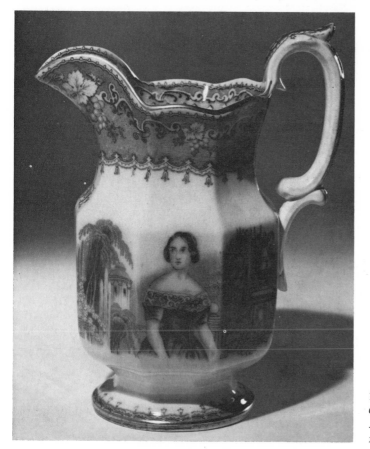

39. *J. & M. P. Bell & Co (printed mark) earthenware with printed portrait of Jenny Lind. A similar example has been reported with date 1850. 8¼ inches high.*

21

Belleek

The Belleek factory in County Fermanagh, Northern Ireland, was established in about 1863 after earlier successful experiments with the local clay. The works were managed by David McBirney and Robert Williams Armstrong under the name McBirney & Co. At first only useful wares were produced, but by the time of the 1865 Exhibition McBirney & Co were able to display Parian china figures and statuettes (stone china and earthenwares were also made). Talented workmen from Staffordshire were employed and the range of objects quickly grew and included the now traditional Belleek marine forms with an attractive iridescent pearl-like glaze, and openwork baskets (Plates 40–5). In 1865 only seventy workpeople were employed of which about thirty were children or apprentices. Within about fifteen years the number of employees had increased threefold.

The earliest wares often have an impressed mark BELLEEK. CO. FERMANAGH, but the standard mark is printed and includes a central tower, a dog, and a harp above the word Belleek (mark no. 326). In the earlier versions the mark is more detailed. After 1891 the words "Co. Fermanagh, Ireland" were added to this mark. The wares are usually very thinly potted or cast and are consequently very light. Several engravings of typical Belleek marine form objects are given in Jewitt's *Ceramic Art of Great Britain* (*c.* 1878 and 1883), and also in my revised 1972 edition. For other examples and illustrations from Belleek catalogues see *British Porcelain, an Illustrated Guide* by G. Godden (Barrie & Jenkins, London, 1974). A good selection of pieces is shown in *The Belleek Pottery* by S. McCrum, a booklet published by the Ulster Museum, Belfast.

The Belleek works are still in production, after several changes of ownership, and many designs of the 1865–75 period are still made and find a ready market.

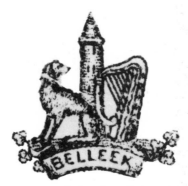

Standard, early Belleek
mark (no. 306).

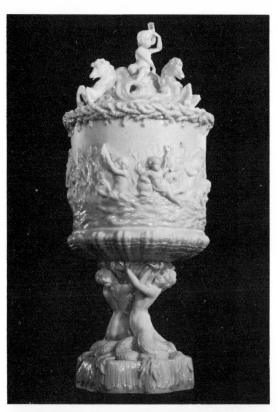

40. *Belleek ice pail and cover in matt and glazed Parian. Designed by R. W. Armstrong and registered in 1868. Printed mark no. 326. 18 inches high.*

41. *Belleek figure, one of a pair in glazed and matt Parian and a typical teapot of marine form (shape registered in 1869). Printed crest mark (c. 1870–80).*

Godden of Worthing

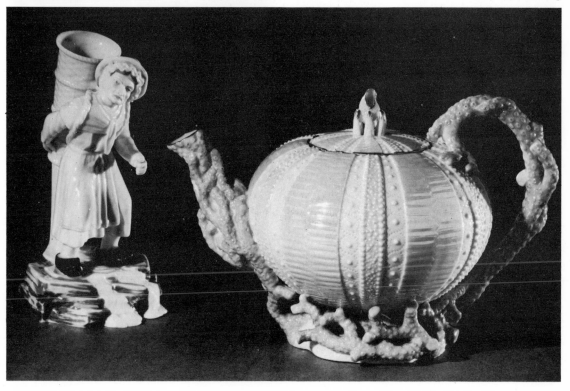

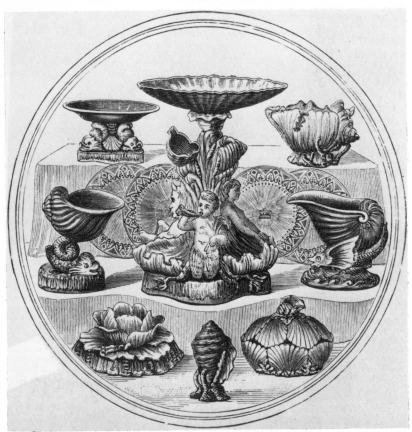

42. Group of Belleek porcelain as shown at the 1872 Exhibition. Reproduced from a contemporary engraving.

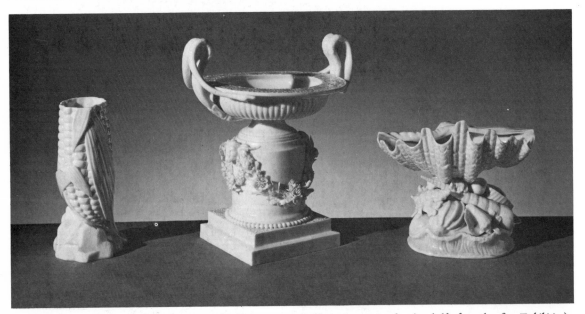

43. Three examples of Belleek ware purchased for the Victoria & Albert Museum in 1871 (probably from the 1871 Exhibition). Tazza. 8½ inches high.

Victoria & Albert Museum

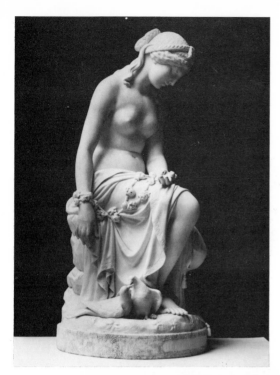

44. *Belleek Parian figure "The Prisoner of Love" (c. 1870),*
25½ inches high. This figure was reviewed in the Art Journal
of February 1871.

Ulster Museum

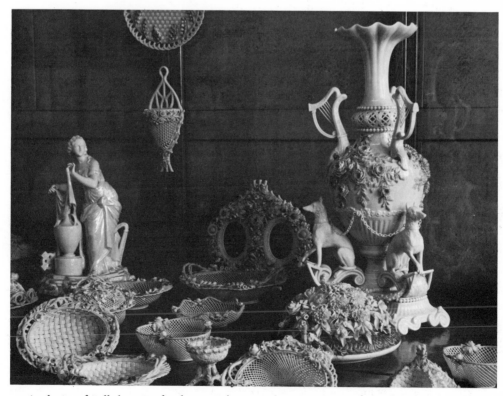

45. *A selection of Belleek wares of early twentieth-century date. Late version of printed mark with "Ireland" or*
"Made in Ireland" added under main mark (no. 327).

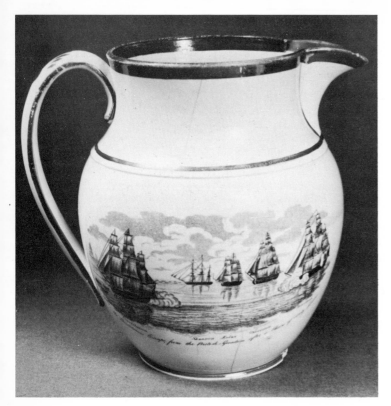

46. *Staffordshire earthenware jug printed by Bentley, Wear & Bourne of Shelton (signed on print) with naval battle, for the American market (c. 1815–23).* $7\frac{1}{4}$ *inches high.*

Willett Collection, Brighton Museum

BEVINGTON AND CO

47. *Bevington & Co, Swansea (impressed marked) unglazed porcelain ram. The initials I W of the modeller Isaac Wood also occur on this rare example (c. 1817–21).*

Victoria & Albert Museum

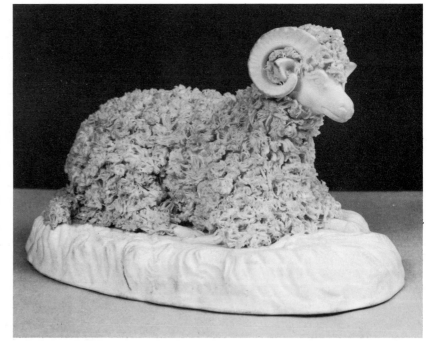

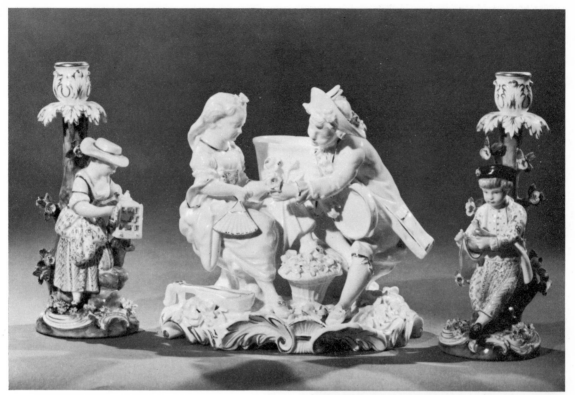

48. *Typical decorative Dresden-type porcelains by John Bevington of Hanley (c. 1872-92), bearing crossed-swords mark with monogram JB below (mark no. 352). Fine floral encrusted vases were also made.*

Godden of Worthing

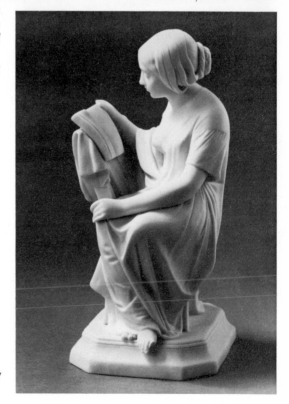

J. AND T. BEVINGTON
49. *Parian figure by James & Thomas Bevington of Hanley (c. 1865-78). Initial mark—J & T B. 12¼ inches high.*

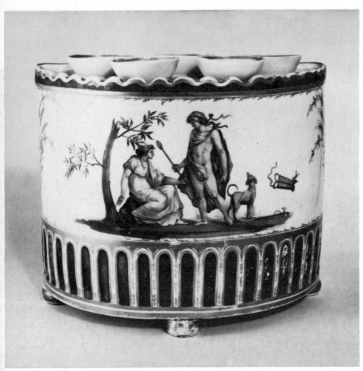

50. *Porcelain bulb pot decorated, by (or for) William Billingsley at Mansfield, in sepia monochrome. Scratched mark on base: "Billingsley, Mansfield, Nottinghamshire" (c. 1799–1802). 6¾ inches high.*

Derby Museum

51. *Porcelain jug and covered cup, decorated by William Billingsley at Mansfield (c. 1799–1802). Marked "Billingsley, Mansfield, Notts", in gold, on jug and "Billingsley, Mansfield", in red, on cup. Jug 7½ inches high.*

National Museum of Wales

Note.—*A jug of similar shape in the Lincoln Museum is marked "Brampton", the site of another Billingsley decorating establishment (see Plate 76).*

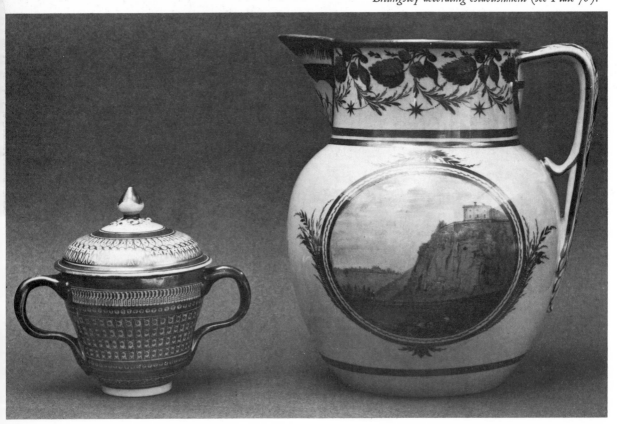

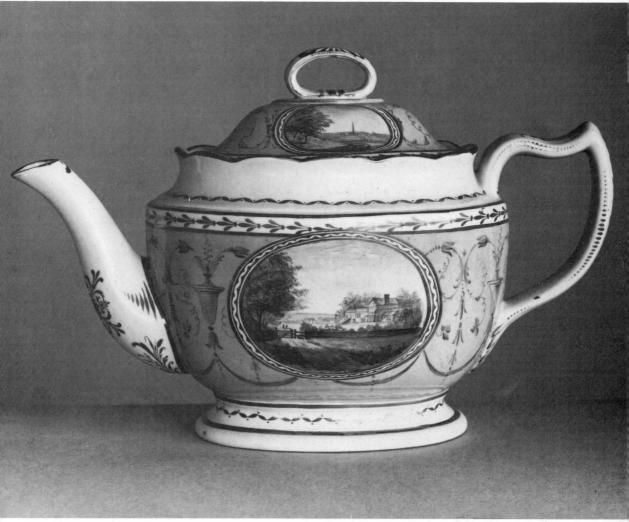

52. *A fine yellow-ground teapot decorated at Billingsley's Mansfield Works. Marked "No 26, Billingsley, Mansfield" and "B26". Billingsley is believed to have been at Mansfield only from 1799 to June 1802.*

Victoria & Albert Museum

The cream jug shown in Plate 456 is decorated with this pattern and also bears the mark, or pattern number, B.26. If the traditional attribution of the cream jug to the Pinxton factory is correct, it would appear that Billingsley used the same pattern book at his several different decorating establishments or factories. It is also possible that Billingsley while at Mansfield purchased undecorated porcelain from the Pinxton factory, with which he was connected before April 1799.

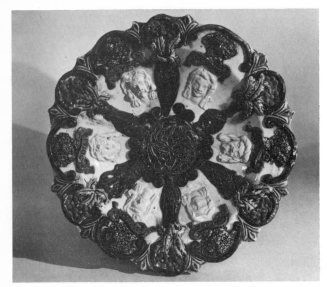

53. *"Castle Hedingham" pottery dish by Edward Bingham (c. 1890). 10 inches diameter. See detail of mark.*

For further information see new 15th edition of Chaffer's Marks and Monograms . . .

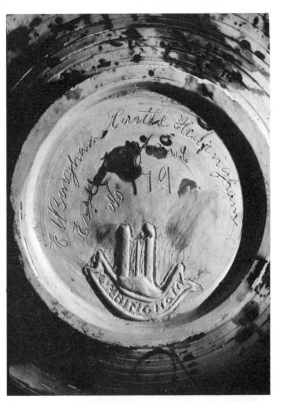

54. *Reverse of Castle Hedingham dish, showing applied castle mark and incised signature, etc.*

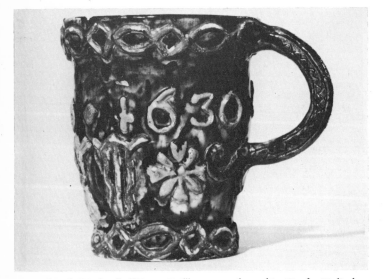

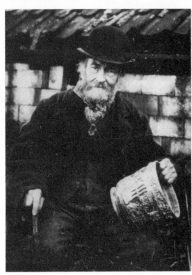

55. *Edward Bingham's "Feare God" mug, made at his Castle Hedingham Pottery. Moulded castle mark, no. 368, with "Made in Essex, England" incised (c. 1890). 5½ inches high. Most Castle Hedingham wares have a very ancient appearance.*

56. *Edward Bingham of the Castle Hedingham Pottery (c. 1900).*

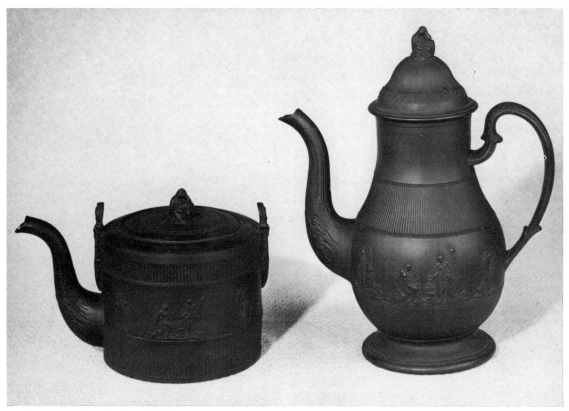

57. *Birch (impressed mark) basalt tea and coffee pot of attractive design. The teapot had a wicker-bound wire loop handle (c. 1796–1814). Coffee pot 12¼ inches high.*

City Museum and Art Gallery, Stoke-on-Trent

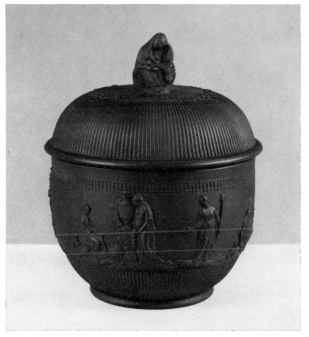

58. *Birch (impressed marked) basalt covered sugar bowl, typical of the 1805–10 period. 5 inches high. Edmund John Birch potted at Shelton from c. 1802 to c. 1814.*

Victoria & Albert Museum

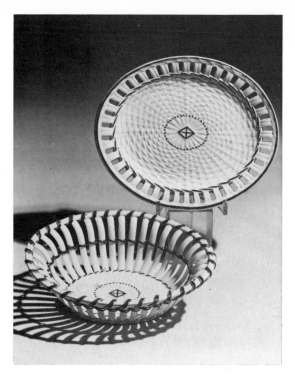

59. *Creamware openwork basket and stand of a type made by most potters (see page xv). This example has the impressed initial mark "B & W" and probably relates to the short-lived partnership of Birch & Whitehead, Hanley (c. 1796). Stand 8½ × 7 inches.*

BISHOPS WALTHAM, HAMPSHIRE

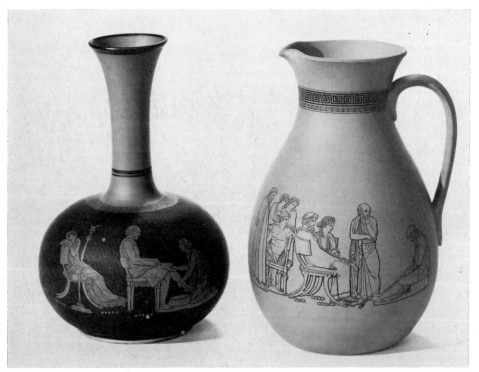

60. *Bishops Waltham (printed mark) terracotta wares with printed motifs. Specimens are very rare as ornamental objects were only produced from February 1866 to December 1867. Jug 6¾ inches high. See page 169 of* Chaffer's *Marks and Monograms,* 15th edition.

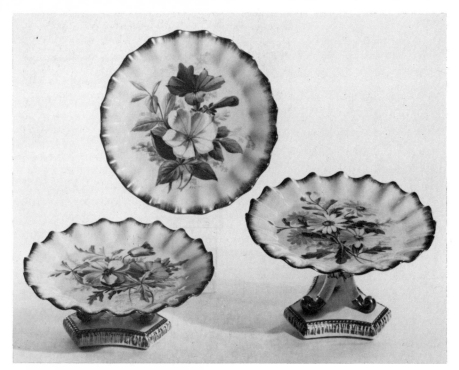

61. *E. J. D. Bodley porcelain dessert service, the forms registered in 1887 and painted by A. Copey. Impressed name mark and printed mark no. 430 (c. 1887–92). Comport 4½ inches high.*

Godden of Worthing

E. BOOTH OF TUNSTALL

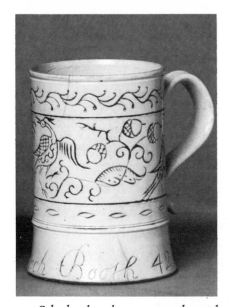

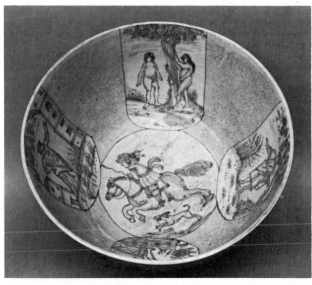

62. *Salt-glazed earthenware mug, decorated with "scratch blue" decoration (see page xv). Signed and dated "Enoch Booth. 1742". 4¾ inches high. Booth was an important manufacturer of salt-glaze and other wares at Tunstall in the first half of the eighteenth century. No true factory mark was used.*

Fitzwilliam Museum, Cambridge

63. *Earthenware bowl by Enoch Booth of Tunstall. Painted in underglaze blue and inscribed "E.B 1743" (see page xv). 10 inches diameter.*

British Museum.

33

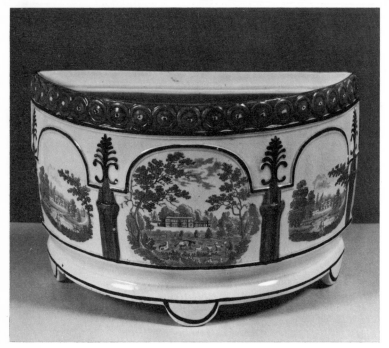

64. *Bott & Co (impressed marked) earthenware bulb pot, with bat printed scenic panels. Other marked specimens show good "silver" lustre decoration. A 1809 directory lists "Thomas Bott & Co, Earthenware Manufact. Lane End"; later directories do not include this firm (c. 1809). 5⅞ inches high.*

Victoria & Albert Museum

E. BOURNE', LONGPORT *c.* 1790–1811

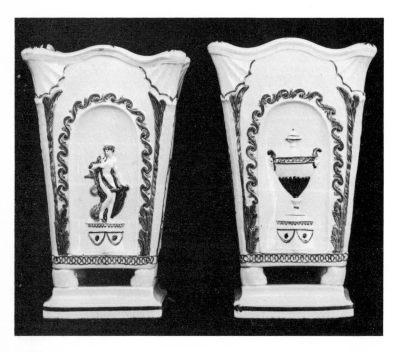

65. *E. Bourne (impressed marked) earthenware cachepots, decorated with Pratt-type raised and coloured motifs (see page xxii). Edward Bourne potted at Longport (c. 1790–1811); marked specimens are very rare. 8¾ inches high.*

D. M. & P. Manheim

The Bow factory was established in the 1740's in the ward of Stratford within the parish of West Ham on the Essex side of Bow Bridge and not, as has been formerly stated, at Stratford-le-Bow. A patent for making porcelain was taken out in 1744 (a second is dated November 1749), but the first evidence we have that porcelain was made on a commercial scale before 1750 is a reference in the 4th edition of Defoe's *Tour of Great Britain* dated 1748: "the first village we come to is Bow where a large manufactory of Porcelain is lately set up. They have already made large quantities of tea-cups, saucers etc. which by some skilful persons are said to be little inferior to those which are brought from China. . . ." At this period, the firm was trading as Alderman Arnold & Co and the works were titled "New Canton", a name which occurs on some small circular inkwells which are sometimes dated 1750 or 1751 (Plate 66).

The Bow porcelain is soft paste and it contains a relatively high proportion of bone-ash so that it is phosphatic when chemically tested. The early wares are of a close compact body and are consequently heavy and not very translucent; most early examples are unmarked—early figures were simply modelled and are often undecorated. A large proportion of early useful wares were decorated in underglaze blue and the enamelled specimens are sparsely decorated, often after imported Chinese prototypes.

After about 1760 the enamelled specimens became more flamboyant, the figures often having floral encrusted bocages at the back and being raised on scroll-footed bases. Such figures are sometimes marked with an anchor and dagger painted in red (see Plates 70–1). The later porcelain was of a rather chalky open texture and is lighter in weight than the earlier. The Bow factory was closed *c.* 1776.

The best modern guide to the Bow factory and its productions is the illustrated catalogue (prepared by Hugh Tait, F.S.A.) to the exhibition of Bow Porcelain held at the British Museum in 1959–60. Interesting articles arising from this exhibition are contained in the *Apollo* magazine of February, April, June, and October 1960 and in the *Transactions of the English Ceramic Circle*, vol. 5, part 4. Information on Bow blue and white porcelains will be found in Dr B. Watney's *English Blue and White Porcelain of the 18th Century* (1963); for Bow figures Frank Stoner's *Chelsea, Bow and Derby Porcelain Figures* (1955); and Arthur Lane's *English Porcelain Figures of the 18th Century* (1961) should be consulted. Hugh Tait's contribution to *English Porcelain 1745–1850* is a very good account of the factory's history. Marks are reproduced in the *Encyclopaedia of British Pottery and Porcelain Marks* (1964). See also the new 15th revised edition of Chaffer's *Marks and Monograms* (1965). A detailed work by Elizabeth Adams and David Redstone is in preparation.

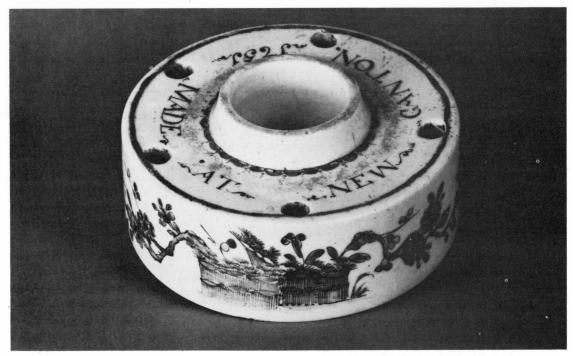

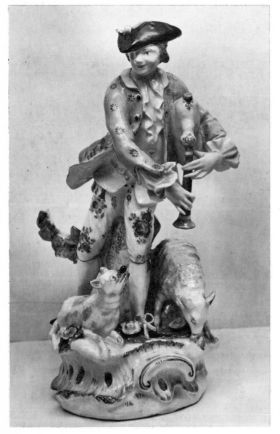

66. *Bow porcelain inkwell. Inscribed "Made at New Canton, 1751". Similar examples are recorded with the date 1750. The name "New Canton" was used by the Bow manufacturers at this period. 4 inches diameter.*

Victoria & Albert Museum

Reproductions of these early documentary inkwells have been reported.

67. *Bow porcelain figure of a shepherd, initialled "IB" and dated 1757 on the bagpipes. This rare dated figure helps to date other figures with this type of base. 10 inches high.*

Formerly in the J. MacHarg Collection

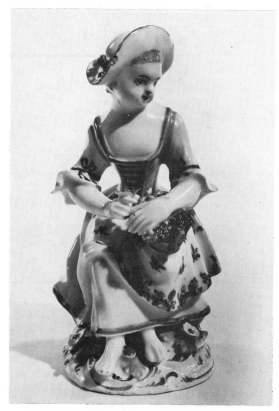

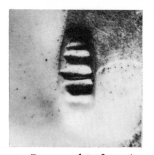

68. *Bow porcelain figure (c. 1755). Pale yellow hat and skirt. Square hole at back of base. Impressed oval "mark" under base (see detail). 5½ inches high.*

Godden of Worthing

69. *Bow porcelain tea-party group, bearing the impressed mark T, attributed to the "repairer" Tebo. See companion mark book (c. 1755–60) 9½ inches long.*

Formerly in the collection of Colonel H. Thynne

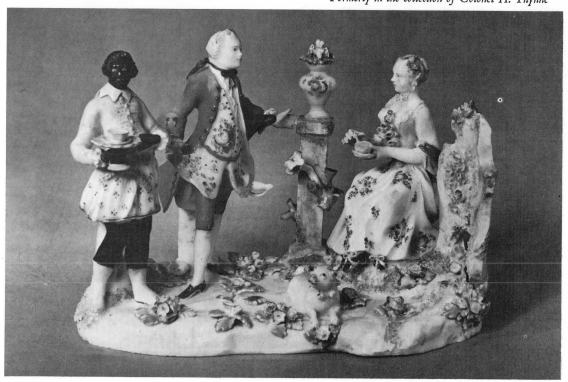

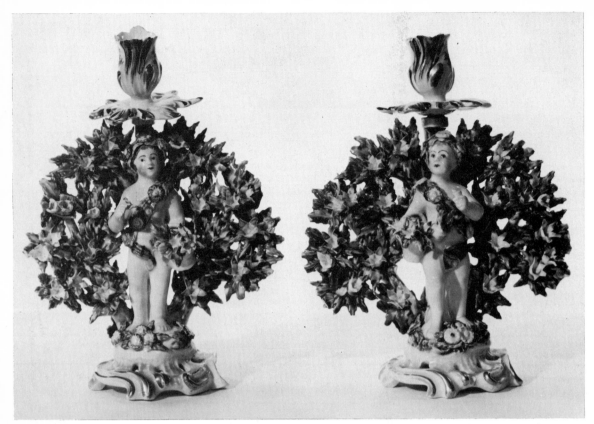

70. *Bow porcelain figure candle-holders, with typical floral background or "bocage" (c. 1760–70). Painted anchor and dagger mark (no. 505) in red. 8½ inches high.*

Godden of Worthing

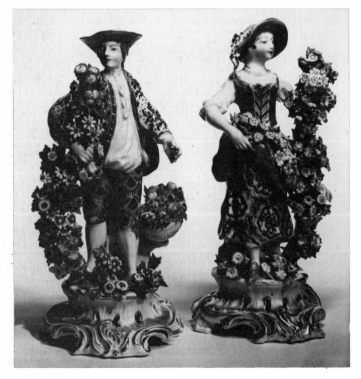

71. *Pair Bow porcelain figures, richly enamelled. Anchor and dagger mark in red (c. 1760–76). 10¼ inches high.*

Godden of Worthing

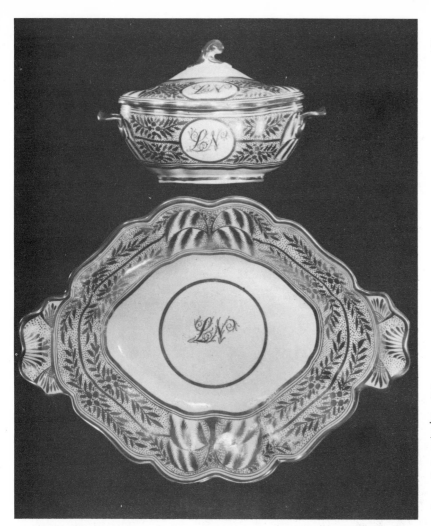

72. Part of a finely gilt Swansea-type porcelain dessert service, with decorator's or retailer's mark "Bradley & Co" (c. 1813–20).

Godden of Worthing

73. Basalt teapots impressed marked "Bradley & Co, Coalport". No manufacturer of this name is recorded at Coalport. These specimens and others bearing this mark were probably made for the London retailer J. Bradley & Co. Directories of 1813–14 list J. Bradley, Colebrook-Dale China Manufact., 54 Pall Mall (c. 1810–15). $4\frac{1}{4}$ inches high.

Victoria & Albert Museum

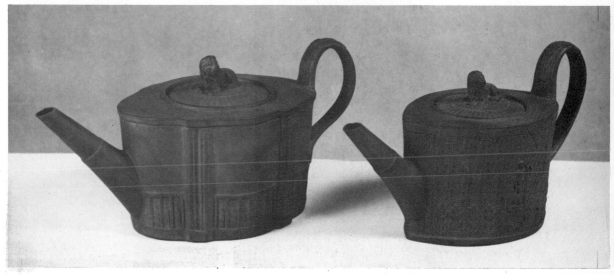

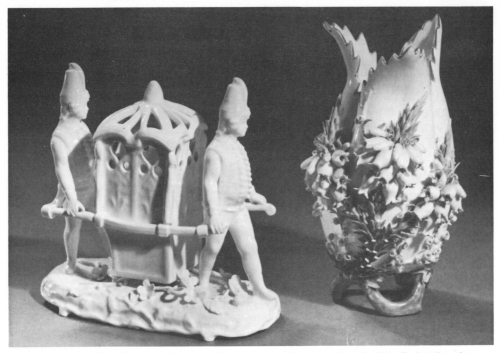

74. *F. D. Bradley of Longton (c. 1876–96) porcelains with impressed marks "Bradley". The white group was registered in 1879. Floral vase 8 inches high.*

Godden of Worthing

BRAMPTON, LINCOLNSHIRE

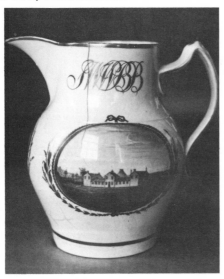

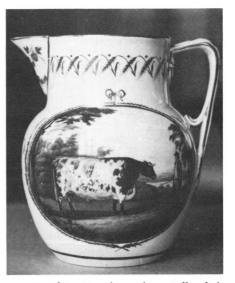

75. *Porcelain jug, dated 1806, decorated at Billingsley's small factory or decorating establish-ment at Brampton, near Torksey, Lincolnshire. The panel depicts the manufactory. Gilt mark or description "Brampt. Manufactory". 7½ inches high.*

Exley Collection, Usher Gallery, Lincoln

76. *Porcelain jug, decorated at Billingsley's Brampton Manufactory (depicted in Plate 75). Very rare gilt mark "Brampton". The form of this jug is the same as the earlier marked "Billingsley, Mansfield" example shown in Plate 51. 7⅝ inches high.*

Exley Collection, Usher Gallery, Lincoln

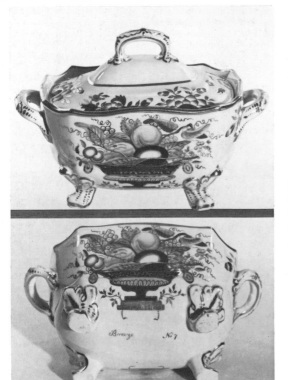

77. *A rare pair of porcelain sauce tureens by J. Breeze of Tunstall, painted name mark as shown. These specimens are well decorated in underglaze blue and overglaze enamels and finely gilt (c. 1805–12). Marked specimens are very rare.*

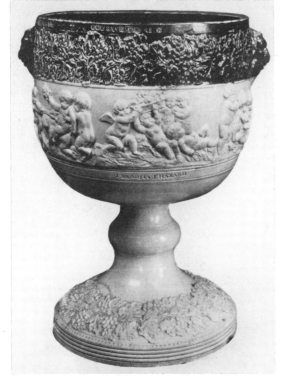

78. *Bristol stoneware goblet made at Bright's Pottery. Rare impressed mark "J Bright. J. Hazard" (c. 1818). 14 inches high.*

Bristol Museum

Bristol Porcelain

The earliest porcelain was made at Bristol in 1749 or 1750 by Benjamin Lund and William Miller of Redcliff Backs, Bristol. Benjamin Lund had taken out a licence to mine soap rock (a constituent of his porcelain) in March 1748–9. Some rare figures are dated 1750, and these and some sauce boats bear the moulded mark BRISTOL or BRISTOLL (see Plates 79, 80). Apart from these name marks, the early Bristol wares do not bear any factory mark, only workmen's private marks.

Early in 1752 the Lund-Miller concern at Bristol was purchased by the partners of the Worcester Porcelain Works and surplus stock was sold in Bristol, although part may have been forwarded to Worcester. Benjamin Lund was in Worcester in February 1753.

The Bristol porcelain discussed above is soft paste and is most attractive, both in the forms and in decoration. Specimens are scarce. For further information the reader is referred to a paper by Aubrey J. Toppin in the *Transactions of the English Ceramic Circle*, vol. 3, part 3, and to an article by H. E. Marshall in *The Antique Collector* (April 1959).

The manufacture of true, or hard-paste, porcelain with its cold glittery appearance and glass-like fracture, was started by William Cookworthy at Bristol about 1770. In 1773 the works at 15 Castle Green, Bristol, were taken over by Richard Champion (& Co). It is believed that the manufacture of porcelain ceased in 1778 and for the next three years objects made earlier were decorated and disposed of. The last sale was held in May 1782, but the Bristol factory may be said to have closed in 1781.

The most frequently found wares are teawares, usually decorated with simple, attractive floral motifs. Figures and vases were also made, as were charming, small, oval unglazed porcelain plaques of armorial bearings, portraits or flowers. A fine selection of wares is illustrated in F. Severne Mackenna's *Champion's Bristol Porcelain* (1947).

The standard Bristol mark is a painted cross, often with a painter's number. The initial "B" also occurs as does a copy of the Dresden crossed-swords mark. Most specimens show wreathing or spiral low ridges on articles which were turned on the potter's wheel (see Plate 88). Reproductions of typical Bristol floral festoon pattern teaware were made or decorated by S. J. Kepple & Sons. They have a *soft* paste body and the glaze is often very crazed; the reproductions often bear the cross mark with the date 1776.

Apart from porcelains, delft-type earthenware, stoneware, and creamware was made by several potters at Bristol. Two reference books—*Two Centuries of Ceramic Art in Bristol* by H. Owen (1873) and *The Old Bristol Potteries* by W. J. Pountney (1920)—give good information on these wares. The Bristol City Museum has a very fine collection of local wares.

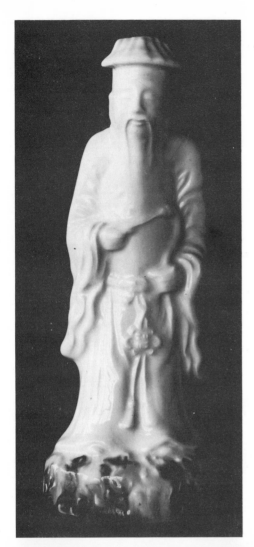

79. "Bristoll 1750" (moulded mark on back of base). Bristol porcelain figure based on a Chinese original. These marked figures are very rare, the name Bristoll also occurs with one l (c. 1750). 7 inches high.

Victoria & Albert Museum

80. Bristol porcelain sauceboat painted in underglaze blue and also with moulded motifs. Marked with the word "Bristoll" moulded in relief (c. 1750). 6¼ inches long.

Victoria & Albert Museum

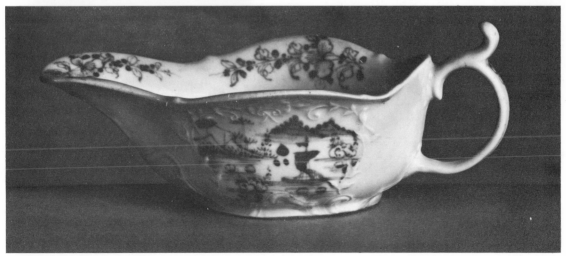

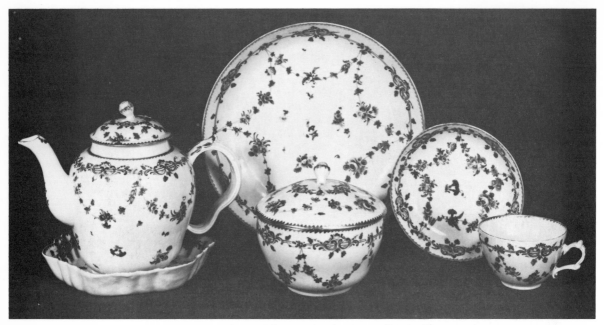

81. *Bristol (hard paste) porcelain teawares of typical forms and style of enamelled floral pattern. Cross mark in blue-grey (c. 1770–81).*

Delomosne & Son

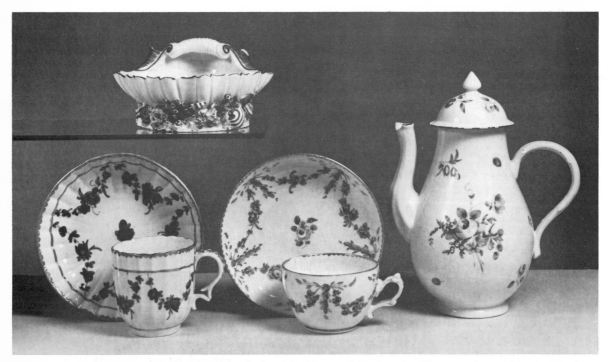

82. *A group of typical Bristol (hard paste) porcelains. The coffee pot, shell salt and middle cup, and saucer bear the crossed-swords mark in underglaze blue. The fluted cup and saucer has the cross mark in blue. The handle forms and gilt dentil borders are often found on Bristol teawares (c. 1770–81). Coffee pot $7\frac{1}{2}$ inches high.*

Victoria & Albert Museum

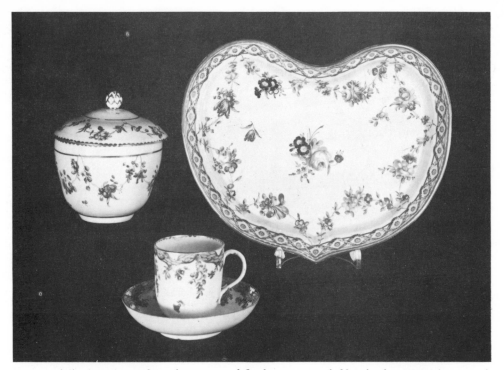

83. *Bristol (hard paste) porcelains showing typical floral patterns. Dish 8¾ inches long. Painted cross mark with "6" in gold (c. 1770–81).*

Delomosne & Son

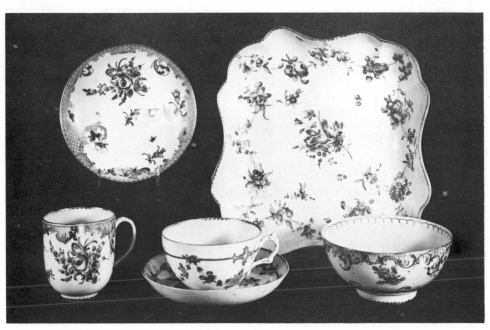

84. *Bristol (hard paste) porcelains of typical forms and decoration. Painted cross marks, with painter's numbers (c. 1770–81).*

Delomosne & Son

45

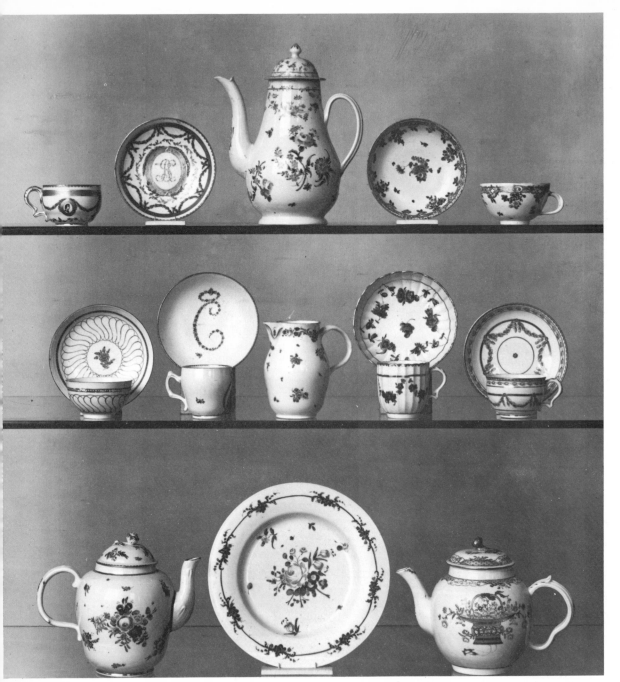

85. *Group of Bristol (hard paste) porcelains from the Allen Collection at the Victoria & Albert Museum. Most specimens have the cross mark with a number. Other pieces have the crossed-swords mark in underglaze blue (c. 1770–80).*

Victoria & Albert Museum

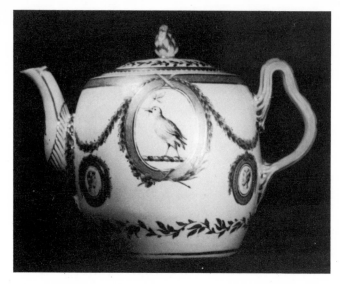

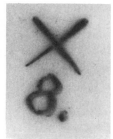

86. *Bristol hard-paste porcelain teapot from the Chough service. Cross mark with number —8, see detail of mark (c. 1775). 6 inches high.*
Bristol City Art Gallery

87. *Bristol hard-paste porcelain teapot, dated 1777. Detail of base shows typical crossed-swords mark in underglaze blue with gilt painter's or gilder's number added over the glaze. 6¼ inches high.*

Bristol City Art Gallery

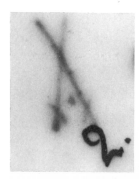

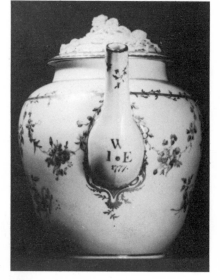

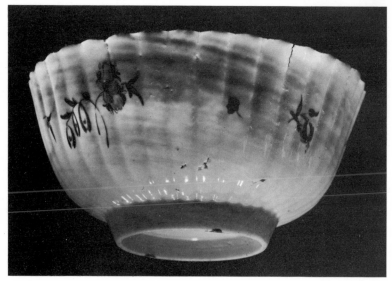

88. *Bristol bowl, showing typical wreathing or spiral ridges, also slight tears in the body. The wreathing may also occur on Plymouth hard-paste porcelain (see page xviii).*

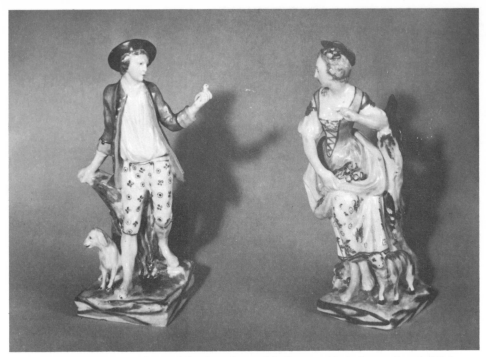

89. *An attractive pair of Bristol (hard paste) porcelain figures, with the impressed mark "To"*
(c. 1770–81).

Albert Amor Ltd

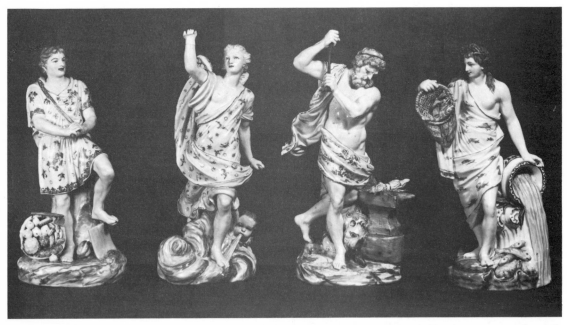

90. *Bristol (hard paste) porcelain figures of the Elements. A letter from Richard Champion, dated February 1772, refers to the modelling of these figures. A similar set is in the Victoria & Albert Museum. "Fire" has the impressed "To" mark (see companion Encyclopaedia of Marks). Fire, 11 inches high.*

Delomosne & Son

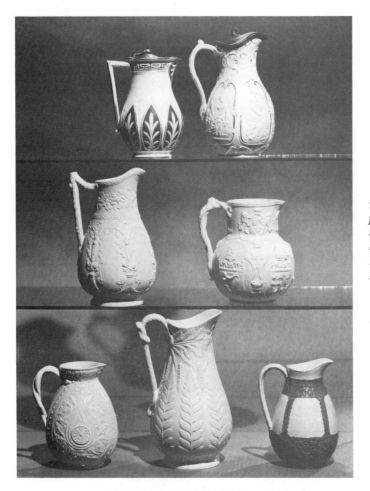

91. *William Brownfield of Cobridge moulded parian jugs, all bearing impressed or moulded initial marks. All these forms were registered by William Brownfield between 1861 and 1868. Many other potters made moulded jugs of similar types.*

PHILIP BURCH

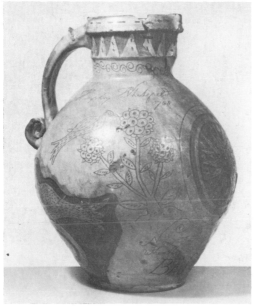

92. *"Philip Burch. Maker, 1788" (incised inscription) earthenware harvest jug, showing typical West Country type of Sgraffiato (incised) decoration (see page xiii). Place-name "Barum" (Barnstaple) under inscription. 12½ inches high.*

Fitzwilliam Museum, Cambridge

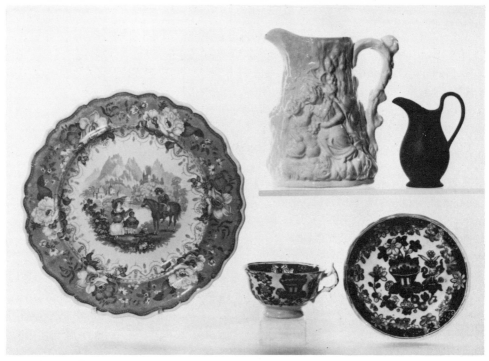

93. *Selection of "C" wares: Blue printed earthenware plate, initial mark of Chetham & Robinson of Longton (c. 1822–37). Moulded jug by Cork & Edge, ornate printed name mark (c. 1855). Basalt creamer of Caughley make, impressed mark "Salopian" (c. 1785–95). Porcelain cup and saucer, printed name mark "Cooke & Hulse" (c. 1835–55). Moulded jug 7¼ inches high.*

JOHN CARTLEDGE OF COBRIDGE, STAFFORDSHIRE POTTERIES

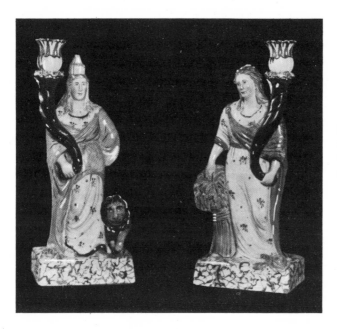

94. *John Cartledge . . . 1800, unique inscription mark. Earthenware candlestick figures of Diana and Ceres. 12 inches high.*

E. W. J. Legg, Esq.

The history of Caughley or "Salopian" porcelain starts when Thomas Turner moved to Caughley, near Broseley, Shropshire, in the middle 1770's. A most important newspaper announcement of 1775 reads: "The Porcelain Manufactory erected near Bridgnorth in this County is now quite completed and the proprietors have received and completed orders to a very large amount. Lately we saw some of their productions which in colour fineness are truly elegant and beautiful and have the bright and lovely white of the much extolled Oriental."

The early Caughley porcelains closely follow those of the Worcester factory, in shape, style of decoration, and in the general type of body. By transmitted light the body is more orange than Worcester and has been described as golden-ochre. Early wares are painted or printed in underglaze blue. The shapes copy Worcester examples—leaf-moulded jugs with mask-head spouts (Plates 95, 99), oval covered butter-dishes and stands with twig handles, openwork baskets of several Worcester types, salad bowls, etc. The early blue printed patterns also seem to be based on those used at Worcester. An exception occurs in the very popular Caughley "Pleasure Boat" or "Fisherman" pattern (Plate 96). The blue printed Caughley porcelains are generally marked with a crescent, a "C" or "S" (or Sx), all printed or painted in underglaze blue. The rarer coloured porcelains are generally unmarked; some dishes, plates, ice pails, etc., have the impressed mark "Salopian"; examples are illustrated in Plates 96, 100. The output of the Caughley factory seems to have been confined to useful ware, mainly teaware. Recent excavations on the factory site have shed light on the later, generally unmarked, Caughley porcelains. Some of the finest overglaze enamel patterns were added at Chamberlain's decorating establishment at Worcester (see page 57). Chamberlain purchased vast quantities of Caughley porcelain in the 1780–95 period, as shown in surviving account and order books. Contemporary prices and names quoted in captions are taken from these sources.

In 1799 Thomas Turner sold the Caughley works, the stock of unglazed goods, and all the implements, fixtures, moulds, and copperplates to Edward Blakeway, John Rose, and Richard Rose "of Coalport, porcelain manufacturers". The new owners continued the factory for about fifteen years, see page 91. The true period of *Turner's* Caughley porcelain manufacture is twenty-five years (1775–99).

For the detailed history of the Caughley works the reader is referred to F. A. Barrett's *Caughley and Coalport Porcelain* (1951). Of particular importance is G. Godden's standard book *Caughley and Worcester Porcelains 1775–1800* (Herbert Jenkins, London, 1969), and see also *British Porcelain, an Illustrated Guide* by G. Godden. Good collections are to be seen in the Victoria & Albert Museum in London, at the Clive House Museum at Shrewsbury and at the old Coalport factory near Ironbridge in Shropshire.

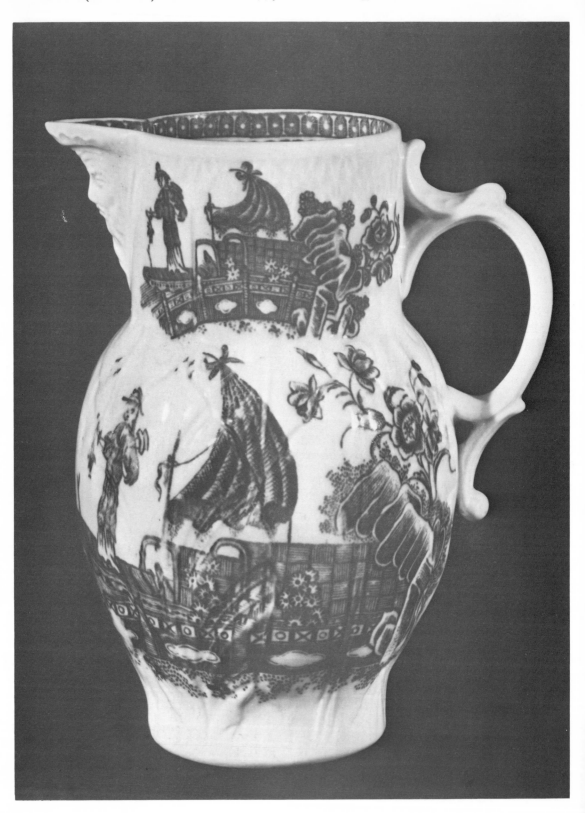

95. *A Caughley mask-head cabbage-leaf jug of typical slender form bearing this factory's version of the Fisherman or "Pleasure Boat" print in underglaze blue. Note the short fat fish held by a tall slender man. "S" mark in blue (c. 1785). 6 inches high.*

Godden of Worthing

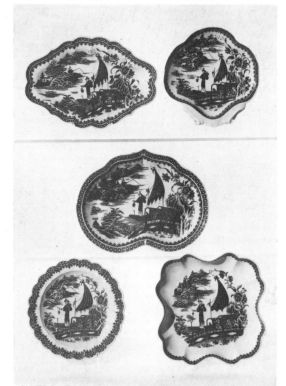

96. *Caughley porcelain dessert service, of the Fisherman pattern, printed in underglaze blue. The dish and plate forms are typical. Impressed "Salopian" mark and printed initial "S" (c. 1785). Plate 8 inches diameter.*

Godden of Worthing

In contemporary records this pattern was termed "Pleasure Boat".

97. *Rare but typical Caughley miniature or "toy" porcelains bearing a standard underglaze blue design found on such pieces. "S" marks in blue (c. 1785). Water bottle $1\frac{9}{10}$ inches high.*

Godden of Worthing

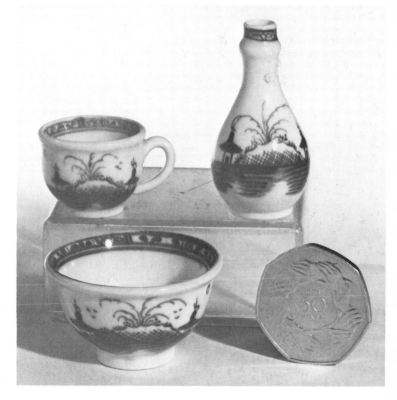

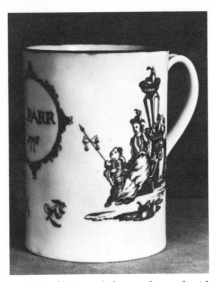

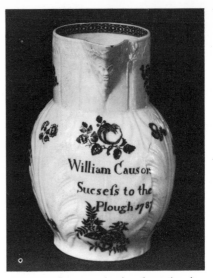

98. *Caughley inscribed mug, decorated with underglaze blue print and painted name and date (1776). Printed "C" mark. 4½ inches high.*

Victoria & Albert Museum

99. *Caughley jug, dated 1787. The shape (copied from Worcester) is generally known as "cabbage leaf, mask head", but in contemporary records they are referred to as "Dutch Jugs". These were made in several sizes and decorated in many designs, underglaze blue, or overglaze enamels, or both.*

Tilley & Co

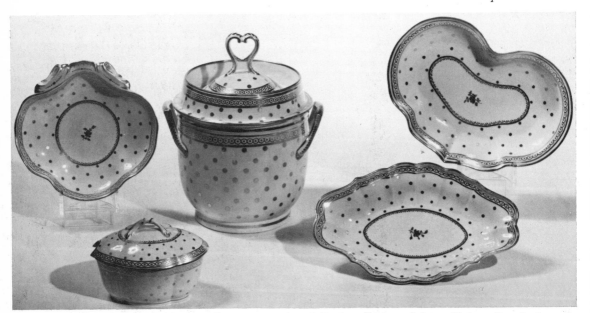

100. *Caughley porcelain dessert service, with rare impressed mark "Salopian". Decorated in gold (c. 1785-90). Ice pail 10¾ inches high.*

Godden of Worthing

Gold patterns were widely used mainly on teawares. Caughley dessert services are rare; unmarked pieces are often attributed to the Worcester factory in error.

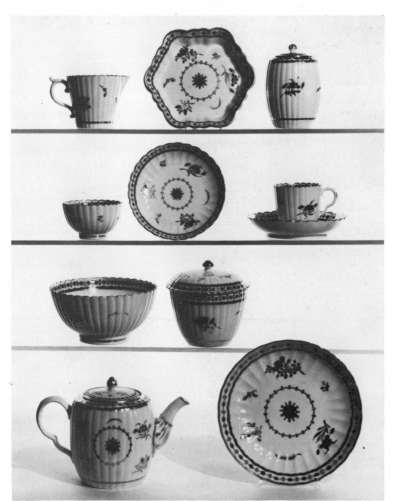

101. *Caughley fluted teaset, showing typical shapes of the 1785–95 period. Underglaze blue design, finished with gilding. "S" mark in blue. Teapot 6½ inches high.*

Godden of Worthing

102. *Fragments found on the Caughley factory site, showing underglaze portions of designs later finished with gilding as in the above teaset. Two pieces in the centre do bear the gilding. The circular object on the bottom row is a porcelain button.*

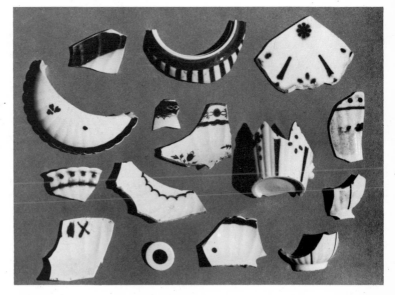

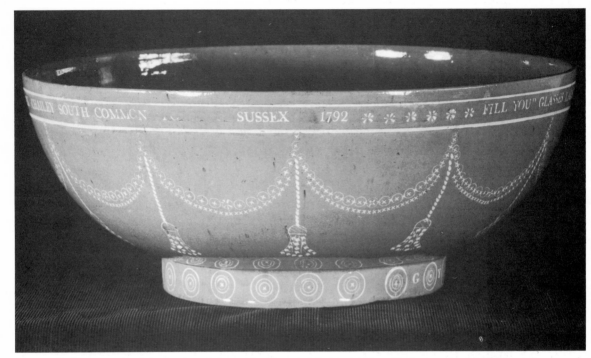

103. *Chailey pottery bowl dated 1792 and decorated with typical Sussex inlaid motifs. Impressed and inlaid inscription around rim—"Fill your glasses lads and lasses round the Maypole frisk and play . . . Tho Alcorn. Chailey South Common Pottery. Sussex. 1792." 13¾ inches diameter.*

Sussex Archaeological Society Museum, Lewes

Robert Chamberlain, a former apprentice at the main Worcester factory established by Dr Wall and continued by the Flights (see page 368), left about 1786 to start his own decorating establishment. At first he and other former Flight painters were content to decorate wares purchased from Thomas Turner of the Caughley works (see page 51).

In 1789 Chamberlain reopened, after alterations, Flight's former retail shop at 33 High Street, Worcester. An entry in John Flight's diary of 28 June 1789 reads: "Yesterday, Chamberlain opened his shop. I was rather surprised as I thought they were hardly ready yet, but they talk of making a flaming shew in about 2 months."

By 1791 Chamberlain decided to manufacture his own porcelain rather than be dependent on Caughley wares. The change-over must have been gradual and for several years Chamberlain and his son, Humphrey, decorated Caughley porcelains as well as their own. The painted patterns were simple; the unique, dated, teapot of 1796 shown in Plate 104 is a typical example of the early form of decoration. Useful wares, particularly tea services, were produced; the shapes are often fluted and oval in form. Marks were rarely used before about 1795, but when they do occur, they appear as written words—"Chamberlains", "Chamberlain Worcester Warranted", etc. These marks often occur inside the cover of a teapot or sugar bowl. Other pieces are unmarked or bear only the pattern number painted in a small, neat manner. The pattern numbers had reached about 170 by 1798, about 225 in 1800, and 1,000 in September 1822.

As the Chamberlain works gained prestige, so the range of their products increased and was no longer confined to useful objects. Richly decorated ornate vases, painted by accomplished artists, became a feature of their manufacture. Before his death in 1824 Humphrey Chamberlain painted some of the finest figure subjects, as did the famous and much-travelled Thomas Baxter. The finest vases were far from cheap; the Prince Regent was charged one hundred and five pounds in 1813 for three pieces painted with figure subjects. Good examples of Chamberlain ornamental ware may be seen in the Victoria & Albert Museum.

In 1811 the patronage of the Prince Regent resulted in the introduction of a new type of porcelain body termed "Regent"; this is comparatively hard and the glaze has a very glossy appearance. The name "Regent" occurs in special printed marks used on this ware. Dessert, dinner and tea services were made in it; marks on the ware sometimes include the words "Regent china". This body was introduced about 1811, but was sparingly used on account of its costly nature and production probably ceased by 1825.

In 1840 the two rival firms, that of Flight, Barr & Barr, and that of Chamberlain, were combined and new workshops erected at the Chamberlain site. The only innovation that was to be continued over many years was a series of double-walled objects, introduced c. 1845; the outer wall was pierced with geometrical designs, see Plate III. The Chamberlain display at the 1851 Exhibition included examples of this "honey-comb" china; also ornamental vases, baskets and services, and decorative china plaques moulded in one piece with the ornate gilt frame also in porcelain.

In 1852, when the Chamberlain Company was wound-up, W. H. Kerr and R. W. Binns formed a new company in which the old spirit was recovered and the name of Worcester porcelain re-established. From this "Kerr & Binns" partnership the present "Worcester Royal Porcelain Company" was formed in 1862.

For further information on Chamberlain wares the reader is referred to R. W. Binns's *Worcester Pottery and Porcelain 1751–1851* (1865 and 1877) and to G. Godden's *British Pottery and Porcelain, 1780–1850* (1963).

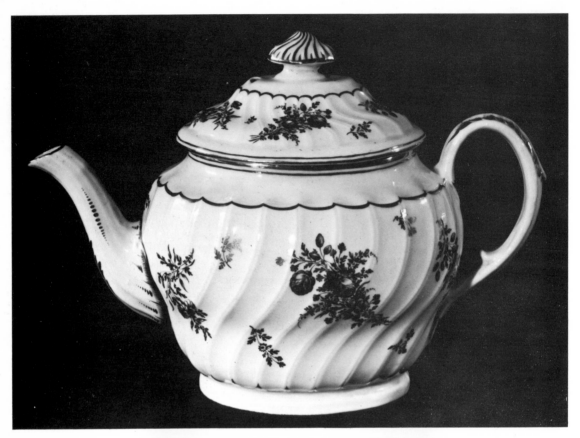

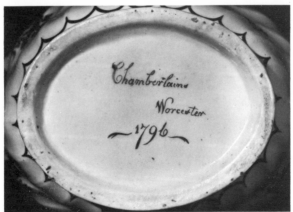

104. *"Chamberlains Worcester" (painted mark, see detail of base) porcelain, an important early dated example. Note pronounced double line effect at the highest point of the flute, other factories produced fluted teawares without this Chamberlain characteristic. Most Chamberlain teawares of this period are unmarked, other pieces are marked inside the cover.*

Godden of Worthing

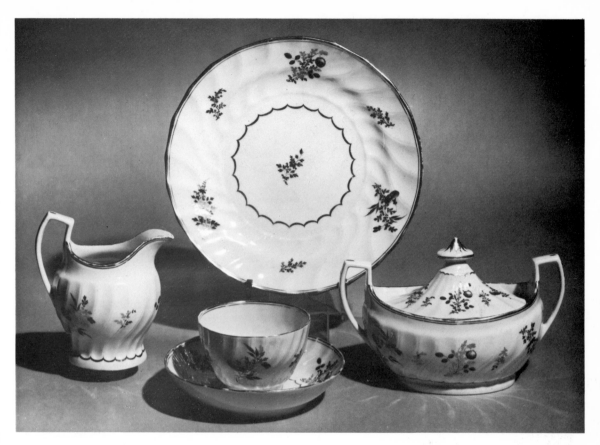

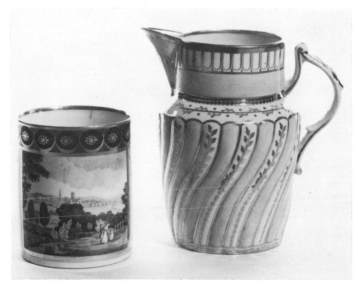

105. *Chamberlain Worcester teawares, showing typical forms, contemporary with the 1796 dated teapot (Plate 104). Marked on the inside of sucrier cover "Chamberlain Worcester Warranted" (written in gilt script). Pattern no. 21. Creamer 5 inches high.*

Godden of Worthing

Chamberlain account books show that tea services of this pattern, no. 21, were sold in 1794 for £4 14s. 6d. and £4 16s. 6d.

106. *"Chamberlain Worcester" (written marks) porcelain mug with fine quality printed view of Worcester and a fluted jug decorated in yellow and gold (c. 1800). Jug 7 inches high.*

Godden of Worthing

Many fine hand-painted as well as printed views of Worcester occur and some scenes show the factory. A "Pint jugg, yellow & gold stripe" was sold by Chamberlains for £1 1s. in August 1796.

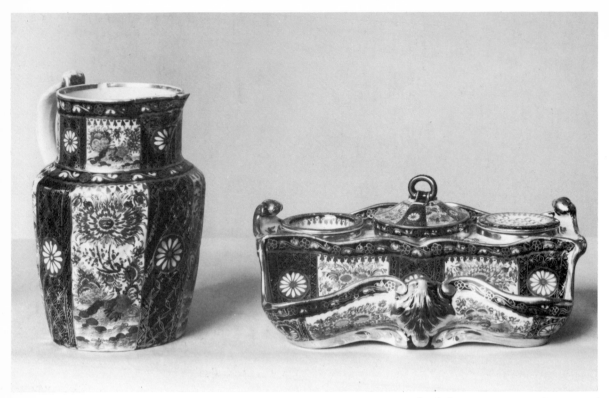

107. *Chamberlain Worcester porcelains painted with colourful so-called "Japan" patterns. Ink-stand marked "Chamberlain's Worcester". Painted in gold, a similar inkstand was sold for £1 11s. 6d. in 1799 (c. 1800). Jug 7 inches high.*

Allen Collection, Victoria & Albert Museum

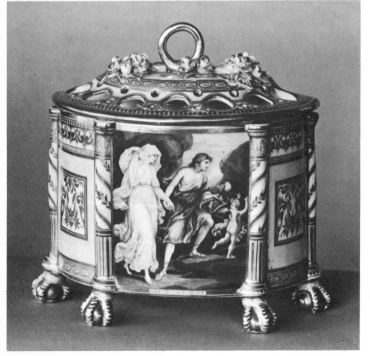

108. *"Chamberlain's Worcester" (painted mark in gold). The fine figure subject panel probably painted by John Wood, Chamberlain's early figure artist. Several "½ circle ornament with piller" are included in Chamberlain order books. One entry of 18 December 1800 reads: "I do (ornament) figures, Orpheus & Euridice, ½ circle shape", the subject depicted on this example (c. 1800). 8½ inches high.*

Victoria & Albert Museum

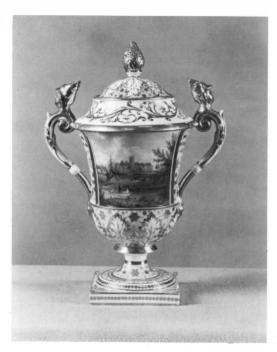

109. *A fine quality Chamberlain Worcester vase and cover. Marked "Chamberlain's Worcester. 155 New Bond St. London" (c. 1811–20). $8\frac{3}{4}$ inches high.*

Victoria & Albert Museum

110. *Part of a fine long Chamberlain Worcester dessert service decorated with raised floral national emblems (roses, thistles and shamrock), called in the 1818 accounts "The New Union Border", on a sage green ground. Hand-painted floral panels. Printed mark no. 842, incorporating address of London shop—155 New Bond Street (c. 1811–25). Ice pails $11\frac{3}{4}$ inches high.*

J. & E. Vandekar

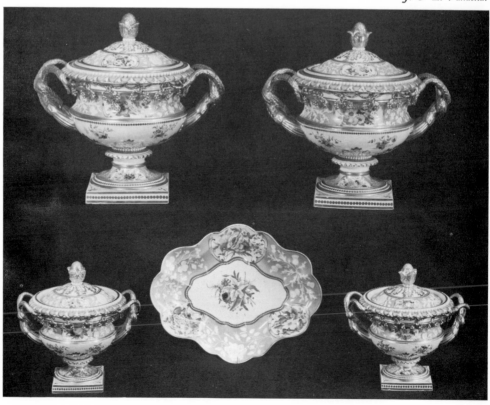

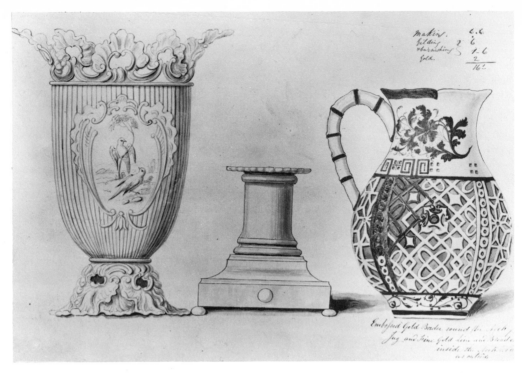

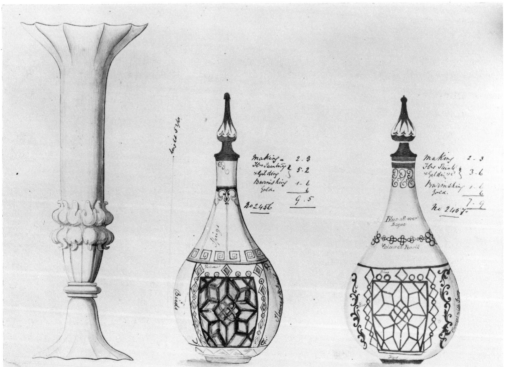

111 & a. *Two pages from a Chamberlain pattern book of the 1840's. Typical double-walled pierced articles are featured with the breakdown of the various manufacturing costs. Similar reticulated wares were illustrated in the Art Union Magazine of March 1846. The French National Sèvres factory produced similar openwork articles.*

Of all English porcelains, that made at Chelsea is the most famous, the most highly priced, and the most valued. Consequently it has been copied extensively, mainly on the Continent, for over one hundred years. Gold anchor marked figures, groups, and animals were reproduced in great numbers and are a danger to new collectors.

The true Chelsea porcelain is of soft paste (as opposed to most copies which are of hard glittery Continental porcelain). The glaze is warm and mellow, the added enamel colours tend to sink slightly into the glaze and become part of it (rather than sit on the surface as with the hard Continental glazes). Where gilding is present it is relatively soft and in the later wares is often tooled to show details in matt and burnished gold; it is never thin or brassy as is the gilding on nineteenth- and twentieth-century reproductions. Especially in the earlier Chelsea wares the porcelain shows slight faults—tears in the body, crazing in the glaze, slight warping in the firing, ground bases, or foot-rims, etc.

When held to the light the Chelsea porcelain often shows lighter spots or "pin holes" and slightly later, irregular patches of larger size termed "Moons" are observed. Plates and dishes often show "spur" or "stilt" marks where the piece was supported during the firing. The underside of a dish shown in Plate 139 illustrates this characteristic.

The historic details of the Chelsea factory and its proprietors are given in most reference books, several of which are listed at the end of this résumé. The following is but a brief summary listing the main periods and characteristics.

The factory was established in or before 1745; the first mark was an incised triangle which, on certain rare jugs modelled as a goat and termed "Goat and Bee" jugs, occurs with the word "Chelsea" and sometimes the year 1745 incised (see Plate 115); one example may be dated 1743, but the last numeral is open to some doubt. These Goat and Bee jugs, as with other triangle marked pieces, are often in white porcelain without any added decoration; marine forms, shell and lobster salts and sauce boats were favoured (see Plates 113, 117, 119–20). It should be noted that the triangle mark was incised into the clay and the strokes should show a slightly ploughed-up edge or have the appearance of being spontaneously incised. Impressed even-sided triangle marks should be treated with the greatest caution. A triangle in underglaze blue is *very* rare (Plate 121). The period known as the "triangle period" is *c.* 1745–9, but at this time another mark was occasionally used: it is a trident piercing a crown painted in underglaze blue (see Plate 122A).

The next period is known as the "raised anchor period", *c.* 1749–52, because the anchor appears moulded on a small raised oval pad (see Plate 126). Sometimes the anchor is picked out in red, at other times both the pad and anchor are left uncoloured. The Chelsea porcelains of this period are most tasteful in form and decoration. The porcelain body was enhanced by simple decoration rather than covered by ground colours or overbearing decoration. It will be observed that the early pre-gold anchor period (1765–9) Chelsea glaze is slightly opaque because of the addition of tin-oxide (as used by the delft ware potters) which gives a milky white appearance to the body. This characteristic (also found on some Longton Hall porcelain) helps to distinguish early Chelsea porcelains from that produced at other mid-eighteenth-century factories and from nineteenth-century reproductions.

The period *c.* 1752–6 is known as the "red anchor period" because the anchor mark was painted in red enamel direct on to the porcelain (the earlier applied raised pad was discontinued). This anchor was of small size (less than a quarter of an inch and often only an eighth of an inch in height) and on figures, groups, etc., it was often tucked away in some easily missed position. Therefore any large anchor marks boldly placed on supposedly Chelsea porcelain should be treated with caution. Apart from anchor-marked reproductions of Chelsea porcelain, several other factories used the anchor mark as their own sign; the most notable example being the eighteenth-century Italian factory at Venice which employed a *large* red anchor. Our own Bow factory also used a red anchor *with a dagger* as a standard mark. Other English porcelains—Derby, Worcester, etc., probably painted by independent London decorators—often had a Chelsea-like red anchor added (see Plate 212) so that in attributing porcelain of the 1752–6 period to Chelsea, the study of the warm mellow body and glaze should come before the mark. As with the earlier "raised anchor" Chelsea porcelain, the red anchor styles of decoration are subdued and tasteful, the forms being often taken from silver prototypes. The red anchor Chelsea figures and groups (Plates 134–7) are considered by many to represent the finest in English porcelain, although several models were copied from Dresden examples.

From about 1756 the general style of Chelsea porcelain became more florid; gilding was extensively used and the former red anchor gave way to one in gold, hence the term "gold anchor period" (*c.* 1756–69). What I have said about the small size of the Chelsea anchor mark is of equal or even more importance in the case of gold anchor wares as this mark has been extensively reproduced (see Plates 678–9). The early semi-opaque glaze with an addition of tin-oxide had been superseded by a clear glaze that was often thickly applied and tended to craze. Bone ash was also introduced into the porcelain body. Figures and groups were often backed by ornate "bocages" of applied leaves and flowers (see Plate 145); ornate ground colours were used on useful as well as ornamental wares (see Plate 141). Many charming small seals and scent bottles were made and are known as Chelsea "Toys". The standard reference book on this important feature of the factory's output is *Chelsea Porcelain Toys* (1925) by G. E. Bryant.

Early in 1769 the proprietors held auction sales of their stock "having recently left off making the same", and later in the year the works, together with all moulds, working materials, etc., were put up for sale and sold in August 1769 to James Cox. William Duesbury, the proprietor of the Derby factory (see page 131), purchased the works from Cox in February 1770, "on or before the 8th. instant". Duesbury continued the works, mainly as a London decorating establishment, although some porcelain was undoubtedly made there, until 1784 when the factory was dismantled and some of the materials, moulds, etc., were transferred to the Derby works. The 1769–84 period is called the "Chelsea-Derby" period. The porcelains were of fine quality, tastefully decorated in the classical style rather than the former florid rococo Chelsea fashion, although the change was not clear-cut and much old stock was decorated and sold after 1769. The body and glaze of marked Chelsea-Derby is superior to that of gold-anchor Chelsea, the porcelain being thinly potted and the glaze clear, close fitting, and normally uncrazed. The former gold-anchor mark occurs on much Chelsea-Derby porcelain, but the main marks of the period were the cursive capital letter "D" with an anchor across the downstroke; the anchor with a crown above also occurs. These marks are in gold. Chelsea-Derby figures, groups and vases, like the Derby examples, normally show three or four unglazed patch marks on their base (see Plates 152, 214).

Constant reference has been made to marks and the way that the various periods are designated by reference to the type of mark used—"red anchor period", "gold anchor period", etc. It would, however, be foolish to suggest that the changes in marking were exact. There was a certain amount of overlap before the new form, or colour, of mark was fully adopted. Much Chelsea porcelain is unmarked and is identified by its similarity to marked specimens such as are illustrated in Plates 112–146.

There is a further class of unmarked early porcelain of Chelsea type, which is referred to as "Girl in a Swing" type after a characteristic group in the Victoria & Albert Museum. These pieces may have been produced at a rival London factory. An interesting paper by A. Lane and R. J. Charleston is printed in the *Transactions of the English Ceramic Circle*, vol. 5, part 3, under the title "Girl in a Swing Porcelain and Chelsea".

For further information on Chelsea porcelains see *Chelsea Porcelain, The Triangle and Raised Anchor Wares* (1948), F. S. Mackenna; *Chelsea Porcelain, The Red Anchor Wares* (1951), F. S. Mackenna; *Chelsea Porcelain, The Gold Anchor Period* (1952), F. S. Mackenna; *English Porcelain Figures of the 18th Century* (1961), A. Lane; new 15th edition of Chaffer's *Marks and Monograms* (1965); and *British Porcelain 1745–1840* (1965), edited by R. J. Charleston. Chelsea marks are reproduced in the *Encyclopaedia of British Pottery and Porcelain Marks* (1964).

Nineteenth-century reproductions of the Chelsea Goat and Bee Jug (see Plate 114) were made at the Coalport factory and at Mintons. The latter bear impressed Minton marks, but the Coalport examples are unmarked or have a triangle *ground* (not incised) into their bases. Although these jugs are too slick and highly finished they have deceived many collectors.

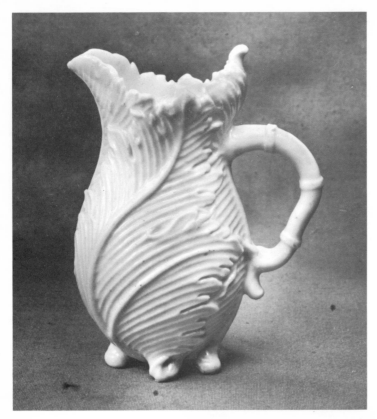

112. *Incised triangle marked Chelsea porcelain jug, showing typical early leaf form in attractive soft paste "friendly" porcelain (c. 1745–9). 5 inches high.*

Sotheby & Co

113. *Rare Chelsea, incised triangle period porcelain sauce boat, one of several models based on marine forms (c. 1745–9).*

Mrs H. C. Isaacson Collection; Seattle

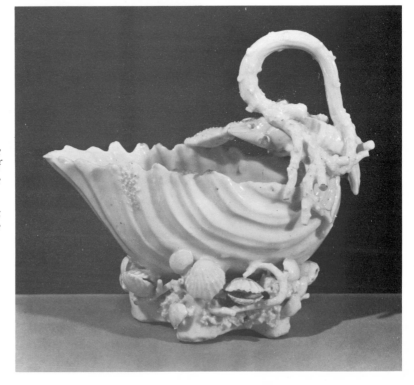

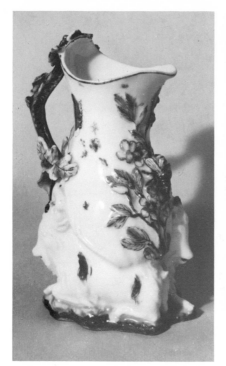

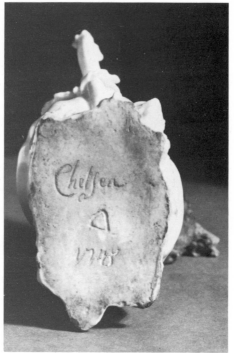

114. *Triangle marked (incised) Chelsea porcelain "Goat and Bee" jug with enamelled details (c. 1745–9). 4¼ inches high.*

Albert Amor Ltd

115. *Base of a "Goat and Bee" jug, showing incised triangle, with place-name "Chelsea" and date 1745(?).*

Rous Lench Collection

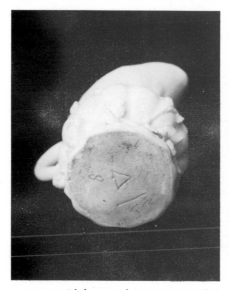

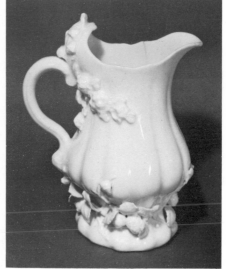

116 & a. *Chelsea porcelain cream jug, with detail of base showing incised triangle mark (c. 1745). 5 inches high.*

Albert Amor Ltd

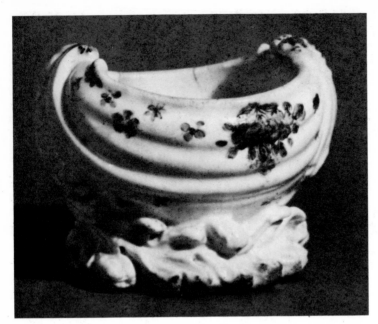

117. *Incised triangle marked Chelsea porcelain salt of shell form. Many early potters favoured shell forms, probably copied from silver examples (c. 1745–9). 2½ inches high.*

Albert Amor Ltd

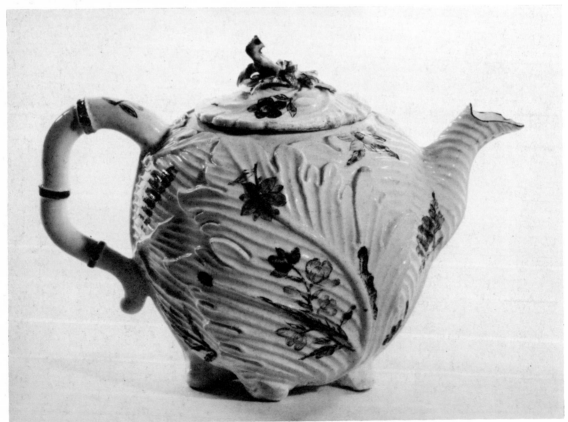

118. *Incised triangle marked Chelsea porcelain teapot of moulded leaf form, enamelled with scattered sprays of flowers, and insects. Undecorated examples are known (see also Plate 112) (c. 1745–9). 5 inches high.*

Godden of Worthing

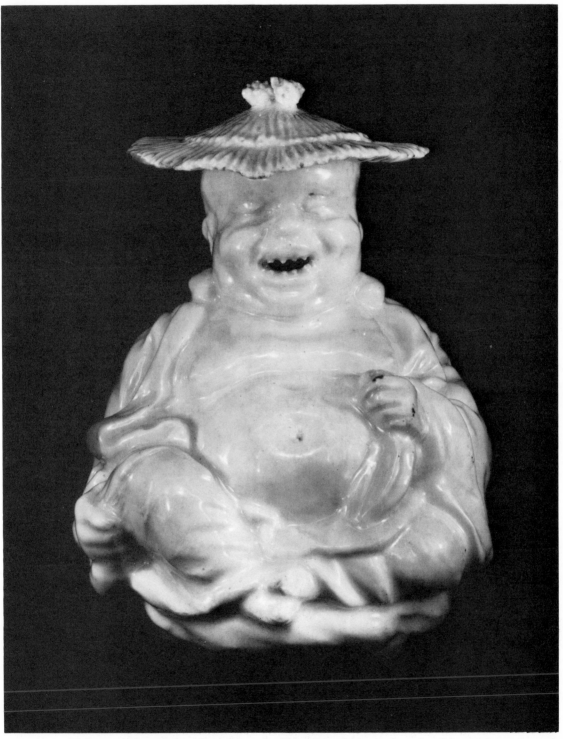

119. *A rare Chelsea covered pot after a Chinese Blanc de Chine original. A typical novelty of the period. Incised triangle mark (c. 1745–9). $6\frac{3}{4}$ inches high.*

Sotheby & Co

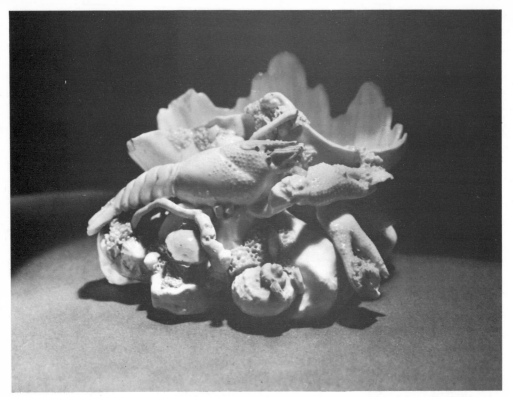

120. *Chelsea porcelain crayfish salt with very rare blue-painted triangle mark (see detail). This mark is normally incised (c. 1745–9). 5 inches long.*

Sir John & Lady Corah Collection

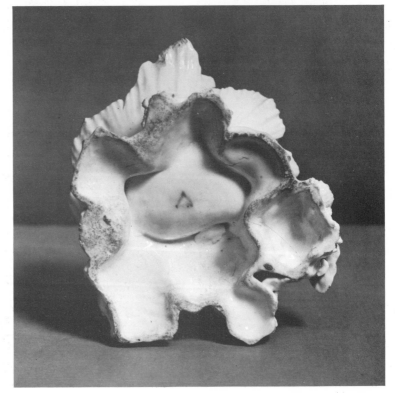

121. *Underside of Chelsea crayfish salt (see Plate 120), showing rare blue triangle mark.*

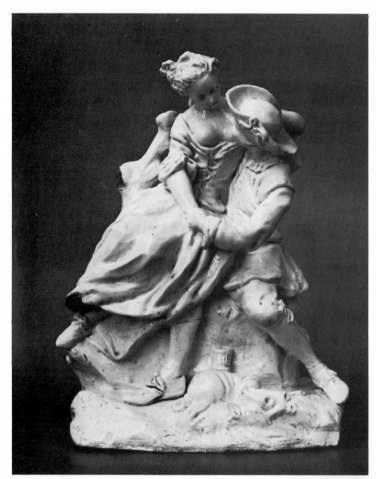

122 & a. *Early Chelsea porcelain group,
The Rustic Lovers. Very rare crown and
trident mark, painted in underglaze blue, as
on cup reproduced (c. 1745–50). 9 inches
high.*

British Museum

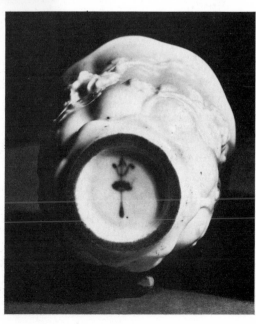

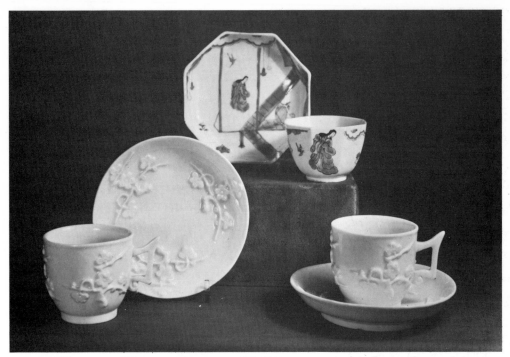

123. *Chelsea porcelain with the raised anchor mark (no. 867). Many early Chelsea porcelains are copied from Japanese or Chinese wares (c. 1749–52).*

Delomosne & Son

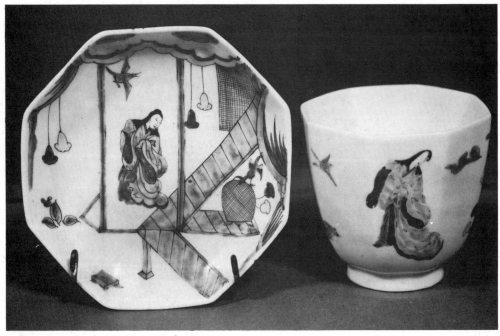

124. *Chelsea (raised anchor marked) tea bowl and saucer, one of several early patterns copied from Japanese porcelains (c. 1749–52).*

Tilley & Co

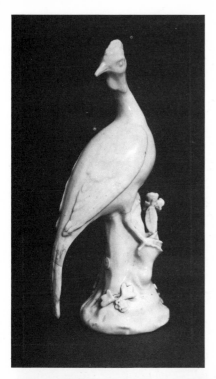

125. *Chelsea porcelain figure, one of several fine bird models, both white and coloured. The raised anchor mark can be seen on the tree trunk support (c. 1749–52). $6\frac{1}{2}$ inches high.*

Tilley & Co (Antiques) Ltd

126. *Raised anchor marked Chelsea porcelain figure of the Chinese Goddess Kuan Yin. The back view shows a typical raised anchor mark on an oval pad (c. 1749–52). $4\frac{1}{4}$ inches high.*

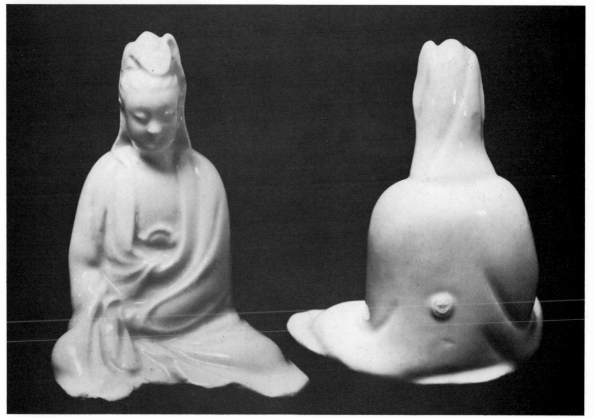

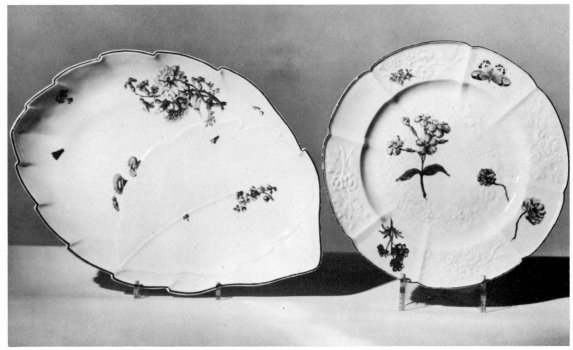

127. *Red anchor marked Chelsea porcelain dish of typical leaf form and a moulded plate of a well-known type. The sparse decoration and simple line edges are characteristic of the 1750–55 period. Dish 12¾ inches long.*

Godden of Worthing

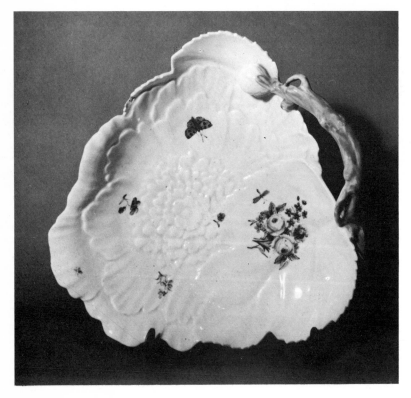

128. *Red anchor marked Chelsea porcelain leaf-shaped dish. Several eighteenth-century factories produced attractive dishes of leaf form (c. 1752–5). 9 inches long.*

Albert Amor Ltd

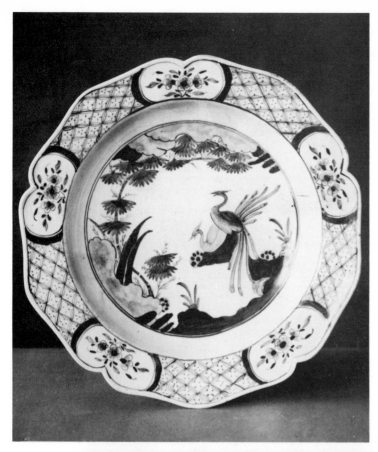

129. Very rare Chelsea porcelain plate, painted in underglaze blue in the Chinese manner and marked with an anchor in blue (c. 1755). 9 inches diameter.

Victoria & Albert Museum

130. Red anchor marked Chelsea porcelain tea bowl and saucer. The simple red or brown line edge is found on early porcelains (c. 1752).

Albert Amor Ltd

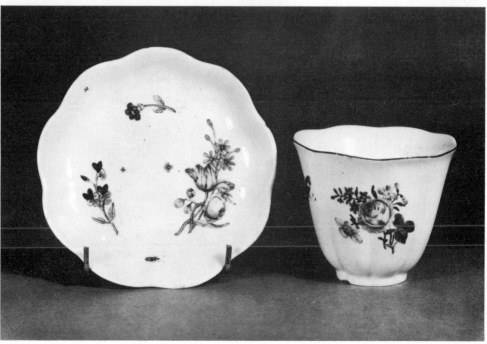

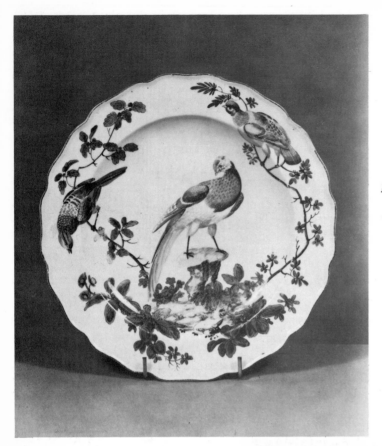

131. *Red anchor marked Chelsea porcelain plate, painted with colourful "Exotic Bird" motifs. Similar Exotic Bird patterns also occur on Derby, Plymouth and Worcester porcelains (c. 1755).*

Albert Amor Ltd

132. *Red anchor marked Chelsea porcelain plate. These botanical plates represent one of the most attractive styles of decoration. All specimens are rare and mainly comprise plates. Teasets are known but are very rare in this style (c. 1755). 9\frac{3}{8} inches diameter.*

Victoria & Albert Museum

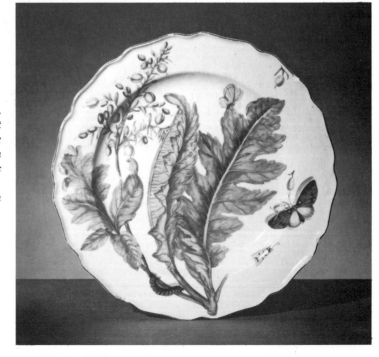

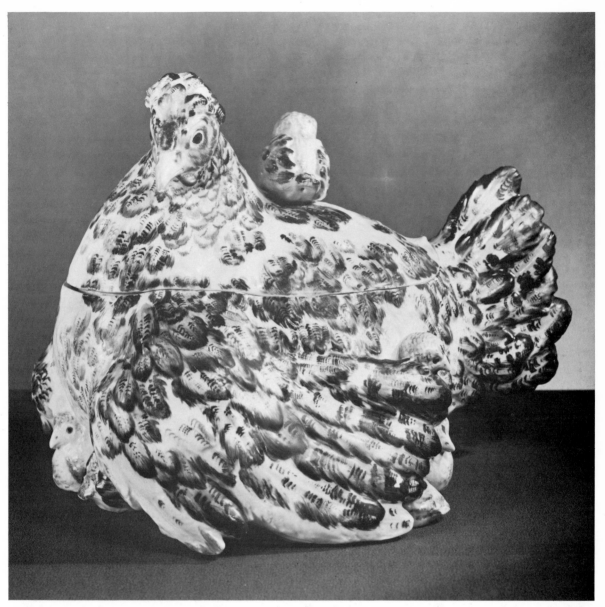

133. *Red anchor marked Chelsea porcelain hen tureen, 13½ inches long. A 1755 sale catalogue of "the last year's large and valuable production of the Chelsea Porcelain Manufactory" includes "a most beautiful tureen in the shape of a hen and chickens, big as life, in a curious dish adorn'd with sunflowers". A further example with the underdish may be seen in the Victoria & Albert Museum (c. 1755).*

Delomosne & Son

Other very fine tureens were made in the form of animals, birds, fish and fowl.

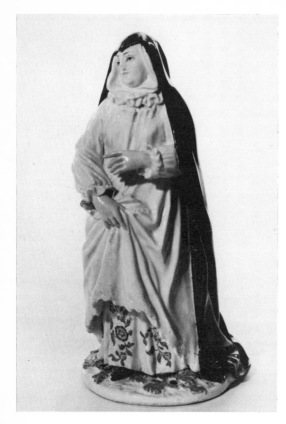

134. *Red anchor marked Chelsea figure of a nun, the subject taken from a German print of 1693. This model is attributed to the Chelsea modeller Joseph Willems by the late Arthur Lane, see* Connoisseur, *May 1960 (c. 1752–6). 6¼ inches high.*

Godden of Worthing

135. *Red anchor marked Chelsea porcelain figures. A rare and very attractive pair, showing the restraint of decoration typical of Chelsea porcelains of the 1752–5 period. About 5 inches high.*

Albert Amor Ltd

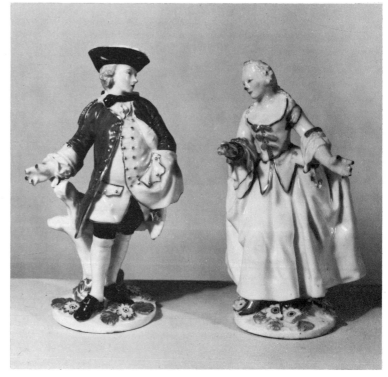

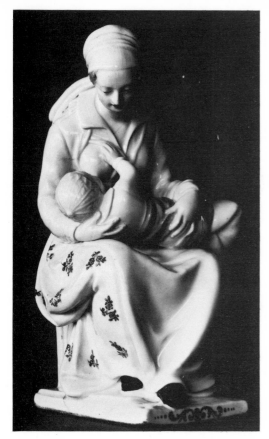

136. *Red anchor marked Chelsea porcelain figure "La Nourice", after a French original. This specimen shows to advantage the charming restraint of decoration on many early Chelsea models (c. 1752–6). $7\frac{7}{16}$ inches high.*

Victoria & Albert Museum

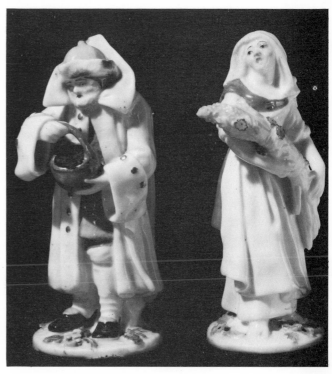

137. *Winter and Summer from a set of the Four Seasons. Chelsea porcelain, red anchor mark (very small) (c. 1752–6). $5\frac{1}{2}$ inches high.*

D. M. & P. Manheim

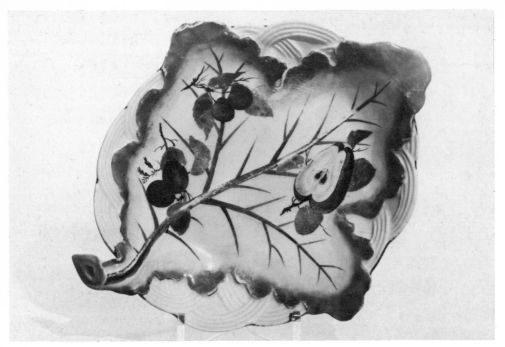

138. *Gold anchor marked Chelsea leaf dish, painted with fruit, etc. (c. 1756–60). 10¾ inches long. See detail of base, below.*

Godden of Worthing

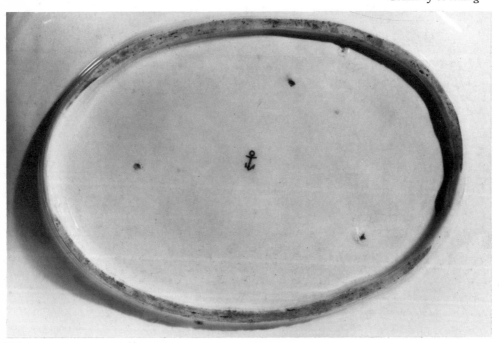

139. *Detail of reverse of gold anchor dish. Note uneven foot rim, ground flat. Three "spur" marks where the dish rested on spurs during the firing; these show as rough blisters in the glaze. Note also the small size of the anchor, a quarter of an inch high. The red anchor can be even smaller. Large anchors should be regarded with suspicion.*

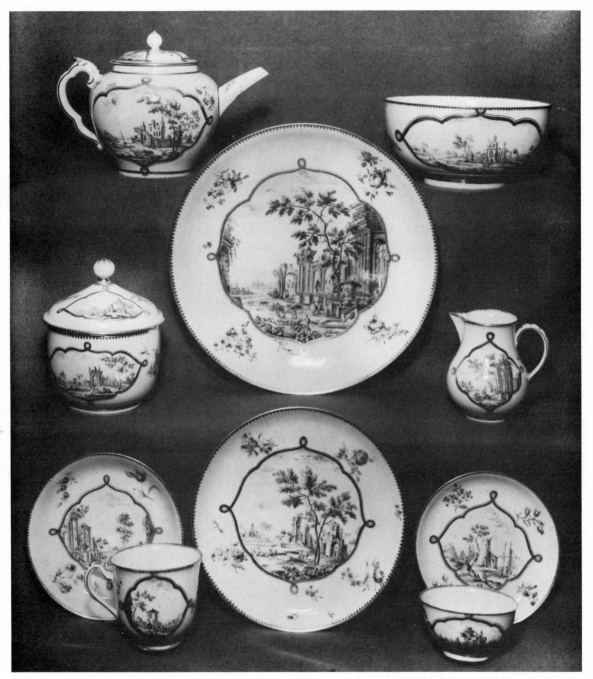

140. *Gold anchor marked Chelsea porcelain teaset (c. 1756–69) of the finest quality painted in puce, in the style of the slightly earlier red anchor period. This "tea equipage" comprises: teapot, cover and stand, sucrier and cover, slop bowl, cream jug, saucer shaped plate, six tea bowls and saucers, and six coffee cups and saucers. Such complete services are now very rare.*

Collection of Mrs F. Shand Kydd

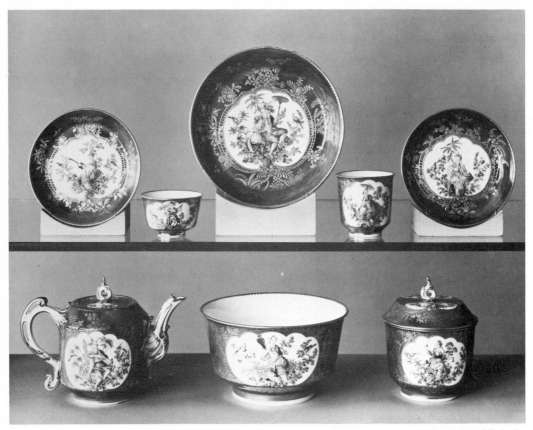

141. Gold anchor marked Chelsea porcelain teaset of the finest quality. Rare claret ground with rich gilt borders, etc., and attractively painted figure panels (c. 1765). Teapot 5¾ inches high.

Victoria & Albert Museum

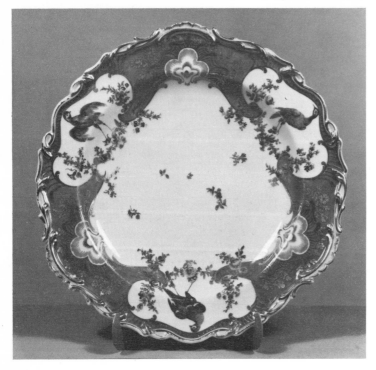

142. Gold anchor marked Chelsea porcelain plate. The border of the rare claret ground with gilt enrichments. The small flowers in the centre cover small blemishes in the glaze, a practice used at other early factories (c. 1756–69).

Albert Amor Ltd

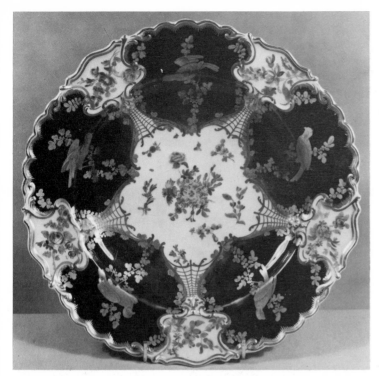

143. Gold anchor marked Chelsea porcelain plate, a fine and typical example of the period 1756–69. Note the rich effect with blue ground and liberal use of gilding. The details of the birds, leaves, etc., are of tooled gold; that is, burnished gold on a matt gold ground.

Albert Amor Ltd

144. Gold anchor marked Chelsea porcelain, a superb set of three covered vases. The flowers painted on a gold ground (c. 1756–69).

Delmosne & Son

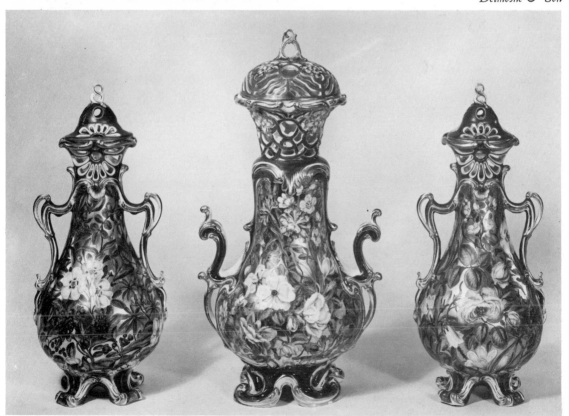

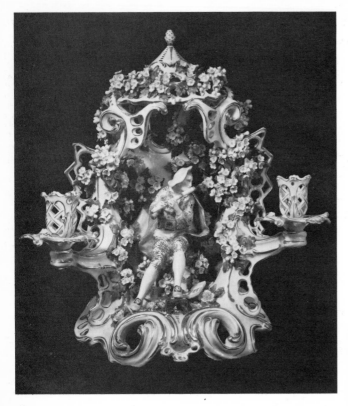

145. *A superb gold anchor marked Chelsea porcelain figure candle-holder (one of a pair). The floral background is known as a "bocage" and is typical of "gold anchor" groups (c. 1756–69).*

Delomosne & Son

146. *"The Imperial Shepherdess". A fine and typical example of gold anchor period Chelsea porcelain (c. 1756–69). 13 inches high.*

D. M. & P. Manheim

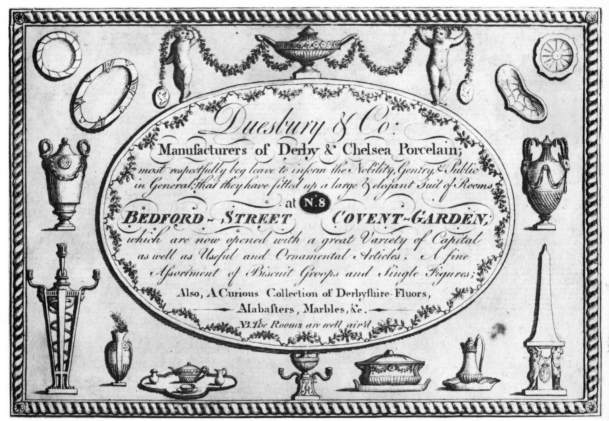

147. *Duesbury & Co trade card of the Chelsea-Derby period, showing typical wares. Note the special mention of "A fine assortment of biscuit groups and single figures" (see Plate 217). The Bedford Street showrooms were opened in June 1773.*

Victoria & Albert Museum.

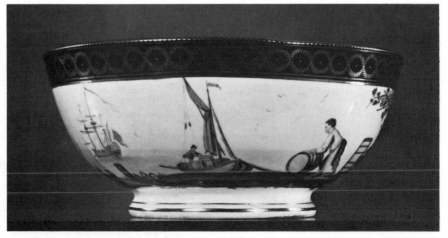

148. *Gold anchor marked "Chelsea-Derby" bowl. The inside painted with the arms of the Cooper's Company. Dated on base 1779. 10¼ inches diameter.*

Schreiber Collection, Victoria & Albert Museum

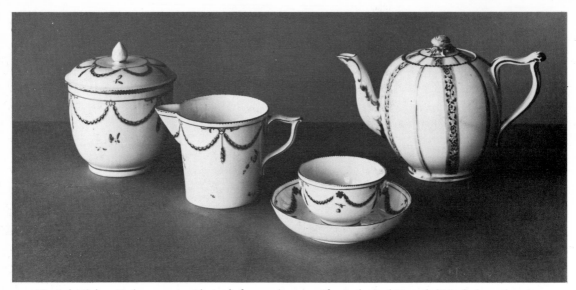

149. *Typical Chelsea-Derby teawares with simple forms and swag motifs. Anchor and D mark (joined) (c. 1769–75). Teapot 5 inches high, creamer 3⅛ inches.*

Victoria & Albert Museum

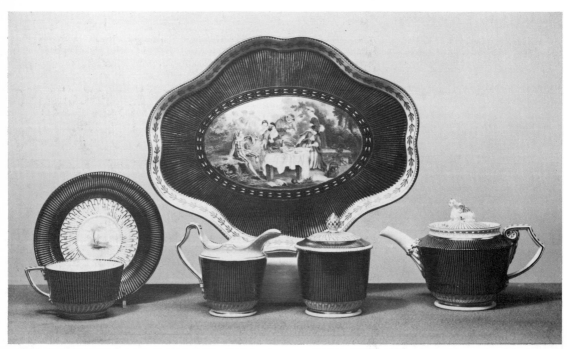

150. *A fine gold anchor marked Chelsea-Derby cabaret set. The tray painted with figure subject after Nicholas Lancret. Note the restrained taste in the shapes. Tray 15 inches long (c. 1769–75).*

Delomosne & Son

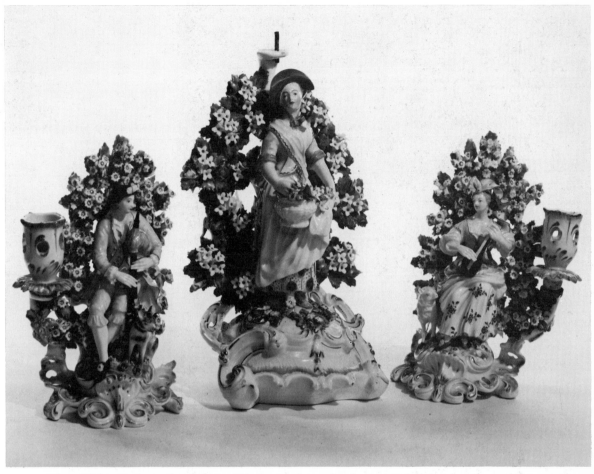

151. *Three Chelsea-Derby candlestick figures. The bases and general style are typical of this class of unmarked (except for "pad marks") figures and groups. Centre figure, candle-holder missing, 10½ inches high.*

Godden of Worthing

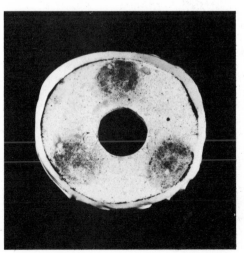

152. *Typical "pad marks" found on Chelsea-Derby and Derby porcelains. The dark marks were formed by the pads used to stop the ware sticking to the kiln shelf.*

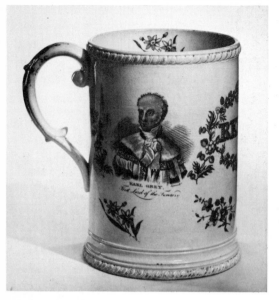

153. *Reform Bill mug of 1832. Printed initial (C & R) mark of Chesworth & Robinson, of Lane End, or of Chetham & Robinson, of Longton. The printed portraits of Lord John Russell and Earl Grey are signed by J. Kennedy of Burslem, Engraver (c. 1832). 6¾ inches high.*

J. CLEMENTSON, HANLEY *c.* 1839–64

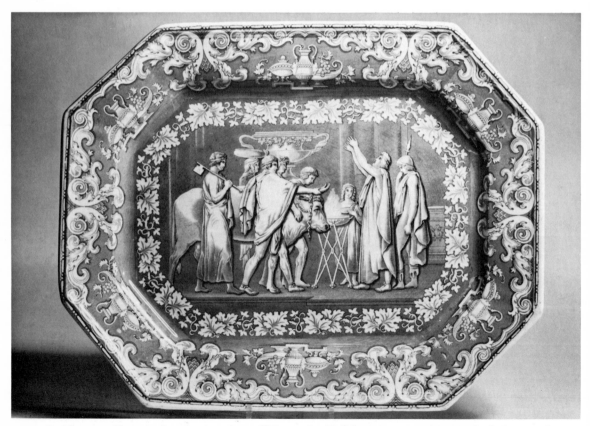

154. *J. Clementson blue printed earthenware platter, "Nestors Sacrifice" (pattern registered in March 1849). Printed name mark (c. 1849–52). 17¾ × 14 inches.*

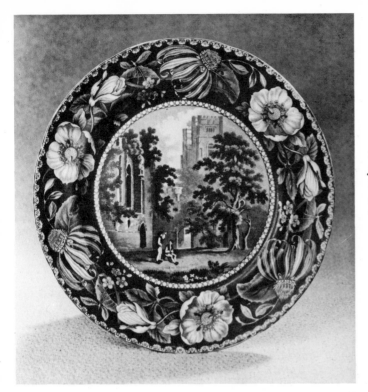

155. *Clews earthenware plate with underglaze print of "Fountains Abbey". Impressed mark "Clews Warranted Staffordshire". Messrs James & Ralph Clews potted at Cobridge from c. 1818 to c. 1834.*

City Museum & Art Gallery, Stoke

156. *J. & R. Clews (c. 1818–34) earthenware plate transfer printed in underglaze blue—"The Landing of Lafayette . . . 1824". This is one of many designs produced by the Staffordshire potters especially for the American market.*

Mrs Frank Nagington

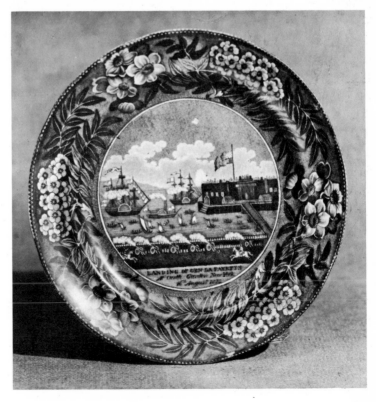

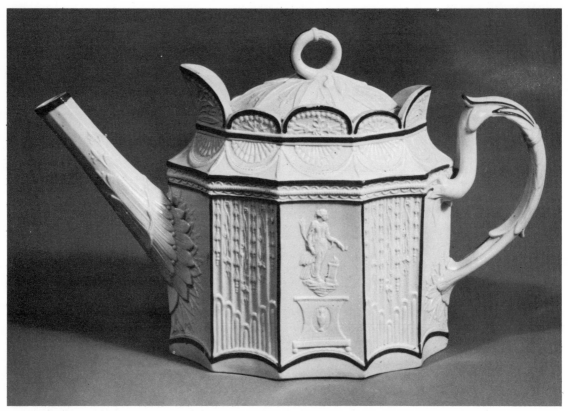

157. *"Clulow & Co. Fenton"* (impressed mark on pedestal) moulded stoneware teapot of a type generally attributed to the Castleford Works, but in fact made by several potters, see page xxiii (c. 1802). Little is known of this firm, but a Robert Clewlow (or Clulow) & Co is listed by A. Meigh with the date 1802. This is the only marked example known.

Courtesy of the Newark Museum, U.S.A.

The name of John Rose is synonymous with Coalport in the history of English porcelain. Born in 1772, he was, according to tradition, apprenticed to Thomas Turner at the Caughley factory which he bought in 1799. He entered into an agreement to purchase land at Coalport on the banks of the River Severn in October 1797 and when he acquired the near-by Caughley factory as a going concern from Thomas Turner in October 1799, he and his partners were described as "of Coalport in the said County of Salop, Porcelain Manufacturers", suggesting that by this date they were producing porcelain at Coalport.

For some fifteen years prior to 1814 John Rose and his partners continued the Caughley works. The original Coalport factory was also continued and some of the Caughley porcelain of the 1799–1814 period was transported to Coalport for the decoration to be added.

Recent excavations on the Caughley factory site have fortunately brought to light unglazed and partly finished factory wasters; these help us to identify the early Coalport porcelains of the pre-1814 period. The discoveries are of the utmost importance as the wares of the period were, with very few exceptions, unmarked and the Coalport porcelains have been attributed to other factories, mainly Chamberlain Worcester, in error. Plates 160–3 show a selection of these fragments or patterns and shapes which match factory wasters found on the site. Much research is being carried out to identify the early, largely unmarked, Coalport porcelains and the result of this will be published under the title *Coalport and Coalbrookdale Porcelains*.

As stated above, the early unmarked wares are similar in general appearance to Chamberlain Worcester ware. This is confirmed by two part-breakfast sets in the Godden Collection (see Plate 158). Two plates bear the very rare painted mark "Colebrookdale", a name sometimes used to identify Coalport porcelain. The pattern comprises a bold formal design in underglaze blue with overglaze enamel painting and gilding (many similar partly finished wasters were found on the site). These two marked Colebrookdale plates, and a further marked example in the Victoria & Albert Museum, have six slight equidistant indentations round the edge. This feature occurs on some signed and dated (1808–9) plates in the Victoria & Albert Museum with fine fruit painted centres by Thomas Baxter, the London decorator. Many unglazed fragments of similar plates were discovered on the Caughley site proving that the many dessert and dinner services having this type of plate with the six indentations are Coalport, not Worcester, as they are now called. A typical example is illustrated in Plate 159.

Some Coalport plates and dishes of the 1810–25 period bear impressed numerals; on plates it is a top-heavy "2". This is most helpful in identifying the otherwise unmarked Coalport porcelains of the period in question (see Plates 164–5). The "2" mark on plates was continued after 1820, as is proved by Plate 167B, which shows a detail of the reverse of a plate with this impressed mark and a printed "Society of Arts" award mark.

In May 1820 John Rose was awarded the Society of Arts Gold Medal for lead-less felspathic glaze, and special large, circular printed marks appear on wares bearing this glaze after 1820. The general potting and decoration of these marked 1820+ wares, in the form of tea and fine dessert services, show a distinct improvement over the 1810 period wares mentioned above (see Plates 167–8).

The Coalport factory specialized in fine porcelains decorated with flowers, etc., in high relief and highly coloured. Such examples are termed "Coalbrookdale" and often bear the marks "C.D.", "C. Dale", "Coalport", or "Coalbrookdale" written in underglaze blue. The "crossed-swords" mark of the Dresden factory also occurs on these wares, but this was also used by other factories, noticeably Minton, on their floral encrusted porcelains.

The Coalport porcelains after about 1835 became more sophisticated. Rich ground colours were introduced and by the 1850's ornate imitations of the finest Sèvres and Chelsea porcelains were being manufactured, often with copies of the original marks. Other ornate and fine quality Coalport porcelains bear marks nos. 954–9. Such wares are shown in Plate 174. A large proportion. of mid-Victorian Coalport porcelain was unmarked, but from 1881 all examples bear a version of the standard mark no. 958. The Coalport Company has changed hands several times and today continues production at Stoke-on-Trent.

For further information on Coalport porcelain of the Victorian era see G. Godden's *Victorian Porcelain* (1961). F. A. Barrett's *Caughley and Coalport Porcelain* (1951) contains much information, but recent research shows that several errors of attribution occur in this book. The present writer's book *Coalport and Coalbrookdale Porcelains* sheds much light on this important but neglected factory.

It should be noted that from 1800 to 1814 John Rose's brother, Thomas, with his partners Robert Anstice and Robert Horton, operated a rival factory at Coalport. They produced porcelains, mainly teawares, which closely followed in shape and decoration those produced at John Rose's factory. These other Coalport porcelains are unmarked, but are identified in G. Godden's book mentioned above. In 1814 John Rose purchased this rival factory on his doorstep and dismantled the Caughley works, so concentrating all his manufacturing processes at Coalport.

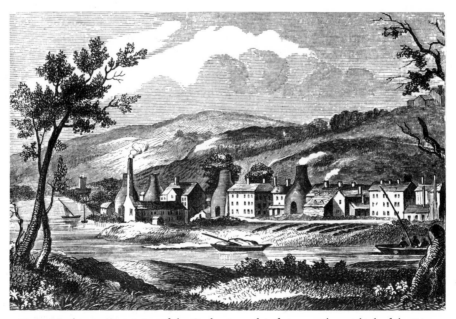

Engraving of contemporary view of the Coalport porcelain factory on the east bank of the River Severn (c. 1820). Reproduced from Jewitt's Ceramic Art of Great Britain *(1878).*

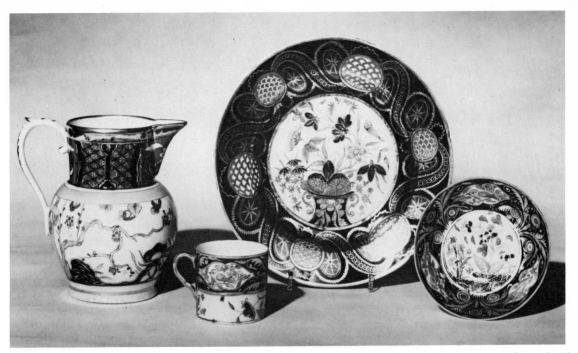

158. Colourful Coalport porcelains of the 1805–10 period. Decorated with rich dark underglaze blue borders, overglaze red and green enamels and gilt enrichments. The plate (with six indentations in the rim) is marked "Coalbrookdale" (see Plate 158. a). The jug is a favourite early Coalport shape. A marked example is in a private collection and one dated 1806 is in the Victoria & Albert Museum. Plate 9½ inches diameter.

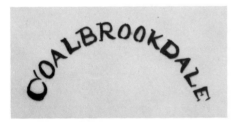

158. a. Detail of red painted mark on plate in Plate 158. This mark is extremely rare as most early Coalport porcelain is unmarked.

159. Marked "Coalbrook Dale" plate with underglaze blue edge. Typical early Coalport shape with six indentations in the rim. Many unglazed fragments of such plates were found on the Caughley site where Coalport blanks were made before 1814. 9⅛ inches diameter.

Victoria & Albert Museum

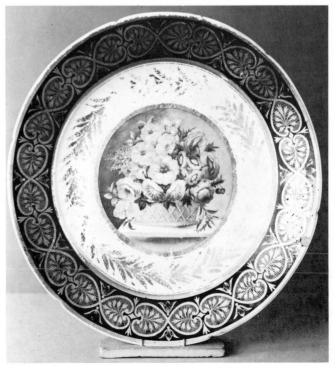

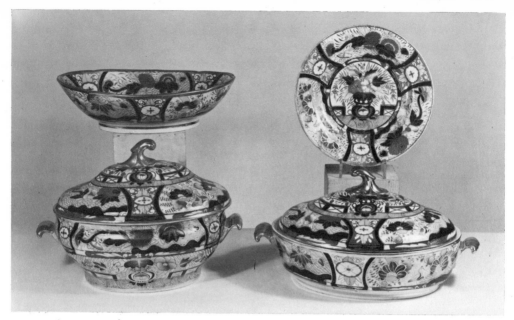

160. *Coalport part dinner service. The forms made and the underglaze blue decoration added at the Caughley factory under John Rose's management before 1814. Many unglazed and glazed fragments of similar tureens, dishes, plates, etc., were found on the factory site as well as pieces bearing the underglaze blue parts of this pattern. Typical early Coalport impressed numbers occur on the dishes and plates of this service (c. 1805–10).*

Messrs Christie, Manson & Woods Ltd

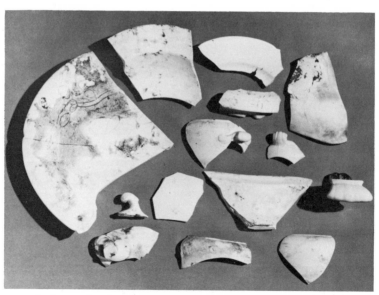

161. *A selection of unglazed Coalport dinner wares of the pre-1815 period found on the Caughley site; illustrating part of a lobed edged dish, part of a lobed edged soup and dinner plate (top). Fragments of soup tureens and sauce tureens, including handles and knobs; matching components of the dinner service shown in Plate 160. To the right of the dish fragment can be seen a piece bearing the impressed number 6. These numbers occur on the lobed edged dishes and refer to the various sizes.*

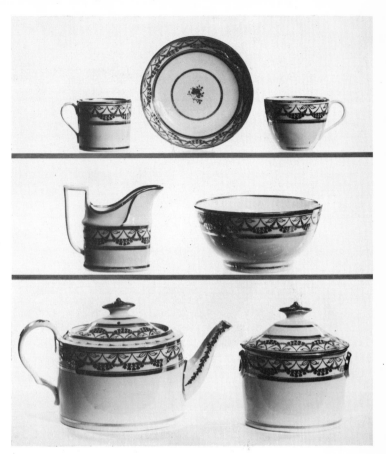

162. *Early Coalport tea service, showing typical forms. Such wares are unmarked but have been identified by unglazed and glazed fragments found on the Caughley factory site where the Coalport blanks were made prior to 1814. The mould for the teapot handle was also found. A sugar basin of this form is recorded with the date 1806. Teapot $9\frac{3}{4}$ inches long, $5\frac{1}{2}$ inches high.*

Godden of Worthing

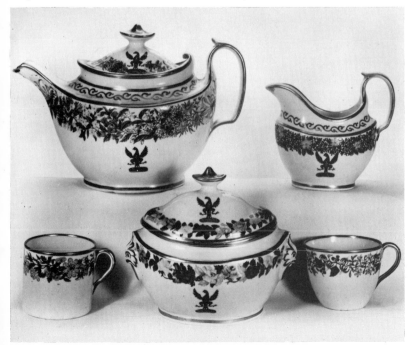

163. *Slightly later Coalport tea service, showing standard shapes of the 1805–12 period. This service was probably decorated outside the factory. Coalport supplied much white ware to independent decorators. A water-colour drawing dated 1810, depicting Baxter's London decorating studio, shows teawares of these forms on the work-bench (see Godden's British Pottery and Porcelain, 1780–1850, Plate 26). Some pieces of this service bear the date 1807. Many unglazed and glazed fragments matching the shapes were found on the Caughley/Coalport site, so identifying these unmarked teawares.*

Sotheby & Co

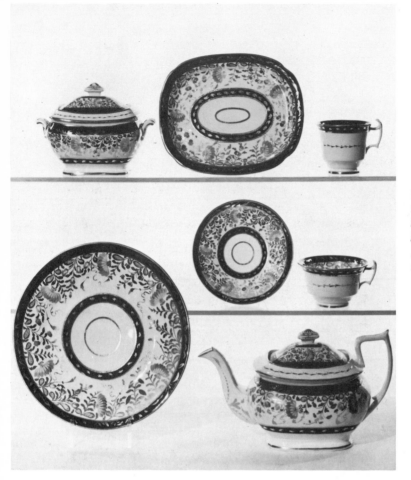

164. *Coalport tea service of the 1810–15 period. The shapes are typical and unmarked except for impressed number "2" on plate. Most Coalport of this period is unmarked. Pattern no. 629.*

Godden of Worthing

165. *Coalport tea service forms. Unmarked, as are most early Coalport wares, except for impressed number "2" on plates and painted pattern numbers (c. 1815–20).*

Godden of Worthing

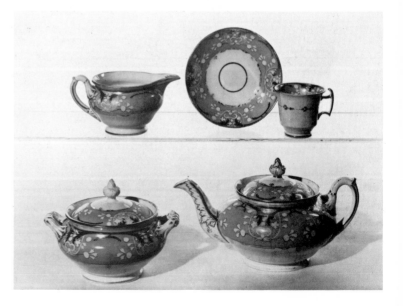

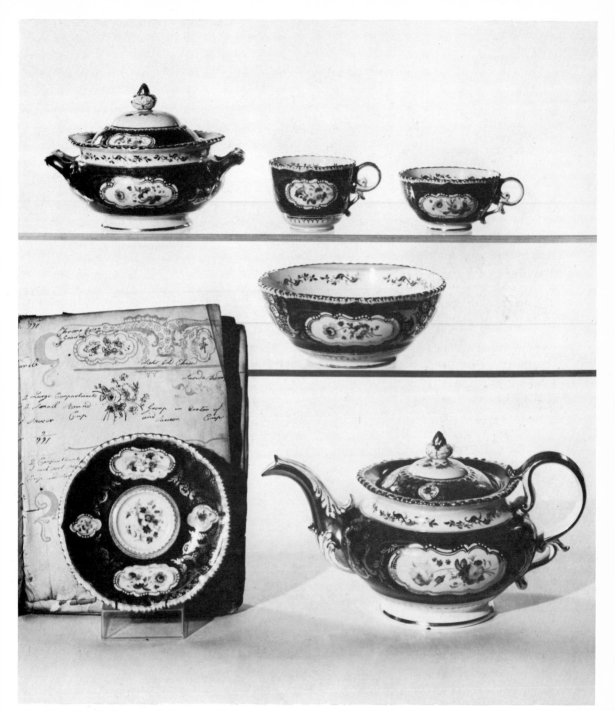

166. Unmarked Coalport porcelain teawares with chrome-green ground, richly gilt and painted with flowers. Attribution checked with factory pattern book (shown behind saucer). Pattern no. 2/200 (c. 1820). Teapot 6 inches high.

Godden of Worthing

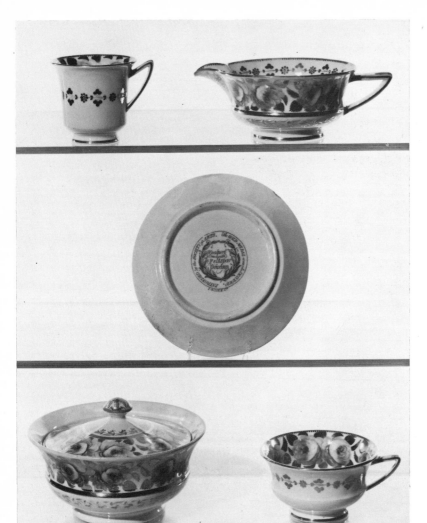

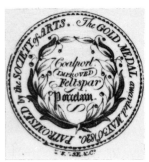

167. a. One of several versions of the 1820 Royal Society of Arts printed mark. Note addition of the word "improved" in the centre (c. 1825).

167. Part Coalport tea service, painted with roses (a pattern also used by Spode and Davenport). Some few pieces have the printed ".... improved Feltspar ..." mark of c. 1820–5. Creamer 2¼ inches high.

Godden of Worthing

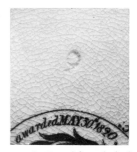

167. b. Detail from the back of a Coalport plate, showing part of the 1820 printed mark with the impressed top-heavy number 2 which occurs on many Coalport plates of the 1805–25 period.

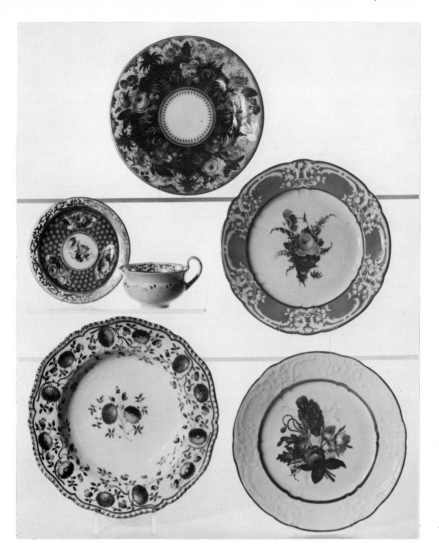

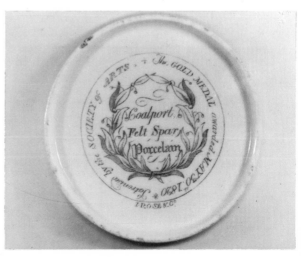

168 & a. *Standard Coalport printed Society of Arts mark used from June 1820 for about ten years.* (Below) *Example bearing this mark.*

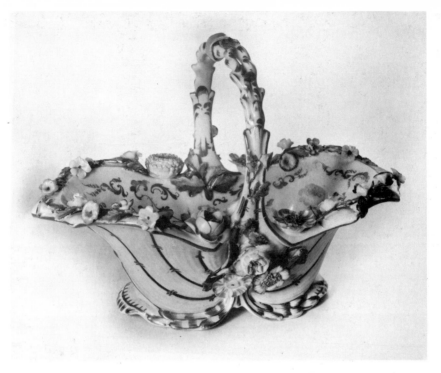

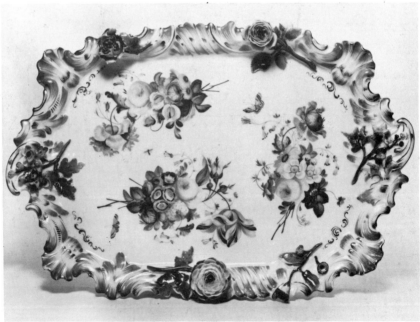

169. *Floral encrusted Coalport porcelains—normally termed "Coalbrookdale". Yellow ground basket bears C.D. initial mark in underglaze blue. 10 inches long. Shaped tray, marked "Coalport" (in writing letters) in underglaze blue. 13 inches long (c. 1820–30).*

Messrs Sotheby & Co

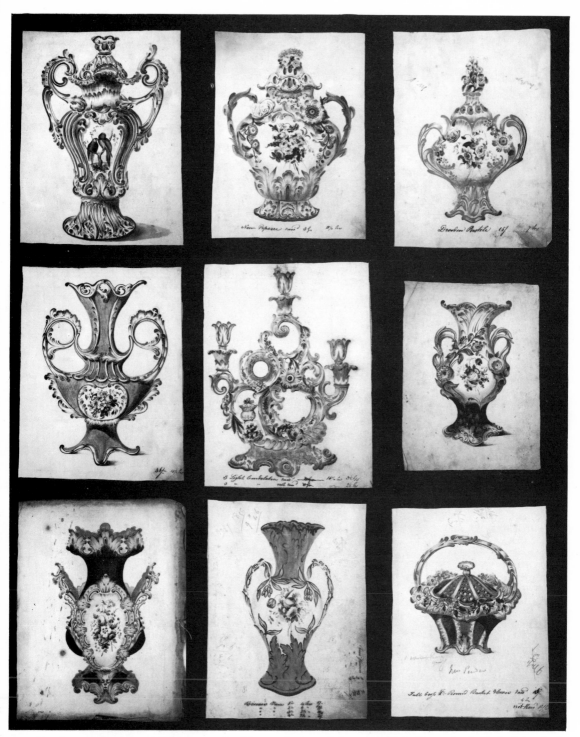

170. *Sample pages showing typical forms, reproduced from a Coalport design or traveller's illustrated order book of the 1830's. Many forms were produced in several different sizes, with or without raised flowers. The floral work was relatively inexpensive—a "Brewer vase" (bottom row, centre) $9\frac{1}{4}$ inches high was 18s. plain and 21s. with raised flowers. Coalport vases, etc., of this period do not normally bear a factory mark.*

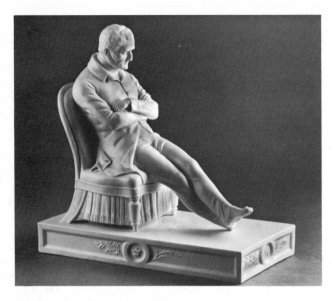

171. Coalport Parian figure of the Duke of Wellington, modelled by G. Abbott. Moulded mark "Manufactured at Coalbrook Dale" (c. 1850). Coalport Parian wares are rare. 10¼ inches long.

Godden of Worthing

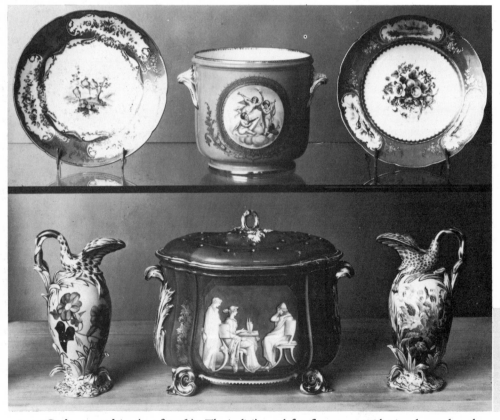

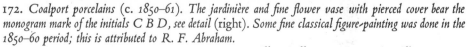

172. Coalport porcelains (c. 1850–61). The jardinière and fine flower vase with pierced cover bear the monogram mark of the initials C B D, see detail (right). Some fine classical figure-painting was done in the 1850–60 period; this is attributed to R. F. Abraham.

Allen Collection, Victoria & Albert Museum

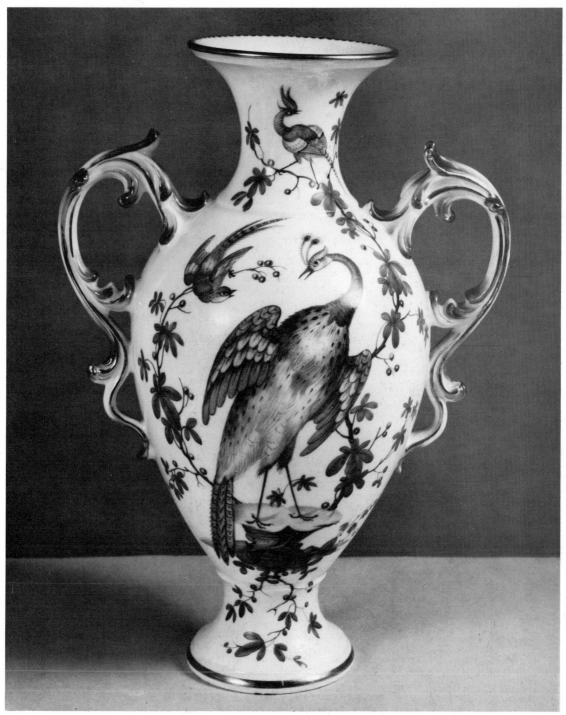

173. *Coalport copy of a Chelsea porcelain vase (c. 1850–60). Marked with an anchor in blue with the letter C above. The Coalport factory made many copies of Sèvres and Chelsea porcelain, to which they added close copies of the original mark. In most cases the mark was painted in a larger size than that on the original. The anchor mark on Chelsea porcelain is less than a quarter of an inch high. 8¾ inches high.*

Victoria & Albert Museum

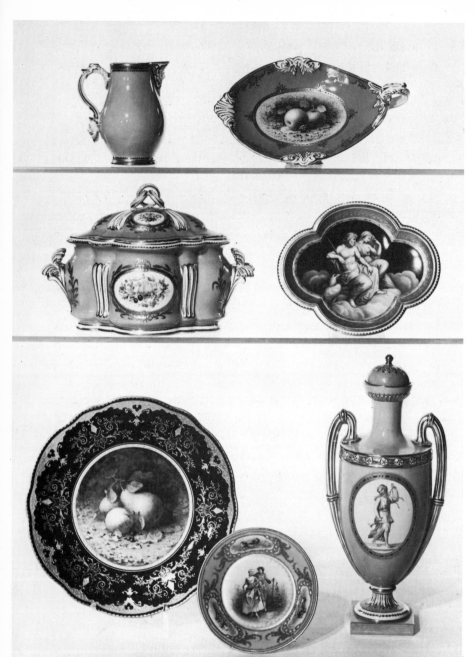

174. *Coalport porcelains (top to bottom, left to right): Pink ground jug, printed ampersand mark (c. 1861–75). Dish painted by F. Howard, printed "Coalport England AD 1750" mark (c. 1900). Covered tureen, gilt ampersand mark (c. 1861–75). Shaped dish, gilt "CBD" mark (c. 1851–61). Fruit plate painted by F. H. Chivers, "Coalport. England. AD 1750" mark (c. 1900). Saucer painted by E. Sieffert, "Daniell" retailers mark in gold (c. 1870). Vase painted with figure panels, gilt ampersand mark (c. 1861–75). This form of Coalport vase occurs in several sizes—one 30 inches high. This example is 11½ inches high.*

Godden of Worthing

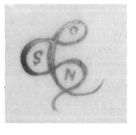

174. a. *Gilt ampersand mark found on much fine quality Coalport porcelain of the 1861–75 period.*

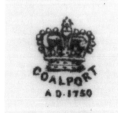

174. b. *Standard printed Coalport mark (c. 1881–90). The word "England" added in 1891 replaced later by "Made in England". The date 1750 is the claimed year of establishment not the date of manufacture.*

William Taylor Copeland succeeded the earlier Copeland & Garrett partnership at the Spode works at Stoke in 1847. The change of ownership did not mean sweeping changes; it was rather a process of concentrating on improving and adapting the best of the old Copeland & Garrett lines. The examples at the 1851 Exhibition included a fine range of Parian figures and groups, richly painted table tops and slabs, vases in great variety, dessert plates with floral, scenic, fruit, and armorial centres and richly gilt borders, cups and saucers, door furniture, trays, and ewers; Parian centrepieces were also displayed .Nearly all Copelands varied products will be found to bear his name incorporated in one of the standard marks.

In the Victorian era the name Copeland was synonymous with Parian (see page xxv); the white, normally unglazed, ceramic body from which hundreds of thousands of figures and groups were produced, both by Copelands and by other manufacturers who sought to emulate Copelands' success in Parian. All Copeland examples bear the impressed name "COPELAND", often with other information such as the date of publication, or the name of the modeller.

Copeland's earthenware and bone china wares of the second half of the century were decorated by several deservedly famous flower painters. C. F. Hurten, a German artist who had painted for the French National Sèvres factory, was engaged by Copelands in 1859. He remained with the firm until 1897 and painted many fine floral plaques and large vases—his paintings are normally signed. Of many other Copeland artists, the figure painting of Samuel Alcock is particularly fine and delicate.

Most Copeland wares bear one of several printed marks incorporating the name "Copeland" (see the companion *Encyclopaedia of Marks*). Some wares after about 1870 bear impressed month and year marks which indicate the period of production; the initial of the month was placed over the last two numerals of the year. All Copelands products are well potted and of good quality. For further information the reader is referred to A. Hayden's *Spode and His Successors* (1925) and G. Godden's *Victorian Porcelain* (1961).

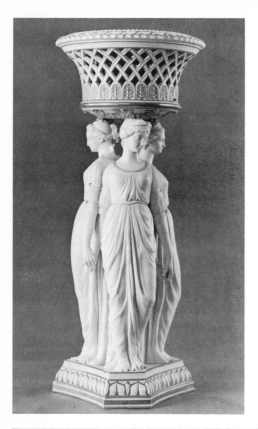

175. *Parian porcelain centrepiece with slight gilt enrichments. Messrs Copelands were renowned for their Parian (unglazed white marble-like) figures and groups. Specimens normally bear the impressed mark— "Copeland" (c. 1850). 20 inches high.*

176. *Copeland porcelain part dessert service with hand-painted scenic centres and moulded borders (dish form registered in May 1852). Printed crossed "C"s and name mark (no. 1073) (c. 1852–5). Dish 12 inches long.*

Godden of Worthing

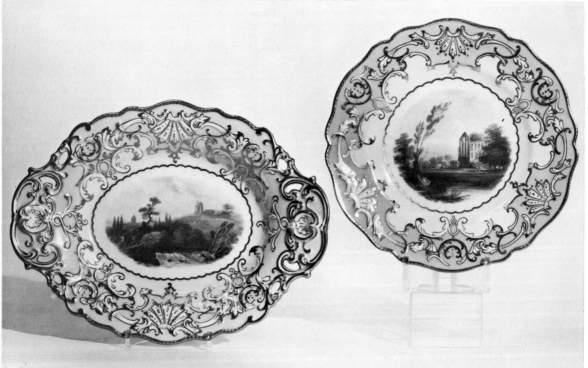

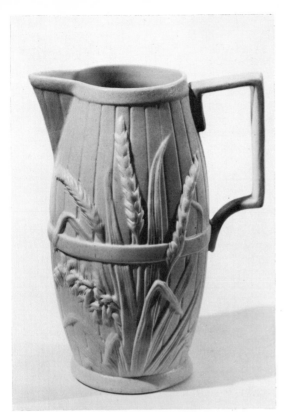

177. *Copeland moulded Parian ware jug. One of many attractive mass-produced jugs. Pattern registered in February 1853. Impressed "Copeland" mark and diamond-shaped registration mark (no. 3224). 7½ inches high.*

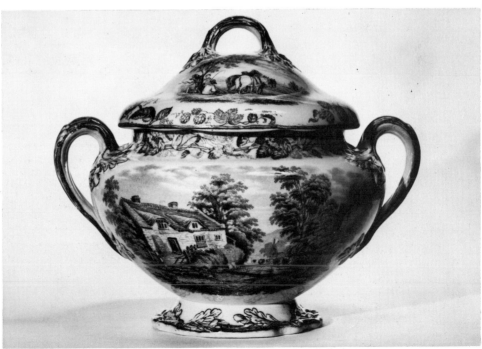

178. *Copeland earthenware tureen with fine quality printed pattern, registered in September 1850. Printed mark "Copeland Late Spode" (c. 1850–3). 11 inches high.*

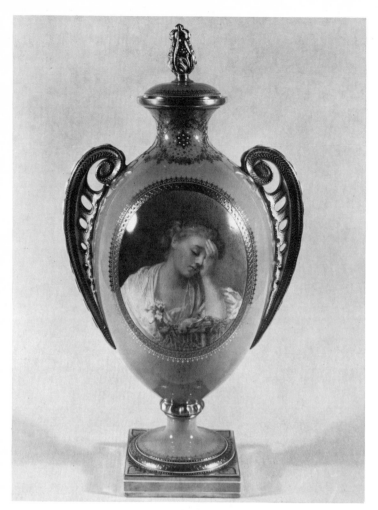

179. Copeland porcelain vase, painted by S. Alcock. Printed "Spode/Copelands China/England" mark of c. 1891–1900.

W. T. Copeland & Sons Ltd

180. Copeland vases, etc., shown at the 1873 Exhibition. Reproduced from a contemporary engraving. These standard forms will be found with many different types of decoration.

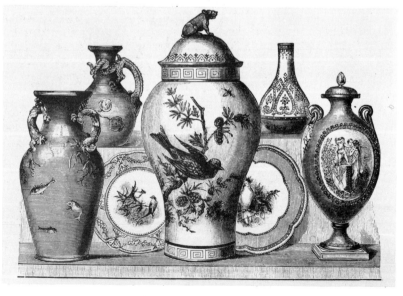

Messrs Copeland & Garrett took over the Spode works early in 1833. They continued the high standard set by Spodes (see page 298). Some decorative porcelain services were produced; a number of examples were painted with landscapes and the floral patterns were of superb quality. The innovations include some fine large models of animals (Plate 185), large plaques, and table and fireplace slabs. The white unglazed Parian body, termed Statuary porcelain, was introduced in the early 1840's and its production was taken up by most Victorian manufacturers.

Messrs Copeland & Garrett produced high-grade porcelains, earthenwares, and Parian ware. The partnership terminated in 1847 and was continued by W. T. Copeland (see page 105). Practically all Copeland & Garrett wares have marks incorporating the name in full or the initials "C. & G."; these all indicate production between 1833 and 1847.

Contemporary quotations relating to Copeland & Garrett wares are included in G. Godden's *Victorian Porcelain* (1961).

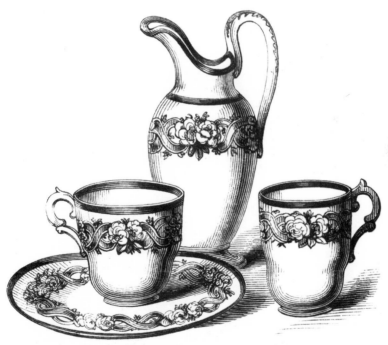

Copeland & Garrett utilitarian pieces "unaided by extraneous ornamentation" (c. 1846). Reproduced from Art Union Journal *of November 1846.*

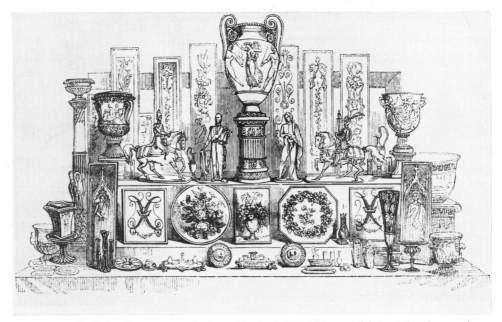

181. *Copeland & Garrett wares shown at the 1845/46 Manchester Exhibition. This shows early Parian vases and a selection of fireplace and other slabs—a speciality of this firm. Reproduced from a contemporary engraving.*

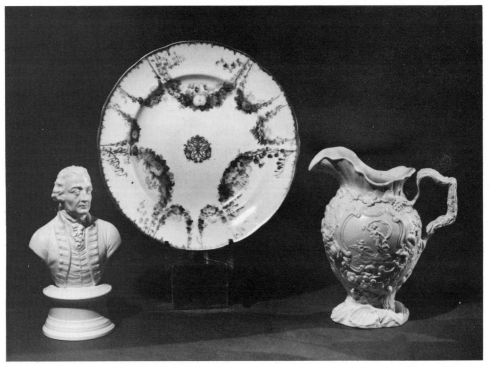

182. *Copeland & Garrett. Bust of Duncan and a moulded jug, both in pre-Parian unglazed felspar porcelain. The floral plate bears a rare ornate gold mark of a shield surrounded with drapes (mark no. 1095) (c. 1833–47). Jug 7½ inches high.*

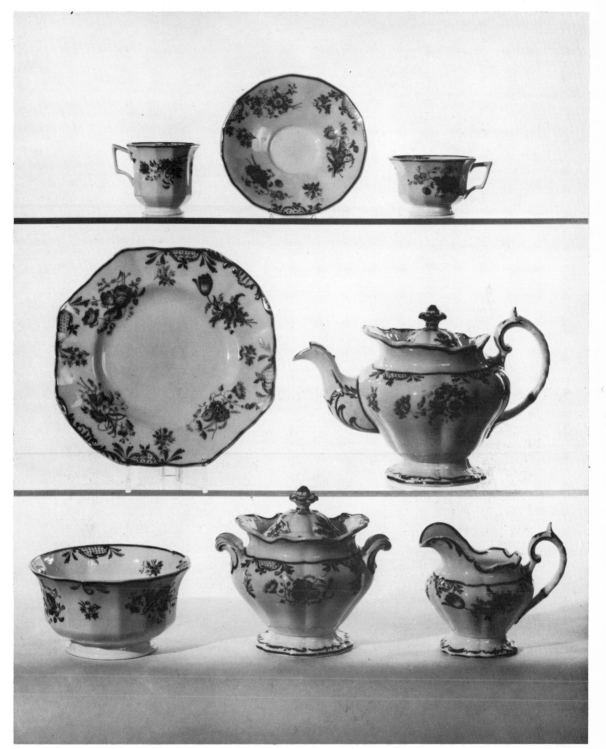

183. *Copeland & Garrett porcelain teaset, showing typical shapes of the period 1833–47. Pattern no. 5083. Printed name mark no. 1093. Teapot 7¼ inches high.*

Godden of Worthing

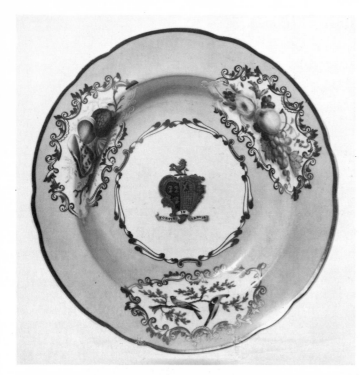

184. Copeland & Garrett porcelain soup plate of the finest quality. Green border with hand-painted panels of shells, fruit and birds. The centre decorated with finely gilt armorial bearings. Printed mark no. 1093 (c. 1833–47).

Godden of Worthing

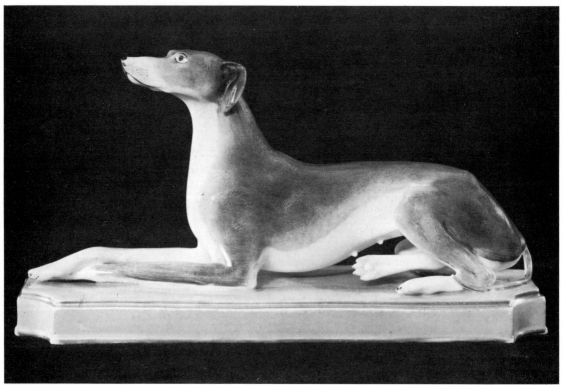

185. Copeland & Garrett porcelain greyhound, one of several fine animal models. Printed mark no. 1091 (c. 1845). 11 inches long.

Godden of Worthing

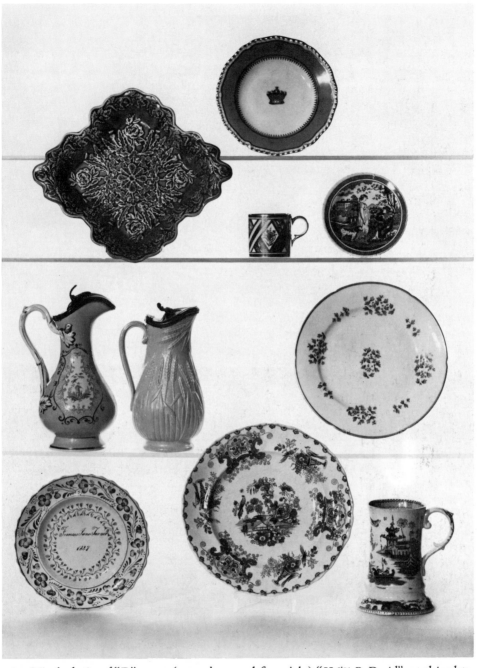

186. *Mixed selection of "D" wares: (top to bottom, left to right) "H & R Daniel" porcelain plate (c. 1827); "Don Pottery" green glazed dish (c. 1825); "Donovan" decorated Derby can (c. 1800); "I Dawson" blue printed plate (c. 1820); "Jas Dixon & Sons" jug (c. 1842); "Dudson" moulded jug (c. 1861); "Donovan" decorated plate (c. 1810); "Davies & Co" earthenware plate (c. 1847); "Deakin & Son" earthenware plate c. 1835); "Daniel & Cork" earthenware mug (c. 1868). 5½ inches high.*

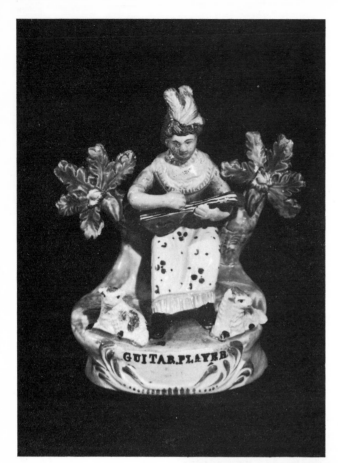

187 & a. *Very rare Staffordshire earthenware figure of a guitar player, bearing the impressed mark of John Dale of Burslem (see below) (c. 1825). 4½ inches high.*

D. M. & P. Manheim

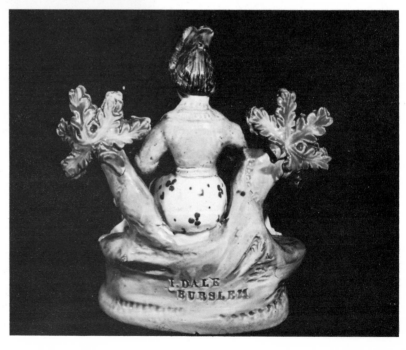

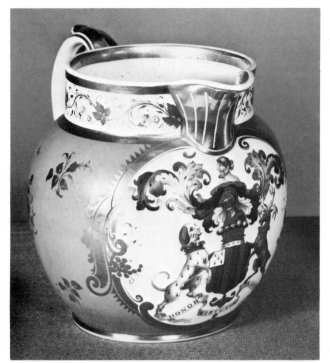

188. *"H & R Daniel, Stoke-upon-Trent, Staffordshire"* (written mark) *porcelain jug, decorated with green ground, richly gilt. The ornate arms are those of Earl Ferrers, and are painted in the finest manner (c. 1826). 4¼ inches high.*

Delomosne & Son

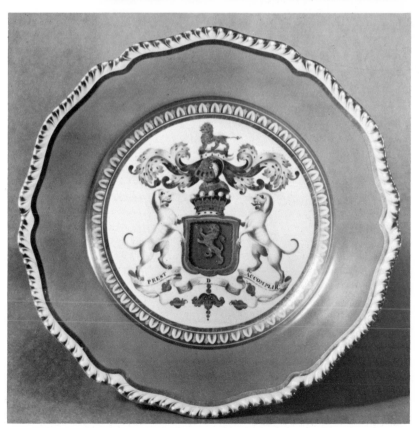

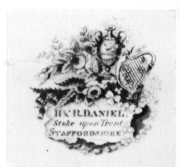

Ornate printed mark of Henry & Richard Daniel (c. 1826–41). This mark occurs on some pieces made for the Earl of Shrewsbury (c. 1827).

189 & a. *"H & R Daniel"* (painted mark) *plate, part of a service made for the Earl of Shrewsbury (c. 1827)— "The most brilliant and costly kind ever manufactured in the district" (S. Shaw, 1829). From c. 1823 to c. 1826 Henry and Richard Daniel traded as Daniel & Son.*

Godden of Worthing

Messrs Davenport

John Davenport took over John Brindley's Pottery at Longport in the Staffordshire Potteries in 1793 or 1794. At first only earthenwares were produced, but in 1801 the manufacture of glass was undertaken as was also that of porcelain at some time prior to 1805. Very good quality "Stone China" was made from about 1805. This is a strong compact opaque earthenware body similar to Spode's "New Stone" (see Plate 196).

John Ward, writing before 1843, noted in his book, *The Borough of Stoke-upon-Trent*, that the Davenports had three separate works at Longport and a further earthenware factory at Newport; "the aggregate of their business, indeed, is of very considerable magnitude, and gives employment to upwards of fifteen hundred hands". The Davenport wares in all their branches were of very fine quality. The various marks include the name "Davenport" (with the exception of the mark "Longport" found rarely on some wares which are probably of Davenport manufacture).

The Davenport works continued to 1887 under various managements. From about 1860, mainly porcelains were produced. The wares from about 1850 are normally marked with the name Davenport. Some very decorative services were made. The standard book on this factory and its products is *Davenport Pottery and Porcelain 1794–1887* by T. A. Lockett (David & Charles, Newton Abbot, 1972).

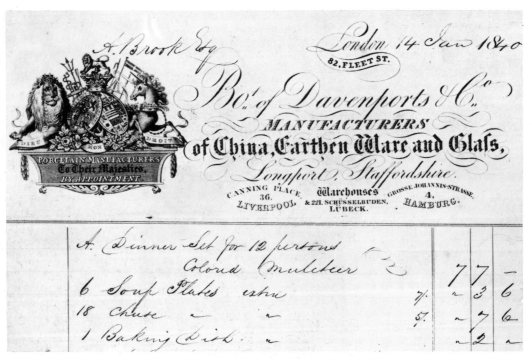

Davenport bill head and account for dinner service shown in Colour Plate V. Note address formerly occupied by James Mist. See Plate 425.

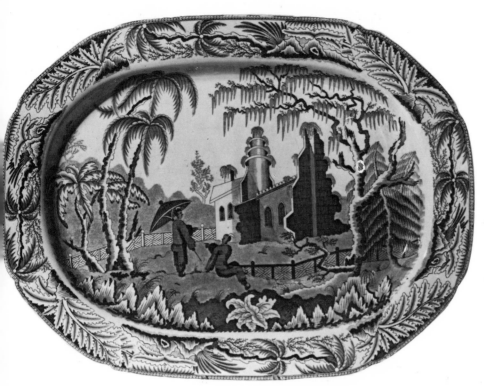

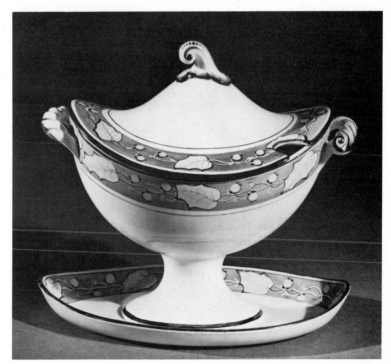

190 & a. Davenport im-
pressed marked earthenware
platter, decorated with underglaze blue print (c. 1795–
1805). The impressed name
mark is of early type with
lower-case letters (see above),
the dish is also thinner
and lighter in weight than
later examples. $20\frac{1}{4} \times 15\frac{1}{4}$
inches.

191. Davenport (early impressed,
lower-case, mark) creamware sauce
tureen and cover, from a dessert service
of the 1800–5 period. The form is
typical of sauce tureens made by other
manufacturers of the period. $6\frac{1}{2}$ inches
high.

Godden of Worthing

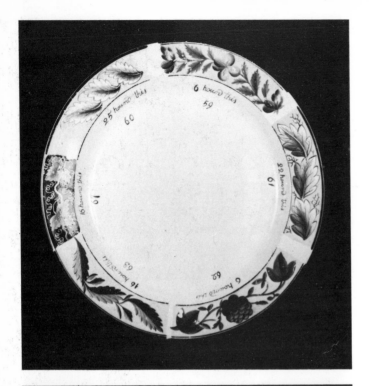

192. *Marked Davenport creamware pattern plates, showing typical painted borders and their numbers. Such pattern plates were supplied to retailers and travellers, so that customers could see a wide range of patterns and choose their services with a minimum of trouble and stock holding. Today such interesting pattern plates are rarely found.*

S. W. Fisher, Bewdley

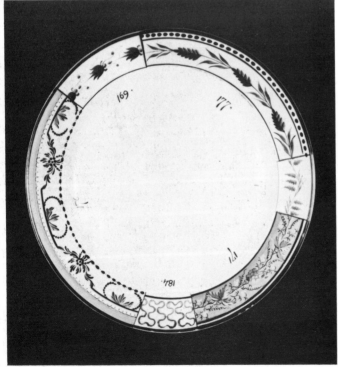

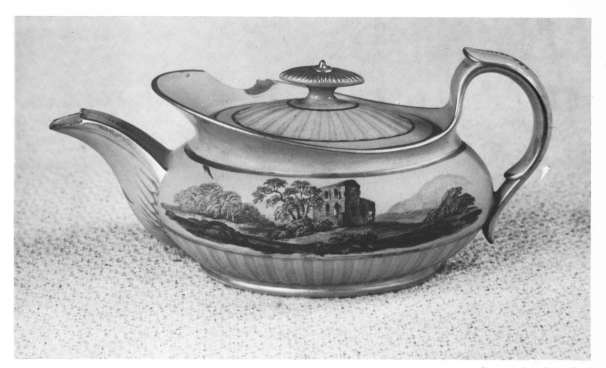

193. *Davenport (impressed mark) earthen-ware teapot of salmon-pink colour with landscape painted in sepia. Many attractive services were made in this style (c. 1805–15). 3½ inches high.*

City Museum & Art Gallery,
Stoke-on-Trent

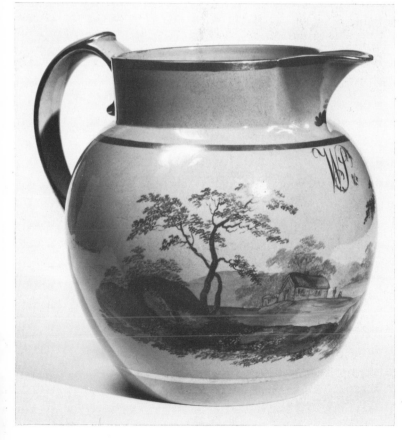

194. *Davenport (impressed marked no. 1181) jug of orange-brown earthenware. A typical example of many fine pieces painted with landscapes, etc., in monochrome (c. 1805–15). 5¾ inches high.*

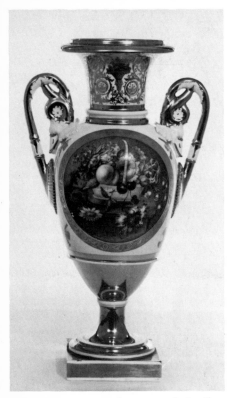

195. *Davenport porcelain vase of the finest quality. The tooled, matt and burnished gilding equals the best French, or Spode, examples. Printed name and anchor mark (c. 1820). 13¾ inches high.*

Godden of Worthing

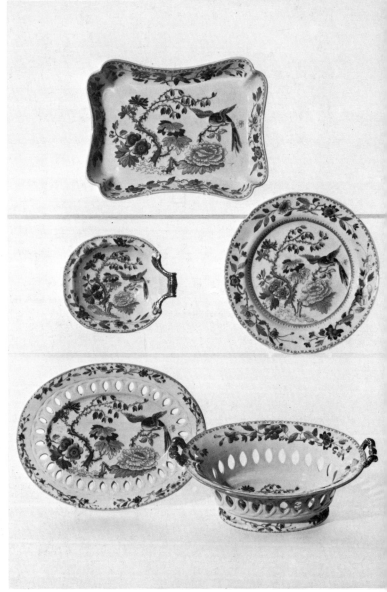

196. *"Davenport stone china" (printed marks nos. 1182 and 1183). Part dessert servic[e] decorated with printed and coloured over Chinese style pattern (c. 1805–20). Baske[t] 10½ inches long.*

Godden of Worthing

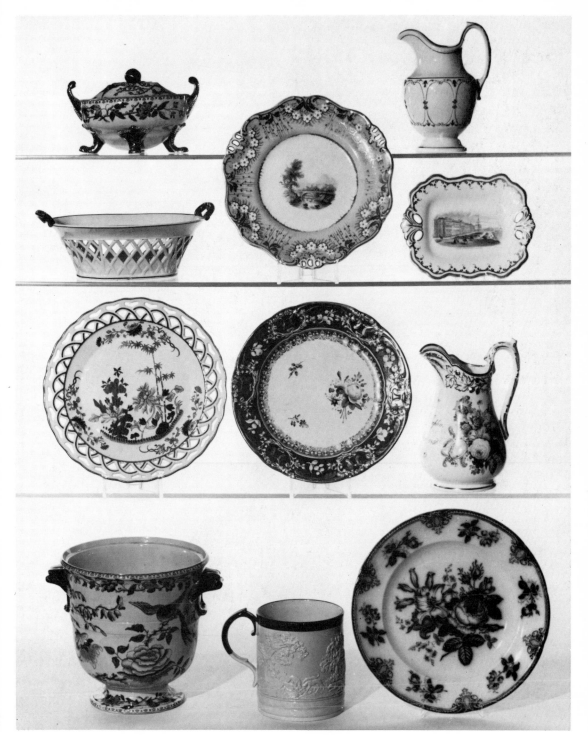

197. *A selection of marked Davenport pottery and porcelain (c. 1805–75). The covered sauce tureen on the top shelf is from a "Stone China" dessert service (c. 1805–15). The moulded stoneware hunting mug on the bottom shelf has impressed anchor and "Davenport" mark (c. 1810–20). Many fine moulded stoneware jugs and mugs were made.*

Godden of Worthing

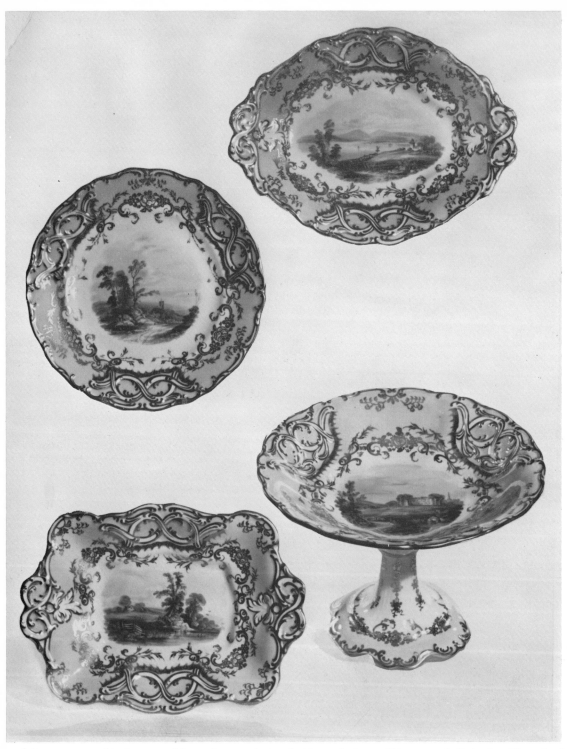

198. *Davenport porcelain dessert set of fine quality. Hand painted with named views, within green and gilt borders. Blue printed mark no. 1191 (c. 1850). Comport 7¾ inches high.*

Godden of Worthing

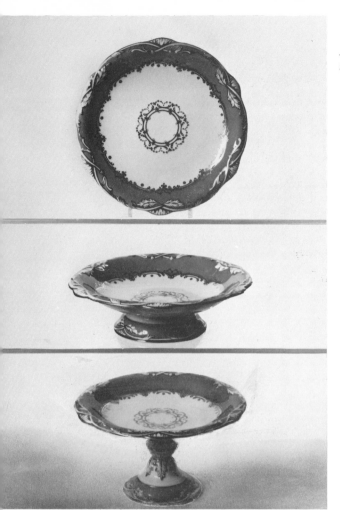

199. *Sample pieces from a Davenport porcelain dessert service. The moulded edge design should be noted as this occurs on many services bearing other painted or printed patterns. Printed mark no. 1191 (c. 1855–70). Comport 4¾ inches high.*

Godden of Worthing

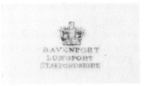

200. a. *Detail of standard printed Davenport mark no. 1194 (c. 1870–87) as occurring on service below.*

200. *Davenport porcelain teaset. Colourful "Japan" pattern (no. 2614). Printed mark no. 1194 (see above). The shapes are typical of the 1870–87 period, when many colourful Derby-type "Japan" patterns were employed.*

Royal Ontario Museum, University of Toronto

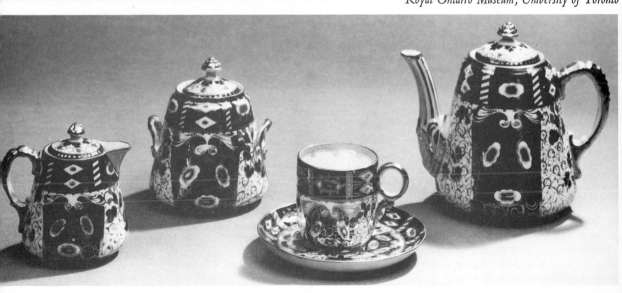

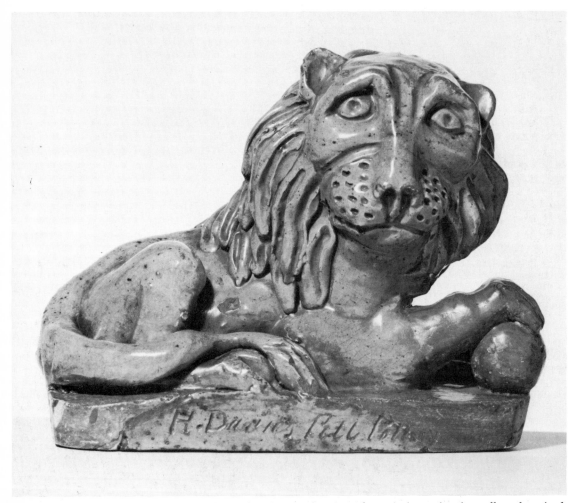

201. *"H Davies. Pill Pottery"* (incised mark). *Red earthenware lion (one of a pair) decorated with a yellow glaze (early nineteenth century). No other marked examples are known. Pill is near Bristol. 7 inches long.*

Fitzwilliam Museum, Cambridge

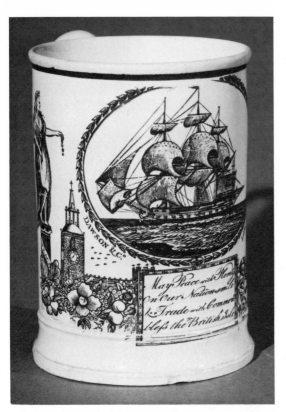

202. *"Dawson & Co, Low Ford" (marked on print) creamware mug of the 1800–10 period. John Dawson (& Co) potted at Sunderland and produced many fine printed patterns. 5 inches high.*

203. *"Dawson" (impressed marked) earthenware plaque. Decorated with coloured over print and typical Sunderland "splash", lustre border (see page xxiv) (c. 1830–50). $8\frac{1}{2} \times 7\frac{1}{4}$ inches.*

Godden of Worthing

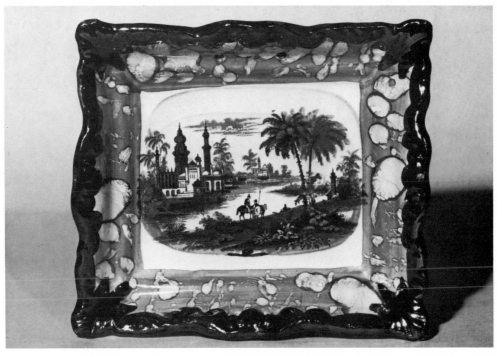

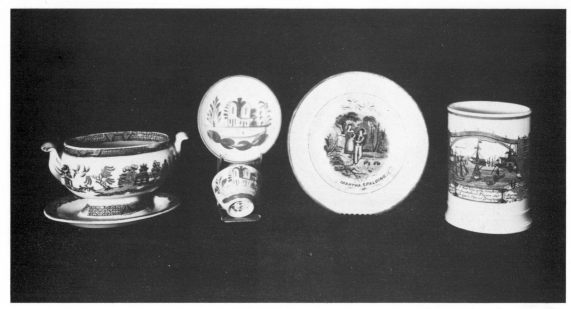

204. *Dawson's earthenwares made at the Low Ford Pottery, Sunderland. Blue printed tureen (cover missing) impressed mark "Dawson" (c. 1820). Lustre painted tea bowl and saucer, impressed mark "Dawson" (c. 1825). Small plate with printed pattern, impressed mark (c. 1845). Printed mug (frog moulded inside) with view of the local Wearmouth Bridge. Printed mark "J Dawson & Co. Low Ford Pottery" (c. 1800). 5½ inches high.*

Sunderland Museum

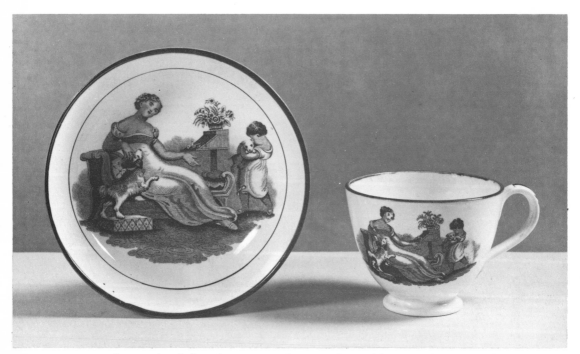

205. *Dawson & Co (impressed marked) earthenware cup and saucer with typical bat printed figure subject of the 1815 period. John Dawson & Co worked the South Hylton and Ford Potteries at Sunderland.*

Victoria & Albert Museum

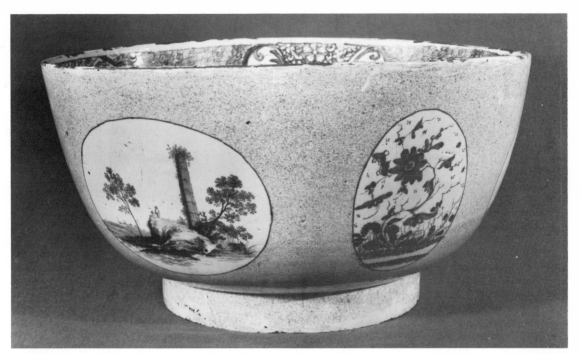

206. *A unique documentary Dublin delft punch bowl by Henry Delamain (died 1757). Interesting letters relating to the firing of Delamain's wares by coal are quoted in Chaffer's* Marks and Monograms, *15th edition. 16 inches diameter.*

British Museum

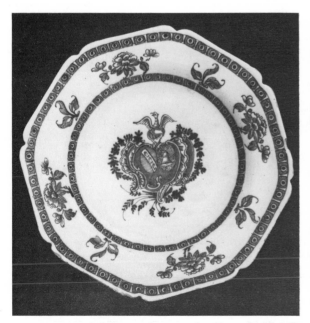 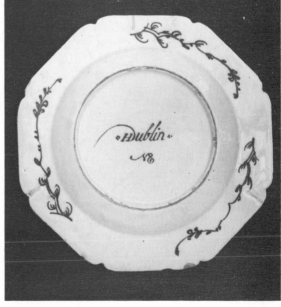

207 & a. *Irish delft-type plate painted in blue and made by Henry Delamain of Dublin (c. 1752–7). See detail of underside for mark. The initials N E should not be regarded as part of the mark.*

National Museum of Ireland

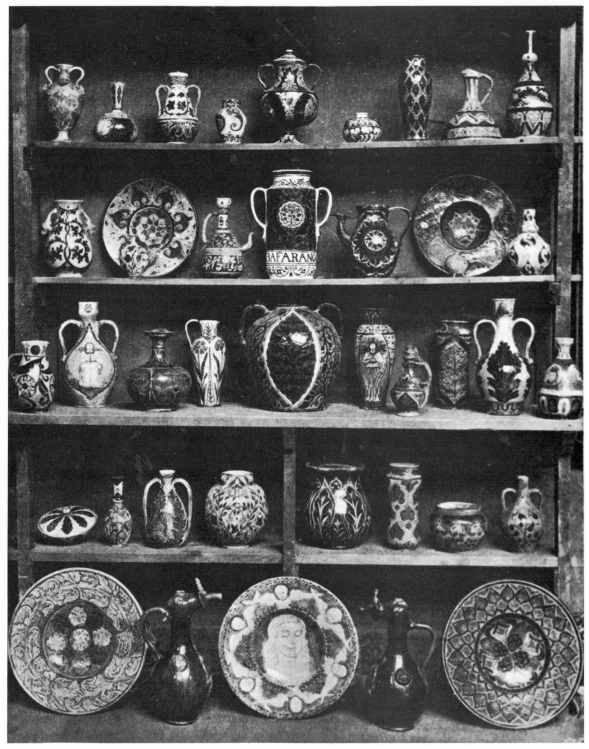

208. *Della Robbia earthenwares of 1896 reproduced from a contemporary photograph. Such wares will be marked with the words "Della Robbia" or with the ship device, mark no. 1228A.*

William De Morgan

William De Morgan (1839–1917), after early training in painting at the Royal Academy School, turned his attention to stained glass and tile painting. He was encouraged in this by his friend, William Morris. His success in tile decoration enabled him to establish his own small pottery and showroom in Cheyne Row, Chelsea, in 1872, where he was able to produce his own tiles, instead of purchasing them undecorated from outside sources as he had done previously.

At this period he was seeking the lost art of Moorish or Gubbio lustres. His fine, bold designs and lustre effects quickly won praise, and vases and plaques were made as well as tiles. Because of the success of this venture De Morgan was forced to find larger premises and in 1882 moved to Merton Abbey where he erected larger kilns. This sufficed until 1888 when he was again forced to move, this time to Sands End Pottery in Fulham. From 1888 to 1898 he was in partnership with Halsey Ricardo, and from then on "& Co" was added to the factory mark. The De Morgan pottery is soft and the glaze is often crazed.

William De Morgan did not enjoy good health and spent the winter months in Florence. While there, he employed local artists to draw, under his supervision, suitable patterns, which were sent back to England and used in the decoration of the pottery. The initials of his chief painters are found on many specimens: they include Charles and Fred Passenger (partners from 1898), Joe Juster, and J. Hersey.

In 1907 ill health forced William De Morgan to retire from the pottery, although pieces were decorated by the remaining artists until 1911. An interesting article by Norman Prouting is contained in the *Apollo* magazine of January 1963. The different De Morgan marks are listed in the *Encyclopaedia of British Pottery and Porcelain Marks*.

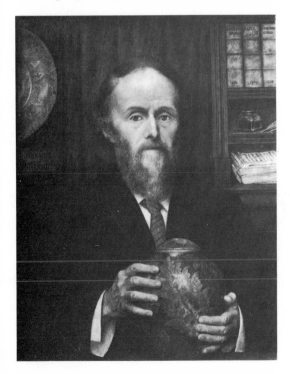

Portrait of William De Morgan (1839–1917). A painting by his wife (in 1909) showing a typical "De Morgan" iridescent glazed earthenware vase—one of the last he made (c. 1898).

Victoria & Albert Museum Photograph

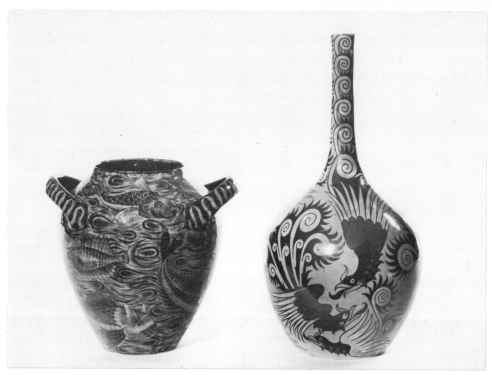

209. *De Morgan earthenware vases showing typical forms and styles of decoration (c. 1885–95). Taller vase has impressed DM—tulip mark (no. 1232). The fish vase bears the painted initials of Joe Juster.*

Godden of Worthing

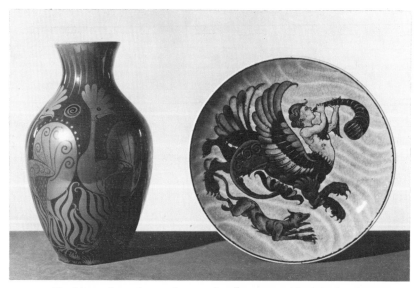

210. *De Morgan lustre decorated vase and a plate decorated by Charles Passenger (c. 1900). Vase 10 inches high.*

Victoria & Albert Museum

The early history of Derby Porcelain is still not fully known. Rare white jugs are marked "D. 1750" and probably represent early trials, perhaps by the mysterious André Planché, who was making experimental porcelain at Derby (at the Cockpit Hill works) in the 1750's.

The story of "Crown Derby" porcelain may be said to commence in 1756 when William Duesbury and John Heath built a new factory on the Nottingham road and traded under the style W. Duesbury & Co. The early porcelains were seldom marked, especially the blue and white specimens, although the anchor marks of Chelsea were sometimes copied on enamelled wares (Plate 212). Early figures usually have three unglazed patches under the base (Plate 214), caused by the pads employed to prevent them sticking to the bottom of the saggar in the kiln. The porcelain is not as translucent as Chelsea or Worcester.

The energetic William Duesbury purchased the Chelsea factory in 1769. The period from 1769 to 1775 is known as the Chelsea-Derby period; some fine decorative wares were made and painted in a rich but tasteful manner, sometimes by former Chelsea artists. Such wares were normally marked with the Chelsea anchor mark (these pieces are thinner in the potting than gold anchor Chelsea examples and the excess of glaze is not present). Other Chelsea-Derby wares bear a gilt mark of a "D" and an anchor (mark nos. 860–2). Porcelain made at the Derby works from about 1770 to 1782 often bears a painted mark, usually in blue, of a crown over the letter "D". These wares are well potted and tasteful; the floral painting is very good.

William Duesbury died in 1786 and was succeeded by his son, also William. The standard mark from c. 1786 had been the crossed batons with a crown above and the initial "D" below. At first the mark was carefully drawn in a puce colour; examples with this are of good quality with a warm, friendly, close-fitting glaze and are normally decorated with restraint. Fine quality figures and groups were made in a white unglazed body, known as biscuit (Plates 215–17). From about 1800 the crowned baton mark was rather carelessly painted and is in red enamel rather than the earlier puce. After 1800 the patterns tend to become heavier in feeling and the glaze is inclined to craze. Most Derby porcelain from 1785 onwards bears one of the standard marks; very little Derby porcelain of this period is unmarked.

In 1810 the Derby works were sold to Robert Bloor, and it can be said that, in general, the firm gradually declined until the closure in 1848. Several marks incorporating the name "Bloor" or the crowned initial "D" were used from c. 1820. Information on Derby porcelains and artists will be found in J. Haslem's *The Old Derby China Factory* (1876), F. B. Gilhespy's *Crown Derby Porcelain*, and *Derby Porcelain* (1951 and 1961). The Derby section of *English Porcelain 1745–1850* (1965) is noteworthy. Much information is summarized in G. Godden's *British Pottery and Porcelain 1780–1850* (1963).

On the closure of the main Derby factory in 1848, a group of the former workmen established their own small works at King Street, Derby. Many of the old traditional Derby patterns and figure models were reissued up to 1935. From 1861 to 1935 the King Street factory used the old Derby crossed batons mark with the addition of the initials S.H. placed one each side of the main mark. Specimens are illustrated in Plates 550–2.

In 1876 a new company was formed and production commenced in 1878 at a factory in Osmaston Road. In 1890 the new company was appointed "Manufacturers of Porcelain to Her

Majesty" (Queen Victoria) and from that date to the present day, the Osmaston Road Derby porcelains have been known as "Royal Crown Derby". Information on the later Derby porcelains and ceramic artists is contained in *Royal Crown Derby* by J. Twitchett & B. Bailey (Barrie & Jenkins, London, 1976). Good collections of Derby porcelain may be seen at the Victoria & Albert Museum in London, at the Derby Museum & Art Gallery and at the Works Museum in the present factory.

Standard Derby mark (c. 1782–1825). Incised on figures and groups (Plates 215–17). Painted in puce, blue or black (c. 1782–1800) on wares such as Plates 218, 221. Painted in red (c. 1800–25) (Plates 222–3, 228).

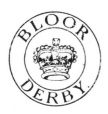

Printed Bloor Derby mark, in red (c. 1825–40) (Plates 230–1).

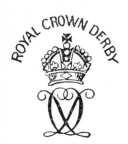

Standard Royal Crown Derby printed mark, without wording (c. 1878–90). With wording as drawn (c. 1891) onwards with the word "England" or in the twentieth century "Made in England" (see Plates 234–7).

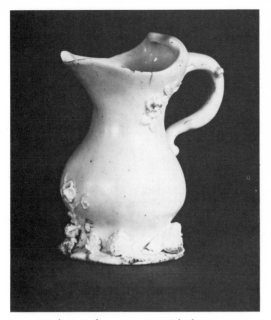

211. *Derby porcelain cream jug with the very rare incised mark—"D./1750". 3½ inches high.*
Victoria & Albert Museum

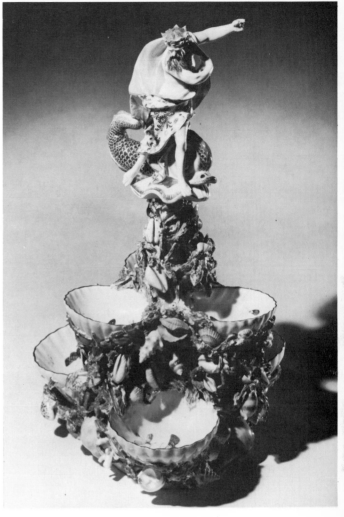

212. *Early Derby porcelain shell centrepiece of un-usually fine quality. Painted anchor mark in red (normally used at Chelsea) and three "pad" marks (c. 1755–60). 16¼ inches high.*
Godden of Worthing

Shell centrepieces, of a simpler nature, were made at several eighteenth-century factories.

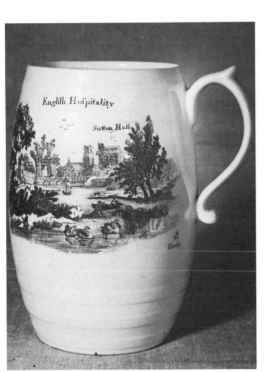

213. *Very rare Derby porcelain mug, printed in black (c. 1768). Signed with the anchor rebus of Richard Holdship and the word "Derby". Holdship was at Derby from 1764 to 1769 and had previously been at Worcester.*
Derby Museum & Art Gallery

133

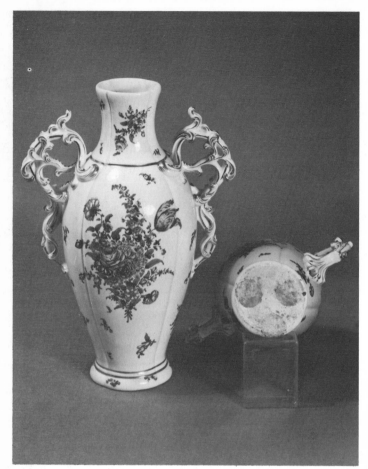

214. *Derby porcelain vase, one of a set of three. Painted with floral sprays, much in the style of contemporary red anchor period Chelsea. Unmarked except for three "pad" marks shown on upturned vase, as three circular dark marks. These pad marks occur on many Derby (and Chelsea-Derby) vases and figures. The marks were caused by pads of clay placed under the objects in the kiln, so that the piece would not stick to the shelf or saggar base (c. 1755–60). 12 inches high.*

Godden of Worthing

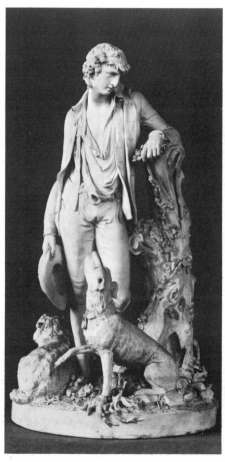

215. *Derby biscuit (unglazed) figure, modelled by W. T. Coffee. Incised crown, crossed batons and "D" mark, with model no. 396 (c. 1794). 13¾ inches high. This figure shows the fine detailed work which is characteristic of the finest Derby biscuit figures and groups (see page xxii).*

Victoria & Albert Museum

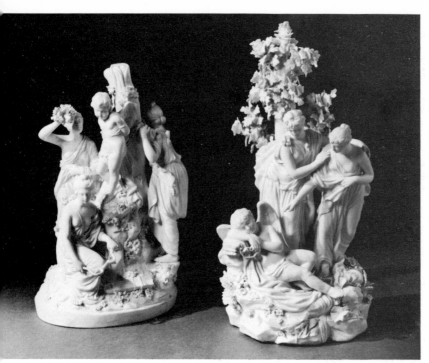

216. Two typical, fine quality Derby biscuit groups of the 1788–95 period. Incised model nos. 379 and 195 with pad marks. The right-hand group (model 195) "Two Virgins Awaking Cupid" occurs in the original price list at £3 3s. When "coloured and gilt" the price was a third less (see page xxii). 12½ inches high.

Godden of Worthing

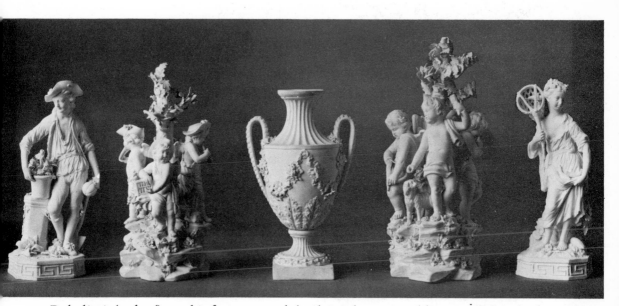

217. Derby biscuit (unglazed) porcelain figures, etc., marked with incised crown crossed batons and "D" marks also model numbers (c. 1785–95). Vase 9½ inches high.

Allen Collection, Victoria & Albert Museum

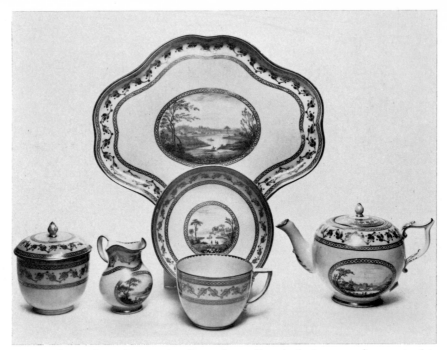

218. *Derby porcelain cabaret service of very fine quality, the landscape panels are painted in puce camaieu, a style of decoration much favoured on Derby porcelains of the 1780–1800 period. Mark no. 1253 in puce. Tray $10\frac{3}{4} \times 8\frac{1}{2}$ inches.*

Sotheby & Co

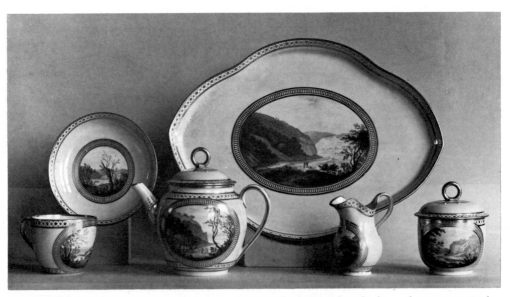

219. *Derby porcelain cabaret service of fine quality. The ground colour is pale pink, the panels—scenes in Derbyshire—are attributed to Zachariah Boreman. Mark crown, crossed batons and "D" painted in blue enamel (c. 1790). Tray $13\frac{1}{4} \times 9\frac{3}{4}$ inches.*

Allen Collection, Victoria & Albert Museum

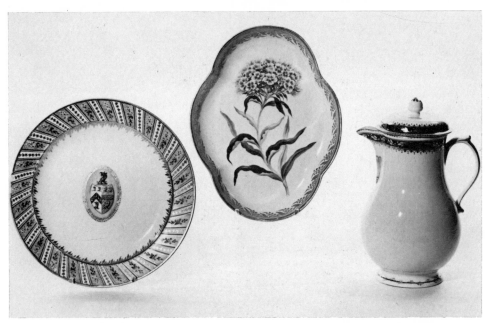

220. *Derby porcelains bearing the crown, crossed batons and "D" mark painted in puce or blue enamel (c. 1790–1800). Many fine Derby services and other wares were painted with botanical specimens.*

Godden of Worthing

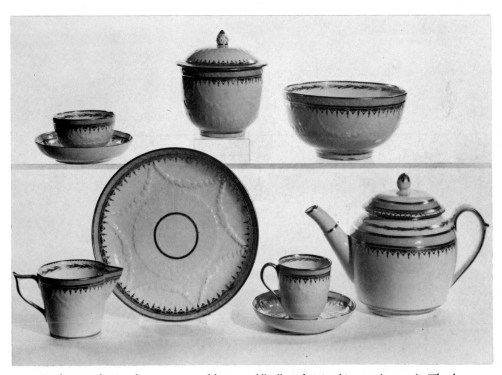

221. *Derby teaset bearing the crown, crossed batons and "D" mark painted in puce (c. 1790). The shapes are typical of puce-marked Derby, as is also the tasteful restrained decoration. Teapot 6½ inches high.*

Godden of Worthing

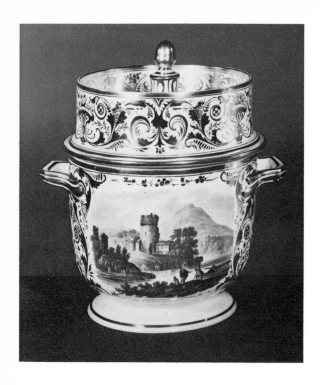

222. *Duesbury Derby porcelain ice pail of typical form and style of decoration. Painted crown, batons and "D" mark, in red (c. 1805–15). 9½ inches high.*

Delomosne & Son

223. *Derby porcelain "Japan" pattern (see page xxii) tea service of the 1810–15 period, showing typical Derby shapes of the period. Teapot 5¾ inches high.*

Godden of Worthing

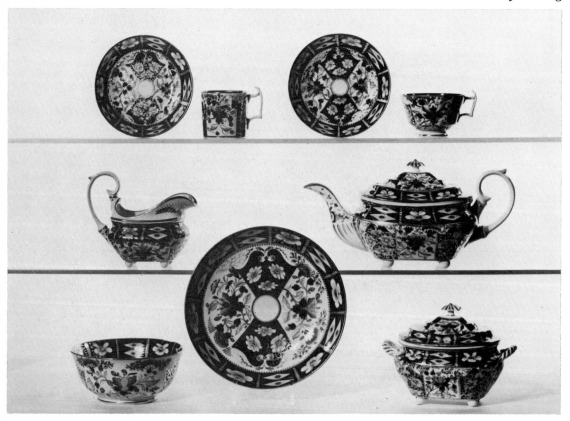

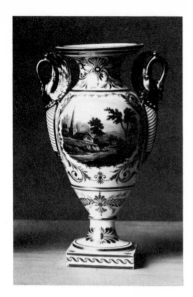

224. *Derby porcelain vase, the landscape painting in the manner of Jesse Mounford. The gilding is typical of Derby porcelains of the 1795–1830 period. Painted mark no. 1253 in red (c. 1820). 8 inches high.*

Victoria & Albert Museum

225. *Selection of Derby porcelain (c. 1800–30). With the exception of the jug on the top shelf and the floral plate on the bottom shelf, both of which bear Bloor Derby marks, all items had the standard crown, crossed batons and "D" mark. Vase (top–centre) 7½ inches high.*

Allen Collection, Victoria & Albert Museum

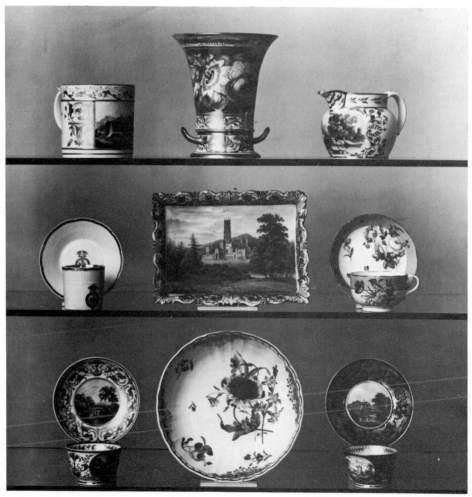

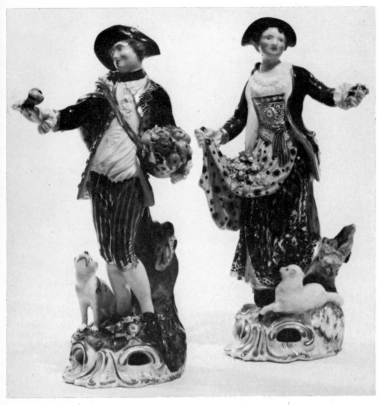

226. *A colourful pair of Derby figures, incorporating underglaze blue with overglaze enamel colours and gilt enrichments (c. 1805–15). Incised model numbers "No 53" and "No 55". 8 inches high.*

Godden of Worthing

227. *Derby porcelain figures (c. 1810–45). Three figures on top shelf (middle) marked with crossed swords in underglaze blue (c. 1810–20). Kneeling children with circular "Bloor Derby" mark (c. 1825–30). Peacock bears late Bloor Derby mark—the word "Derby" on a ribbon with crown above (c. 1830–48). Other figures have incised model numbers only. The tailor and his wife on goats are marked "No 62" (c. 1820). $5\frac{3}{4}$ inches high.*

Allen Collection, Victoria & Albert Museum

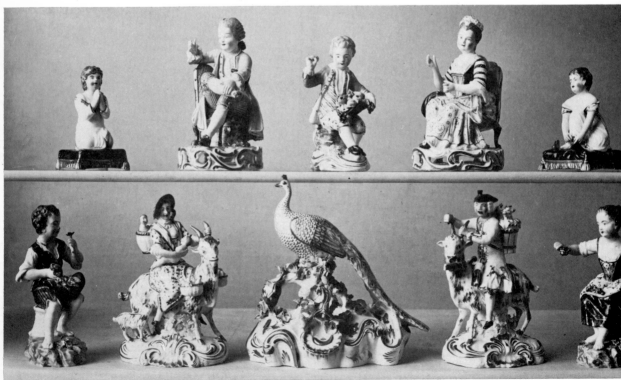

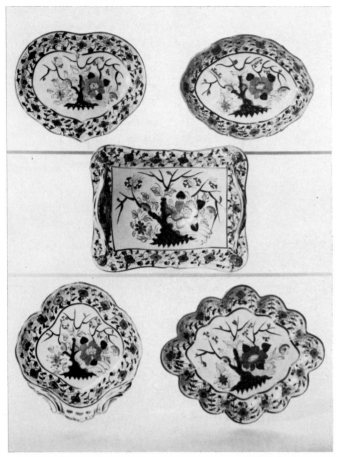

228. *Selection from Derby dessert service, showing typical dish forms of the 1810–20 period. The centre dish is on a raised foot—not shown. This "tree" pattern is typical of the Derby "Japan" patterns decorated in underglaze blue and overglazed red with gilt enrichments. Red mark no. 1253.*

Godden of Worthing

229. *Derby porcelain figures of the four seasons. Mark crown, crossed batons and "D" painted in red (c. 1810–20). 8¼ inches high.*

Allen Collection, Victoria & Albert Museum

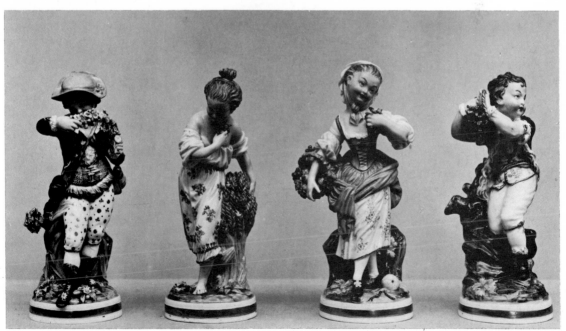

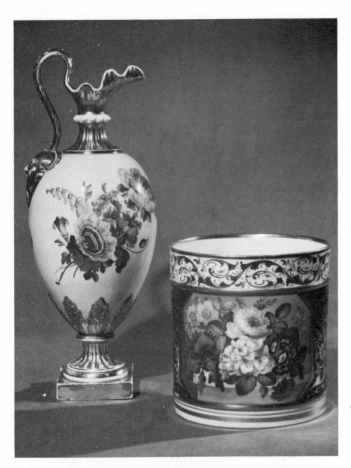

230. *Bloor Derby ewer. Also a finely painted and gilt mug, circular name mark (no. 1259) (c. 1825–35). Ewer 11 inches high.*

Godden of Worthing

231. *A superb set of Bloor Derby porcelain vases, finely painted with flowers in the style of Thomas Steel and richly gilt. Circular printed "Bloor Derby" mark (c. 1820–35). Centre vase 29½ inches high.*

Delomosne & Son

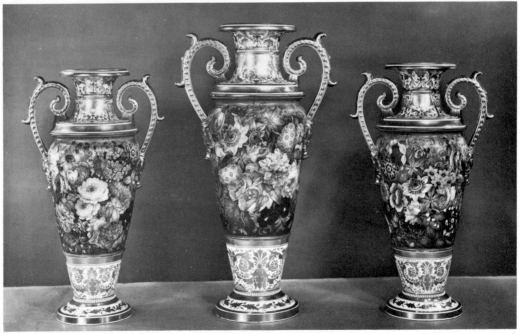

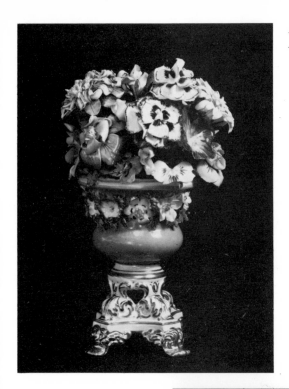

232. *Bloor Derby floral encrusted pot (one of a pair) of fine quality. Printed mark no. 1261 (see below) (c. 1825–30). 6½ inches high.*

Delomosne & Son

232. a. *Printed Bloor Derby mark no. 1261 (one of four standard marks of the 1820–48 period) (c. 1825–40).*

233. *Bloor Derby group, showing rare combination of matt white unglazed ("biscuit") body with glazed and richly decorated porcelain. A decorative example of the much maligned Bloor period prior to 1848. Mark no. 1261 (see above). 8¼ inches long.*

Godden of Worthing

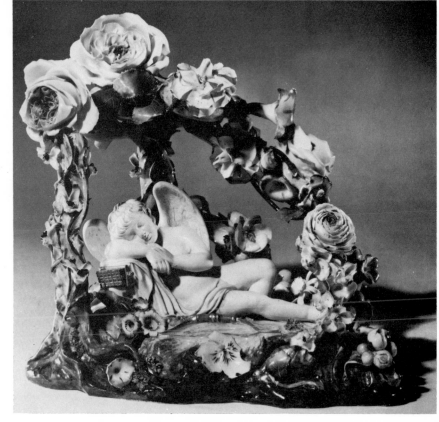

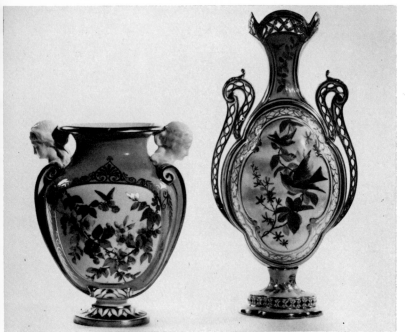

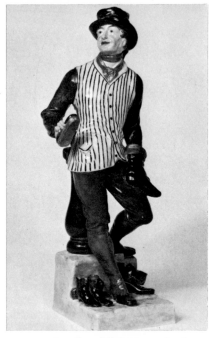

234. *Derby porcelain vase of pre-"Royal" period with simple printed mark, no. 1268 (c. 1878–90). 9¾ inches and 15½ inches high.*

Godden of Worthing

235. *A well-modelled Crown Derby (pre "Royal") figure (c. 1880). Mark no. 1268. 12 inches high.*

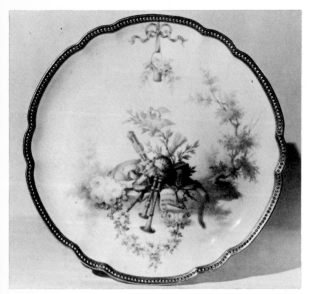

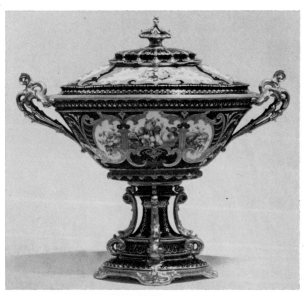

236. *Royal Crown Derby plate, painted by the former Sèvres artist—Desire Leroy (c. 1895). Printed mark no. 1270.*

237. *Royal Crown Derby covered vase-bowl of fine quality. Flower panels signed by A. Gregory, richly gilt over a deep blue ground (c. 1905). Printed mark no. 1270.*

In 1751 a partnership was formed by William Butts, John Heath, Thomas Rivett, and Ralph Steane to make pottery (not porcelain) at Cockpit Hill, Derby. By 1770 John Heath had become sole owner and in 1764, with William Duesbury (of the Derby porcelain works), acquired details of Richard Holdship's printing process as practised at Worcester. In 1779 John Heath became bankrupt, and in March 1780 the whole stock-in-trade was sold by auction.

A vast amount of cream-coloured earthenware must have been produced at this pottery, but only a few rare examples with printed decoration are marked. Two of these can be seen in Plates 238–9, others are illustrated in the *Transactions of the English Ceramic Circle*, vol. 3, part 4, and vol. 8, part 1 (1971). These marked examples and the characteristic teapot forms enable some of the other enamelled Cockpit Hill creamwares to be identified. See D. Towner's *Creamware* (1978).

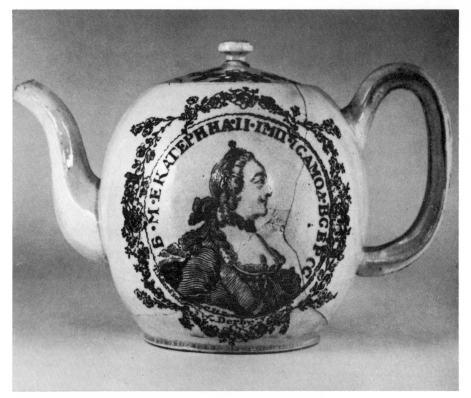

238. *Unique Cockpit Hill creamware teapot, decorated with black printed pattern taken from a Russian rouble coin (1765). Signed in print, "T Radford Sc. Derby". This form of teapot (with pierced knob) occurs with other rare signed Cockpit Hill prints (c. 1765–70)*
Derby Museum

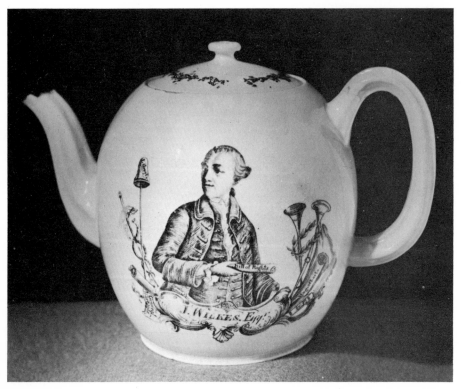

239. *Cockpit Hill, Derby creamware teapot, bearing a hitherto unillustrated print signed by Thomas Radford. The reverse side shows a seated "Britannia" (c. 1770). 5 inches high.*
Brighton Museum

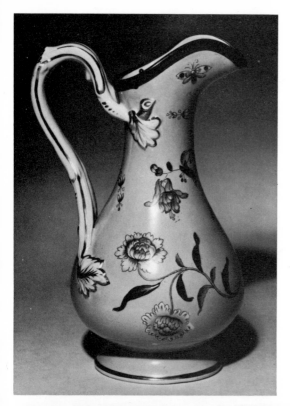

240. *"James Dixon & Son" metal mounted Staffordshire earthenware jug, with printed name mark and date 22 September 1842. Many other jugs bear the name of this firm of mounters.*

DOE AND ROGERS, DECORATORS

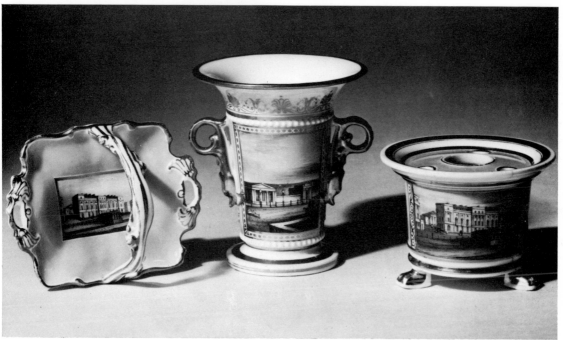

241. *Worcester porcelains painted by the local independent decorators—Doe & Rogers and bearing their written name marks (c. 1820–40).*

L. Godden Collection

147

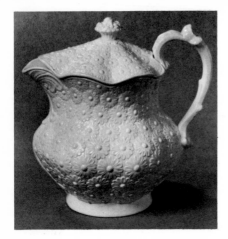

242. *Don pottery moulded jug and cover. Relief moulded name mark (no. 1313) (c. 1820–30). 9¾ inches high.*

Godden of Worthing

243. *"Don Pottery" footbath with fine underglaze blue printed pattern (c. 1820). Impressed mark "Don Pottery" also printed crest mark (no. 1314). This Yorkshire pottery produced many well potted and transfer printed specimens. 9¾ inches high.*

Godden of Worthing

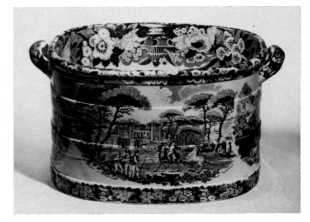

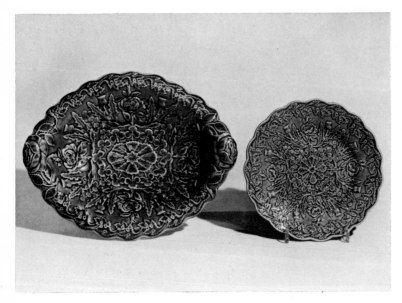

244. *Part of a moulded and green glazed earthenware dessert service with the impressed Don Pottery name and crest mark (c. 1820–5). Dish 11½ × 9 inches.*

Godden of Worthing

"They have given large value to common things—made precious a material of little worth, creating indeed, what may be justly described as a new art."

From *c.* 1820 to 1854 Messrs Doultons traded as Doulton & Watts. An earlier partnership traded under the style Jones, Doulton & Watts, but no mark was used. Stoneware jugs and ornamental bottles bear impressed "Doulton & Watts" marks, but the main concern of the factory was in the production of utilitarian wares. From 1854, on the retirement of John Watts, Henry Doulton continued as Doulton & Co.

In 1862 Henry Doulton, on the advice of John Sparkes (Head of the Lambeth School of Art), made experiments in decorated pottery. At first these were not successful, but in 1867 progress had been made in this department and examples of decorated wares were included in the 1867 Paris Exhibition. The advent of the 1871 Exhibition at South Kensington really marks the beginning of Doultons Art Pottery—students from the near-by Lambeth School of Art being employed to decorate the ware. In the field of salt-glazed stoneware the names that achieved lasting fame were George Tinworth for his fine sculptured stoneware vases, figures, groups, and religious plaques, and Hannah Barlow and her sister Florence for their fine animal and bird studies incised into the unfired stoneware. Items by these and other Doulton artists are illustrated in Plates 246–52 and represent typical examples of their work.

An interesting feature of the Doulton wares is that each example bears the personal mark of the decorator as well as the factory mark and, in many cases, the date of manufacture. The Doulton wares made at Lambeth have two qualities—that of being relatively inexpensive and at the same time being individually designed and executed.

The salt-glazed stoneware was but one of the many bodies used by Doultons. Several of the early examples were decorated on the so-called "Faience" body—a somewhat heavily potted creamware much used in decorative plaques and vases. Other Doulton bodies were "Impasto" (introduced in 1879), "Silicon" (1880), "Carrara" (1887), "Marqueterie" (1887), and the "Chine" ware in which various fabrics were impressed into the soft body, giving a woven pattern. Doultons also specialized in architectural terracotta work and tiles, and the output of this department ranged from the facings and decorative features of important buildings to mantelpieces and hearths.

A student visiting Messrs Howell & James's stock of Doulton wares in 1876 writes: "the general effect of the gallery exceed my expectations, and there were so many nice things to look at, I found it puzzling to know what to purchase. The shape of the vases etc. was good and the designs and colouring broad in effect. The whole exhibition does great credit to the Doulton factory, and to the students from the Lambeth School of Art (principally young ladies I am told) who design for it. This new industry struck me as being of great artistic merit." The personal marks of the leading Doulton decorators are reproduced on pages 216–19 of the companion *Encyclopaedia of Marks*.

In 1882 the manufacture of high-grade porcelain was commenced at a separate factory at Burslem, but much of this Doulton porcelain was produced after 1900 and continues to the present day. The production of stoneware at Lambeth ceased in March 1956.

Further information on Doulton's varied products will be found in Desmond Eyles's *Royal Doulton 1815–1965* (1965). Some information on the Lambeth artists is contained in G. Godden's *Antique China and Glass under £5* (1966).

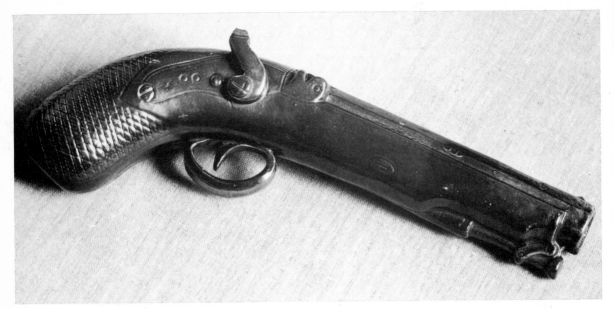

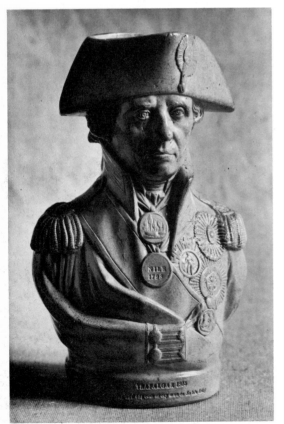

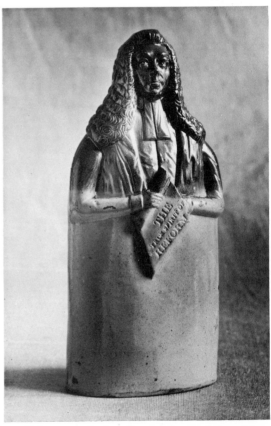

245. a. b. c. *Impressed marked "Doulton & Watts" (1820–54) moulded stoneware bottles, often made in several sizes. Many other different models were produced (not only by this firm). "The true spirit of reform" bottle (right) dates to the early 1830's. 14 inches high.*

Messrs Doulton & Co Ltd

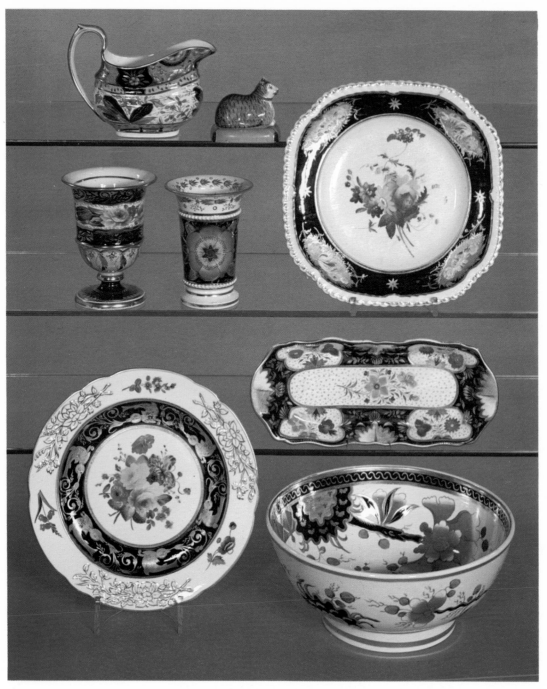

COLOUR PLATE I

A selection of fine quality porcelain by Charles Bourne of Fenton. Each piece bears the pattern number under the initials C.B., e.g. $\frac{C.B.}{233}$ on the bowl. The cat (and other animal models) is very rare (c. 1817–30). Bottom plate $8\frac{3}{4}$ inches diameter.

Godden of Worthing

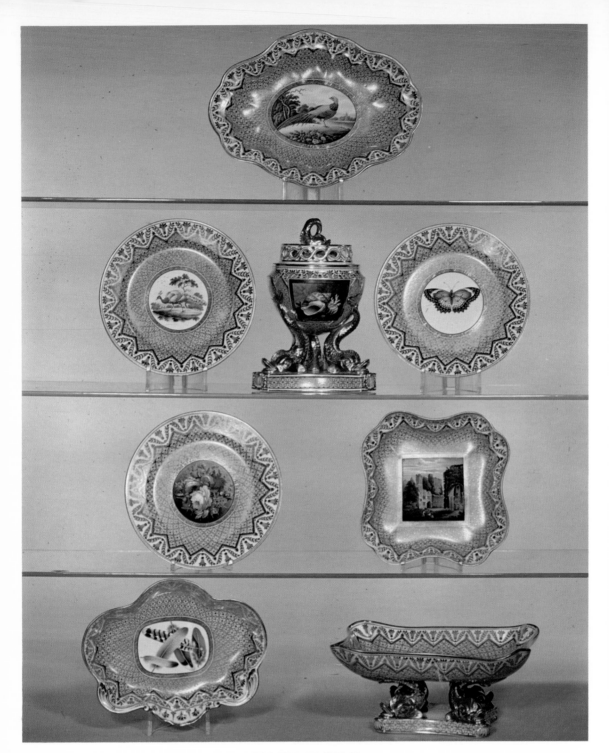

COLOUR PLATE II

Part of a superb Chamberlain Worcester dessert service showing various forms of decorative panel. The shell, butterfly and feather subjects are rare. Printed mark "Chamberlain Worcester Porcelain Manufacturers to H R H The Prince Regent" (c. 1815). "Dolphin cream bowl", centre. 9¼ inches high.

Godden of Worthing

The Chamberlain account books of the London Bond Street retail shop record the sale of "1 complete dessert, rich fawn & gold with different subjects. £84–0–0" in November 1815. The rare centrepiece (lower right) was sold to the same buyer separately in 1816: "1 dolphin centrepiece, fawn & view. £9–9–0". Apart from one similar service supplied to the same buyer, no other Chamberlain service (without ice pails) approaches the cost of this magnificent set. To gauge its equivalent present-day cost one could fairly multiply the 1815 cost by ten.

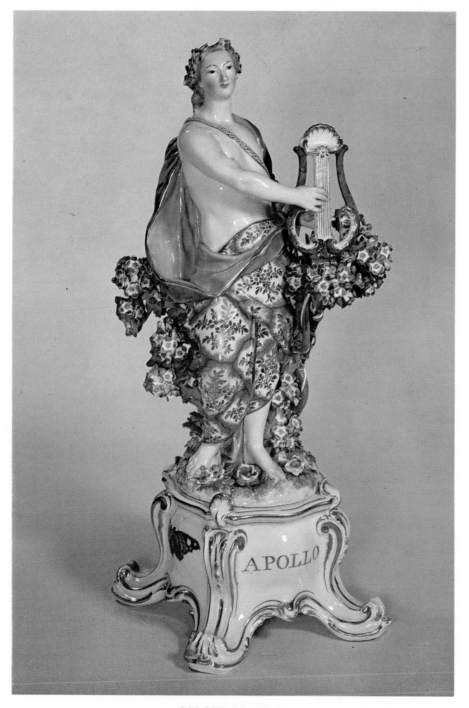

COLOUR PLATE III

Gold anchor marked Chelsea porcelain figure of Apollo, on loose base (c. 1765–9). 16 inches high.

Godden of Worthing

It is interesting to see that the stock in trade of Thomas Turner, china-man, when sold by Mr Christie in July 1767 included—"a beautiful Chelsea enamelled figure of Apollo, on a pedestal. £2."

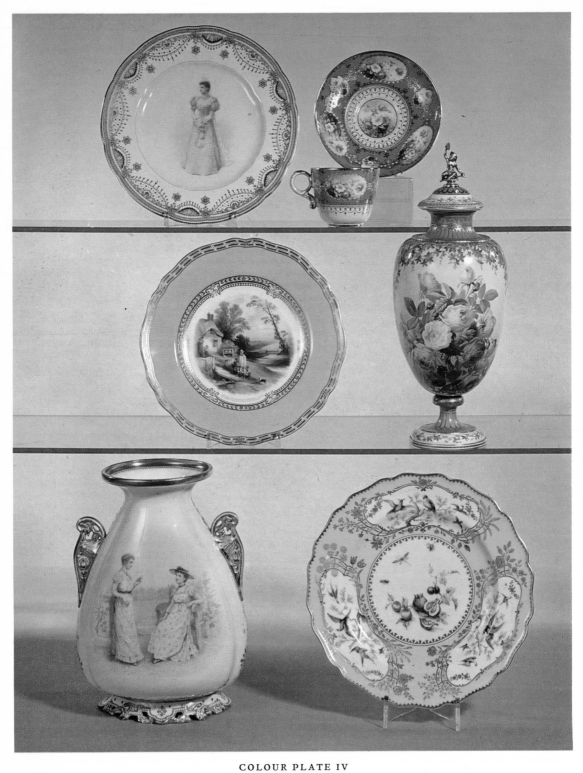

COLOUR PLATE IV

Selection of Copeland porcelains. Top plate and bottom vase are painted by Samuel Alcock. Floral vase by C. F. Hurten,
bottom plate by C. B. Brough (c. 1875–1900). Alcock vase 10½ inches high.

Godden of Worthing

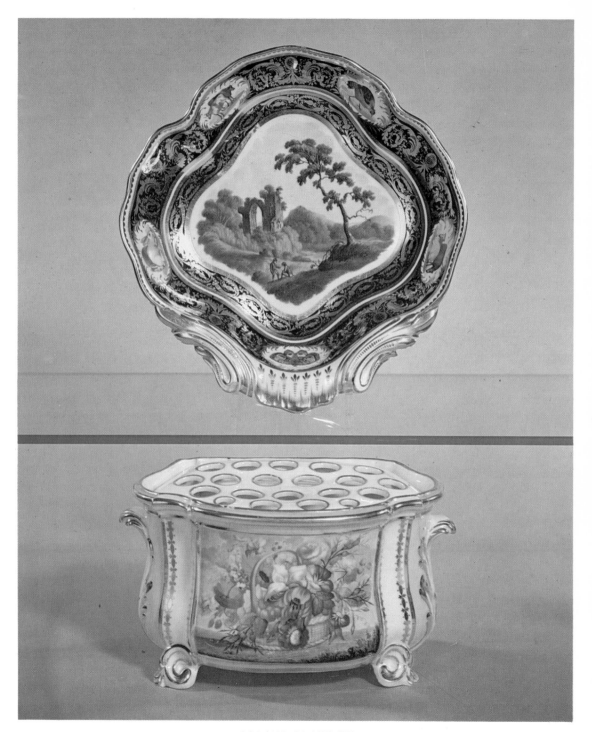

COLOUR PLATE VII

Derby porcelain dish (from a dessert service) painted with typical landscape centre, the whole of the finest quality. Red mark no. 1253. (Below) Bulb pot, with loose cover, showing Derby flower painting at its best. Mark no. 1253, painted in puce (c. 1782–1800). 8 inches long.

Godden of Worthing

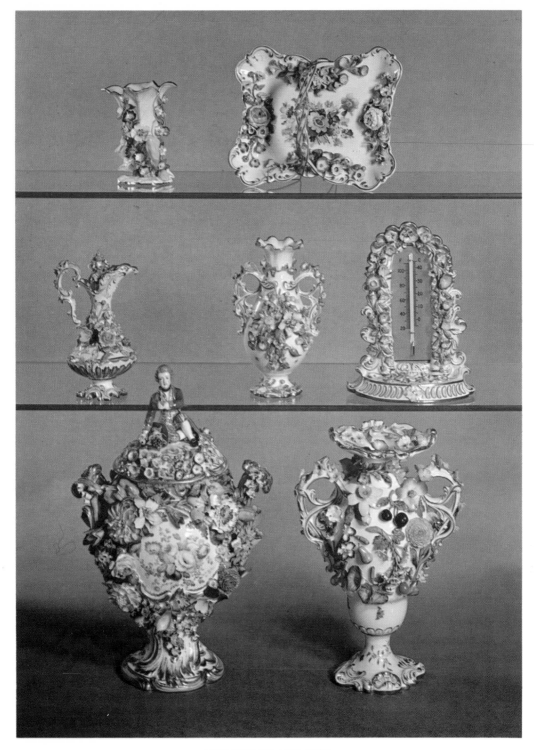

COLOUR PLATE VIII

Minton floral encrusted porcelains matching shapes in the factory pattern books. Such pieces bear a copy of the Dresden crossed-swords mark (c. 1830–40). Vase and cover $11\frac{3}{4}$ inches high.

Godden of Worthing

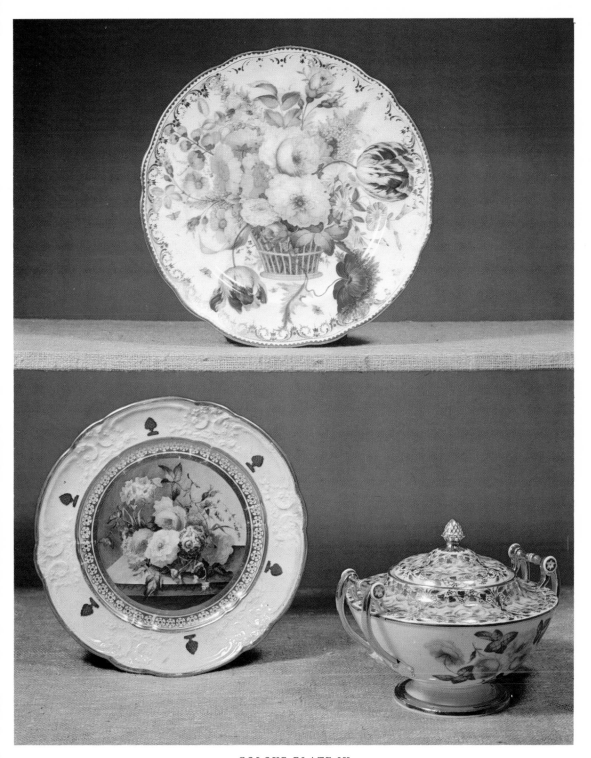

COLOUR PLATE IX

Nantgarw porcelains of fine quality and translucency. Some of the ornate designs were added by London decorators. Impressed marks "Nantgarw" (c. 1817-22).

Victoria & Albert Museum

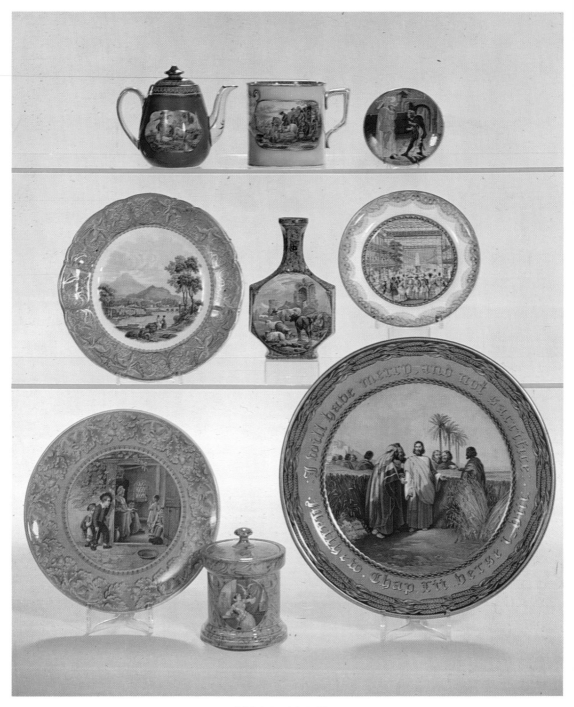

COLOUR PLATE X

Selection of multi-colour prints by F. & R. Pratt of Fenton. The large platter—Christ in the Cornfield—was engraved by Jesse Austin and was a subject shown at the 1851 Exhibition (mark no. 3148) (c. 1850–60). 13 inches diameter.

Godden of Worthing

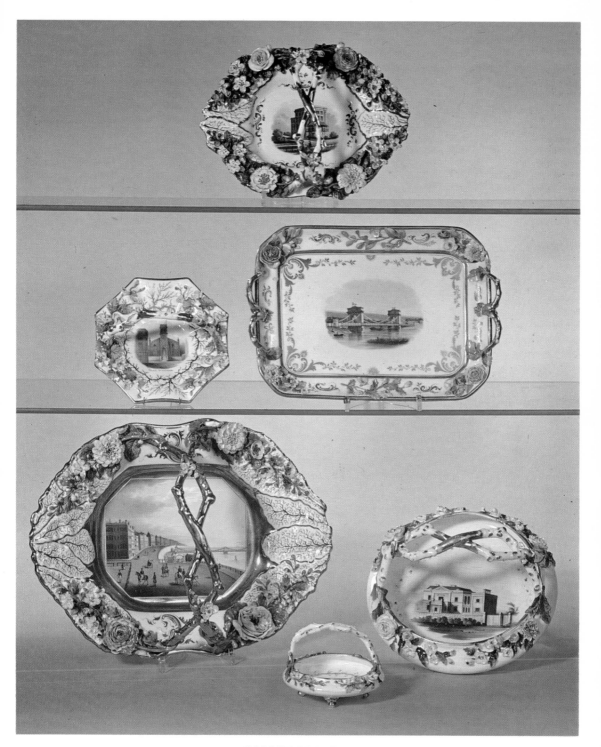

COLOUR PLATE XI

Rockingham porcelain floral encrusted baskets, etc., painted with Sussex views—Brighton, Hastings, Shoreham and Worthing. Similar examples will bear other views or subjects. Printed Griffin marks—nos. 3358 and 3359 (c. 1826–37). Large Brighton basket $13\frac{1}{2} \times 10$ inches.

L. Godden, Esq.

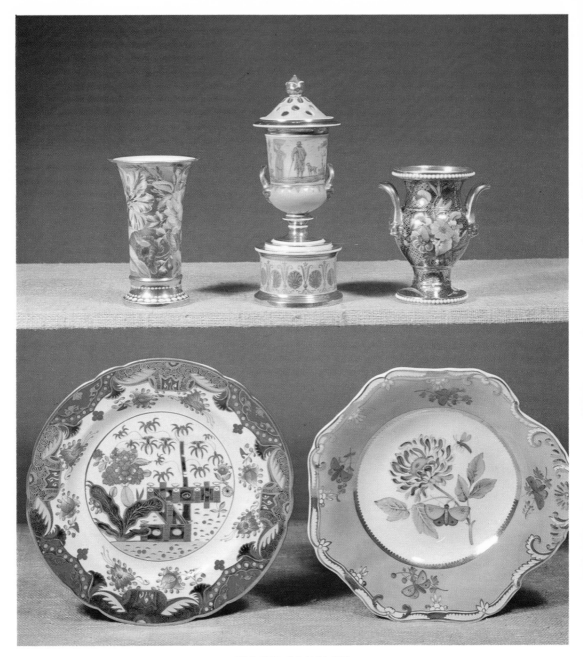

COLOUR PLATE XII

Spode porcelains (c. 1810–20). Left-hand plate a popular "Japan" pattern (see page xxii). Right-hand dish from a fine quality dessert service. Right-hand vase of the popular 1166 pattern. Centre yellow ground vase $7\frac{1}{2}$ inches high.

Victoria & Albert Museum

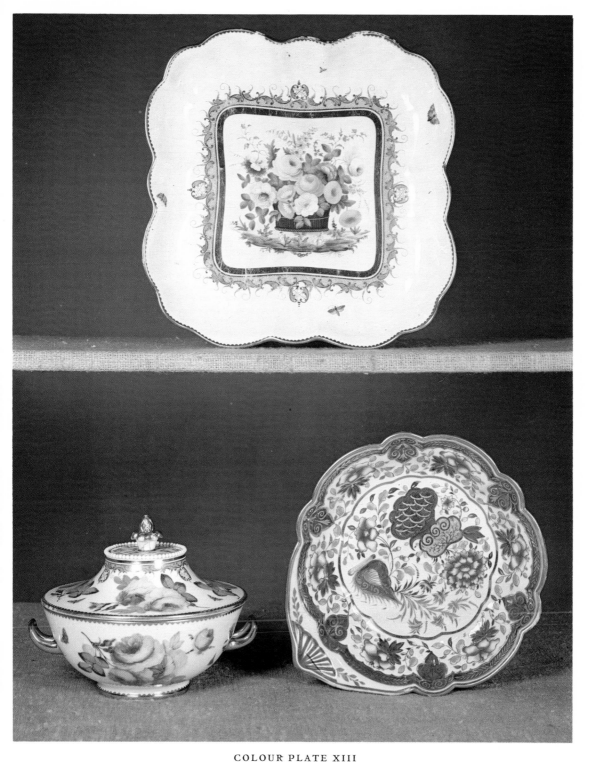

COLOUR PLATE XIII

Swansea porcelains, showing fine flower painting and a typical "Japan" pattern dish, from a dessert service (c. 1814–22). Square dish 9½ inches.

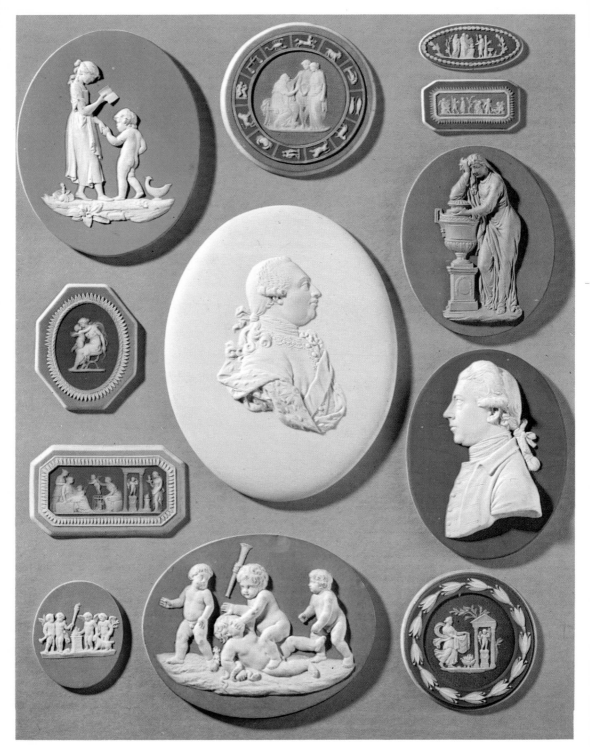

COLOUR PLATE XIV

Wedgwood (and Wedgwood & Bentley) jasper ware plaques, showing typical subjects and colours, the three colour examples are rare. All specimens marked "Wedgwood" except standing figure with urn which is Wedgwood & Bentley (c. 1769–80) and a rare colour—perhaps a trial piece. Large centre plaque of George III, 5 × 4 inches.

Godden of Worthing

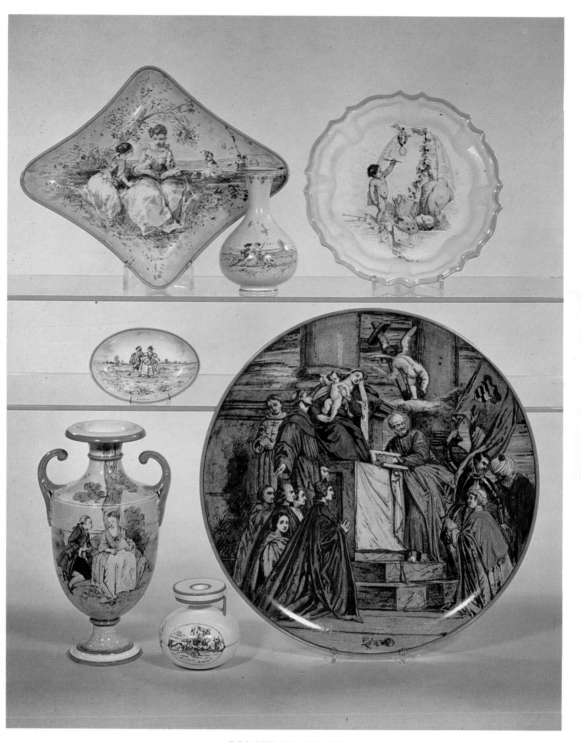

COLOUR PLATE XV

Wedgwood creamwares painted by Emile Lessore (see page 340). All examples are signed and the objects bear Wedgwood's impressed name mark and year letters. Large footed dish after Titian's "Pesara Madonna" (c. 1861). $14\frac{1}{2}$ inches diameter.

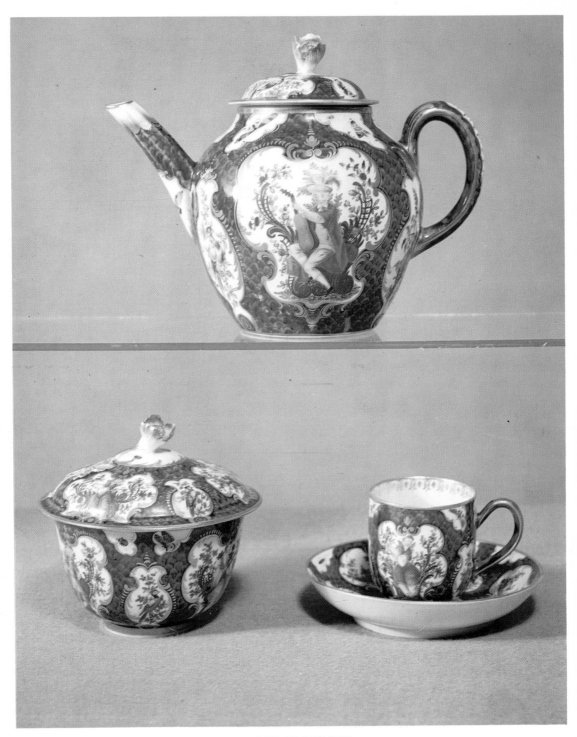

COLOUR PLATE XVI

First, or Dr Wall, period Worcester porcelain teawares with typical scale-blue ground. Reserve panels of Watteau-type figures (a very rare form of decoration), exotic birds and insects. Blue "square mark" (see Plate 650a) (c. 1770–5). Teapot 6¼ inches high.

Victoria & Albert Museum

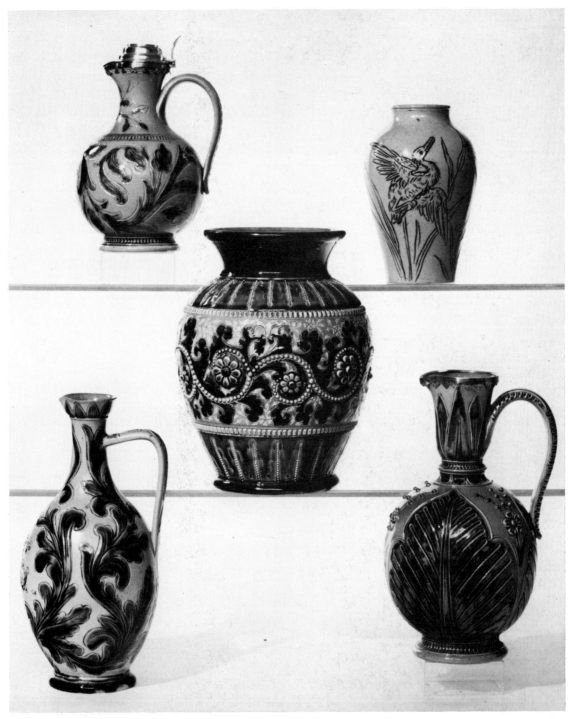

246. *Typical Doulton (Lambeth) stonewares* (top to bottom, left to right): *Jug with simple pattern by Arthur Barlow (initial mark ABB) (c. 1873). Vase with early, simple incised pattern by Hannah B. Barlow (see detail of monogram and mark) (dated 1873). Vase with incised pattern by George Tinworth, monogram mark (1884). 8¾ inches high. Jug decorated by Arthur Barlow in 1879. Jug by Arthur Barlow, silver rim "hall" marked in 1872. All with impressed mark no. 1340 and artist's initials.*

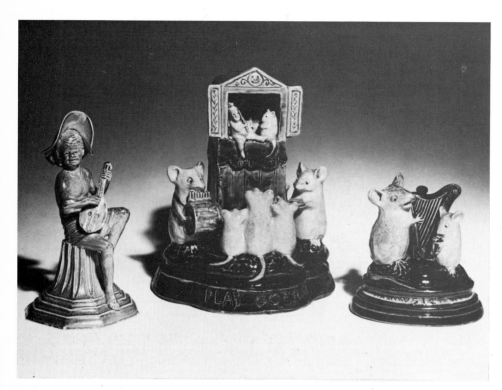

247. *Doulton (Lambeth) stonewares modelled b[y] George Tinworth and signe[d] with his incised initial mono[-]gram (c. 1885–1900). Punc[h] and Judy group 5¾ inche[s] high.*

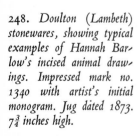

248. *Doulton (Lambeth) stonewares, showing typical examples of Hannah Barlow's incised animal drawings. Impressed mark no. 1340 with artist's initial monogram. Jug dated 1873. 7¾ inches high.*

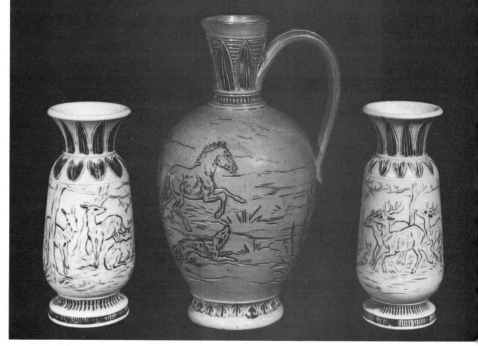

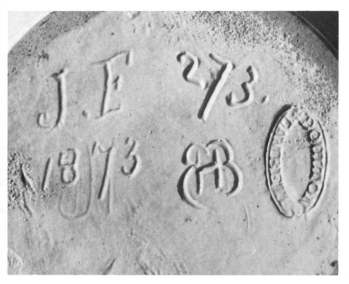

249. *Detail from base of Doulton stoneware jug (Plate 248, centre), showing oval factory mark (right), incised monogram of artist—Hannah B. Barlow—and date of manufacture—1873. Also with other decorator's initials.*

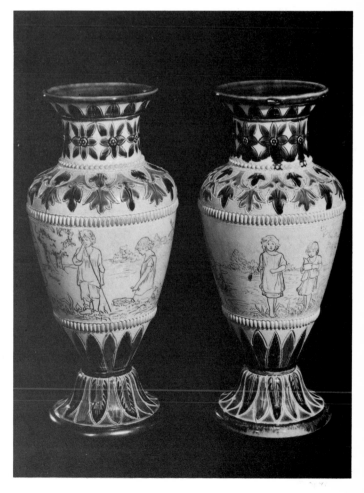

250. *(Right) Doulton (Lambeth) stoneware vases with incised figure subjects by Mary Mitchell. Impressed mark no. 1340, dated 1879. 10¼ inches high.*

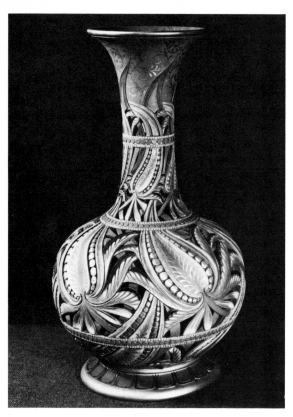

251. (Left) *Doulton Lambeth silicon (impressed marked) vase, the carved and painted decoration by Miss Edith D. Lupton. Signed with initials (see companion mark book) and dated 1888. The word silicon in the mark relates to the type of earthenware body. 13⅛ inches high.*

Victoria & Albert Museum

252. *Doulton (Lambeth) earthenware vase painted by J. H. McLennan. Impressed mark no. 1343 with "England" (c. 1891–1900). 16 inches high.*

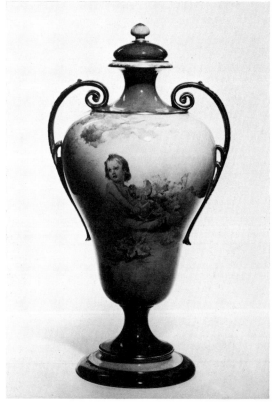

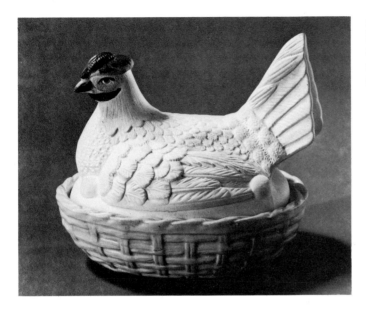

253. *Dudson (impressed marked) earthenware hen on nest. Similar "nest eggs" were made by many Staffordshire potters from c. 1850, but marked examples are very rare (c. 1860). 6 inches high.*

Godden of Worthing

254. (Below) *James Dudson's jasper wares in the Wedgwood style, reproduced from an 1886 advertisement. These wares are sometimes impressed marked "Dudson".*

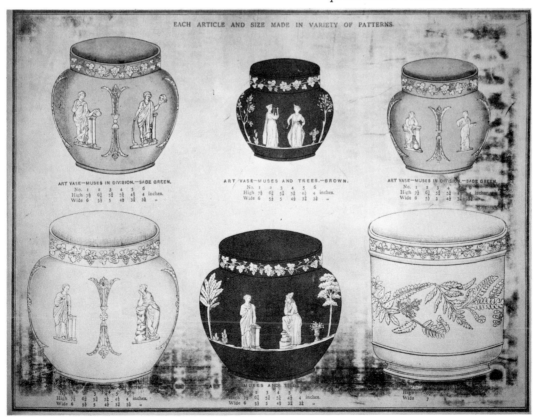

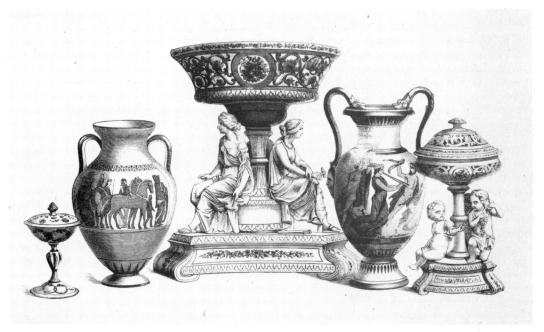

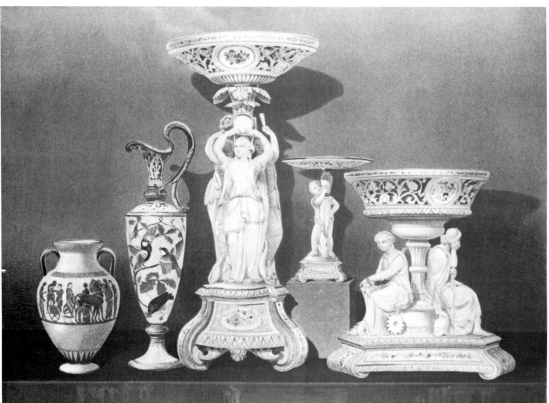

255. a. b. *Sir James Duke & Nephews (Hill Pottery, Burslem, Staffordshire Potteries) porcelains (reproduced from contemporary engravings) shown at the 1862 Exhibition. As most wares from this firm are unmarked and often pass as the products of better-known firms, these illustrations are therefore important documents.*

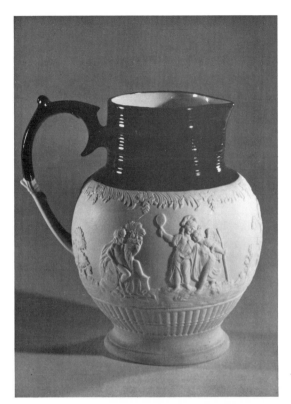

256. *Castleford stoneware jug, impressed mark D D & Co/ Castleford/Pottery* (c. 1800). *7 inches high.*

Godden of Worthing

257. *Castleford moulded teapot with impressed mark "DD& Co. Castleford"* (c. 1800–20). *4¾ inches high.*

Victoria & Albert Museum

Moulded teapots of this type with painted blue enamel lines, and often with hinged or sliding covers are traditionally attributed to the Castleford Works, but very few are marked and several other firms made pots and other wares of this type (see page xxiii). Apart from these white wares the Castleford Pottery made good creamwares and black basalt wares of Wedgwood type.

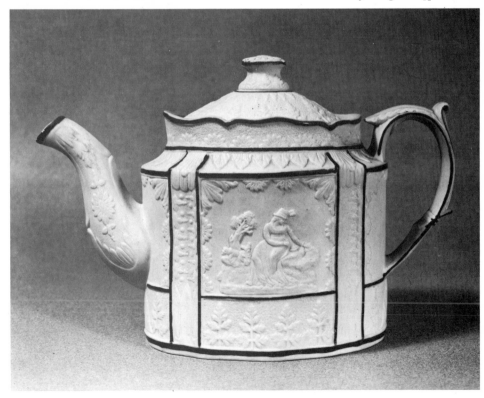

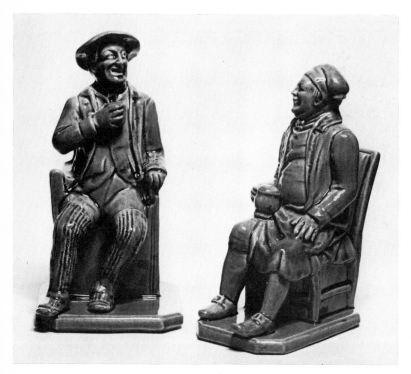

258. *"Dunmore" (impressed mark) earthenware figures. Marked specimens of Peter Gardner's Dunmore Pottery made at Airth, Scotland, are rare (c. 1860). 8 inches high.*

Godden of Worthing

259. *Dunmore Pottery with circular mark—"Peter Gardner. Dunmore Pottery". This Scottish pottery was established in 1860, late nineteenth century. Covered box 11¾ inches high.*

Glasgow Art Gallery & Museum

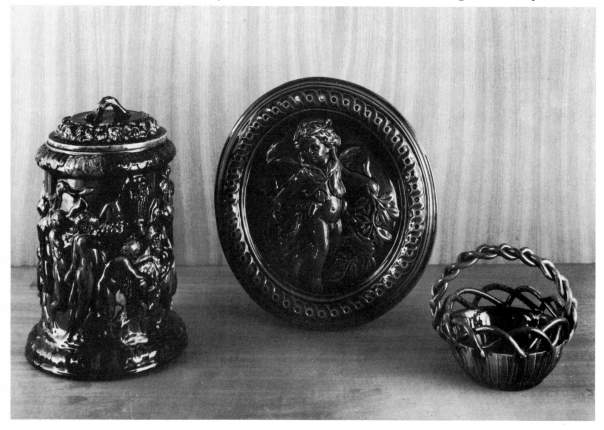

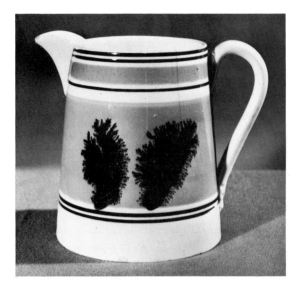

260. Edge Malkin & Co (impressed marked) earthenware jug with typical "Mocha" decoration (see page xvii) (c. 1871–90). 5⅞ inches high.

City Art Gallery & Museum, Stoke-on-Trent

J. AND T. EDWARDS, BURSLEM c. 1839–41

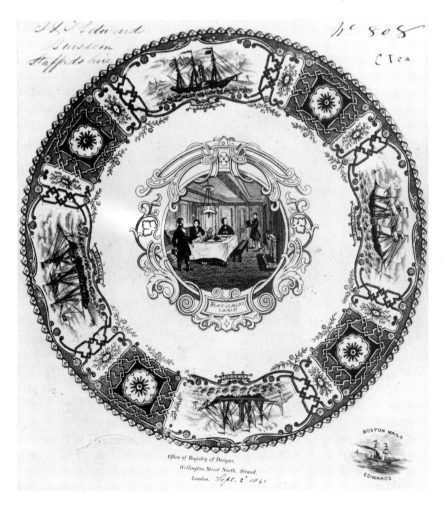

261. J. & T. Edwards "Boston Mails" print. A pattern registered in September 1841 and used on dinner wares. This is a pull from the original copper plate, the "Edwards" mark can be seen in the right bottom corner.

Patent Office Design Registry

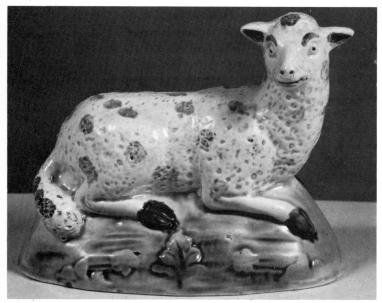

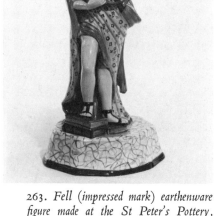

262. *Fell (impressed mark) earthenware lamb with semi-translucent coloured glazes. Thomas Fell established the St Peter's Pottery at Newcastle upon Tyne in 1817, but this example would appear to be of an earlier date.* 4⅜ *inches high.*

Victoria & Albert Museum

263. *Fell (impressed mark) earthenware figure made at the St Peter's Pottery, Newcastle upon Tyne (c. 1817–20). Marked examples are very rare.*

Godden of Worthing

N.B.—*Some early-looking marked "Fell" figures and groups with translucent coloured glazes would seem to be of twentieth-century date.*

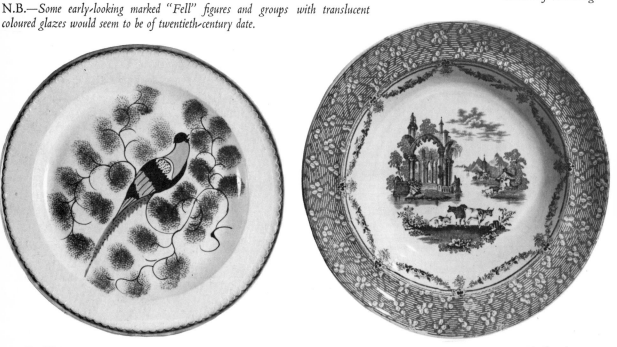

264. *"Fell" (impressed mark) earthenware plate of a very attractive naïve style of decoration, with sponged foliage (c. 1817–25). Other potters made similar patterns; most specimens are not marked.*

Victoria & Albert Museum

265. *Thomas Fell & Co's blue-printed earthenware plate, bearing impressed mark "T Fell & Co" over an anchor, also printed mark with initial mark—"T F & Co" (c. 1870–90).*

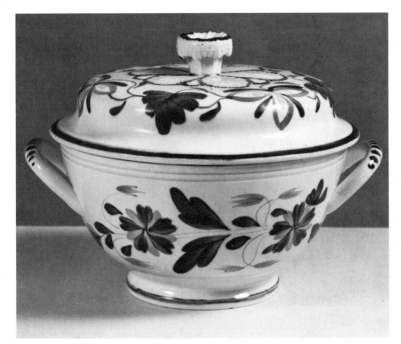

266. *Ferrybridge (impressed marked) earthenware covered sugar bowl, painted in an attractive free style. Marked examples from this Yorkshire pottery are rare (c. 1804–10). 4¼ inches high.*

Victoria & Albert Museum

WILLIAM FIFIELD, BRISTOL DECORATOR c. 1810+

267. *Bristol earthenwares decorated by William Fifield. Puzzle jug, 7 inches high. Miniature barrel dated 1835. Many other Bristol barrels are recorded and are often dated. Circular plaque, signed on reverse with initials and dated 1830 (see detail). 4 inches diameter. Several drawings, landscapes, figure subjects and flower studies by William Fifield and his son are preserved in the Victoria & Albert Museum.*

Bristol City Art Gallery

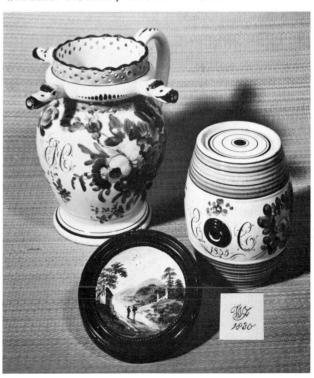

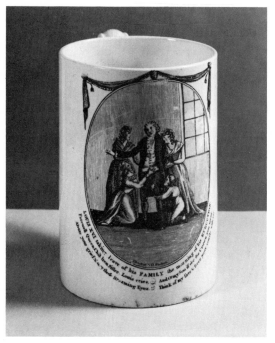

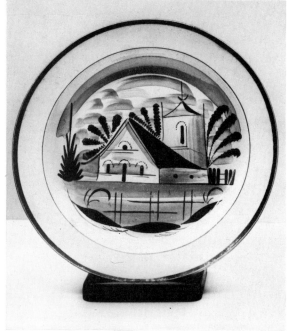

268. *Staffordshire creamware mug, decorated with printed pattern "Louis XVI taking leave of his family", engraved by Fletcher & Co of Shelton. Signature mark at bottom of print (c. 1786–1810). 4⅝ inches high.*

Victoria & Albert Museum

269. *Newcastle earthenware plate, decorated with pink lustre formal scene (see page xxiv). Impressed mark, Ford & Patterson (c. 1820–30?). 8½ inches diameter.*

Laing Art Gallery, Newcastle upon Tyne

T. FORESTER AND SONS

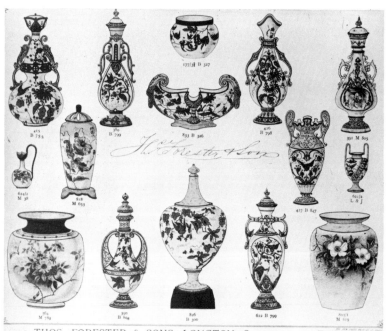

270. *Thos. Forester & Sons' advertisement of 1890, showing typical vase forms and patterns of the period. The marks will include the initials "T F & S".*

THOS FORESTER & SONS. LONGTON, STAFFORDSHIRE, ENGLAND.

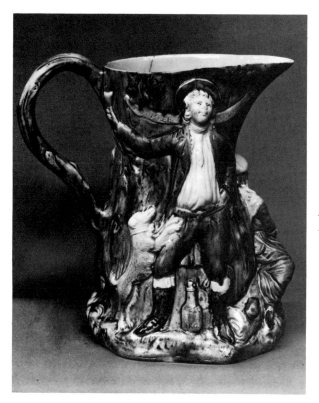

271. *"Fair Hebe" moulded earthenware jug with initials R G on bottle. These initials are attributed to Robert Gardner of Fenton. This form of jug was modelled by J. Voyez in 1788. For reverse side, see Plate 18 (c. 1790) 9½ inches high.*

Victoria & Albert Museum

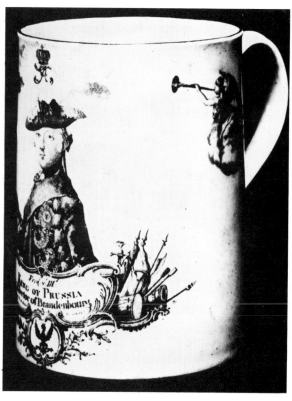

272. *Liverpool porcelain mug, signed (under print of Frederick III of Prussia) "Gilbody maker. Evans Sc" (c. 1755–61). 4¾ inches high. This is believed to be a unique signed specimen by this Liverpool potter, but Dr Watney has suggested that the porcelain is Worcester, printed, not made at Liverpool.*

City of Liverpool Museum

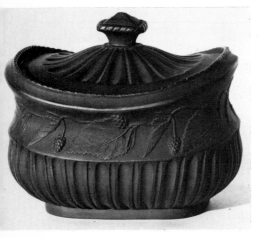

273. J. Glass, Hanley, impressed marked basalt covered sugar of moulded pattern (c. 1822–30). $4\frac{1}{2}$ inches high.

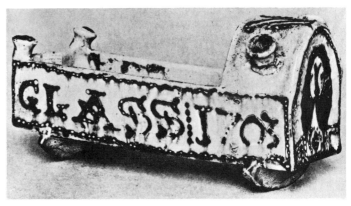

274. Slip decorated (see page xii) earthenware model of a cradle by Joseph Glass of Hanley (dated 1703). 10 inches long.

Fitzwilliam Museum, Cambridge

THE GODWINS

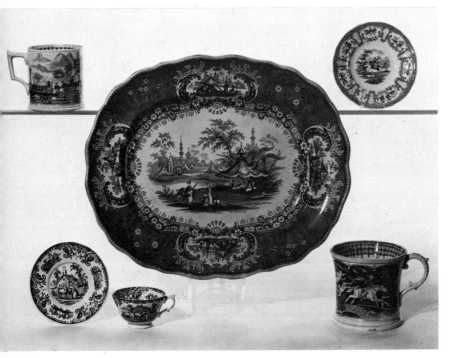

275. Printed earthenwares by the Godwins (top left to bottom right): Railway mug by J. & R. Godwin of Cobridge (c. 1845–55). Small plate by Benjamin Godwin of Cobridge (c. 1834–41). Platter "Medina" pattern by Thomas Godwin of Burslem (c. 1834–40) (mark no. 1731, formerly attributed to Thomas Green). Cup and saucer by J. & R. Godwin (c. 1845–55). Mug "Tam-o-Shanter" by Thomas Godwin (c. 1840–54). All with printed initial marks, except last item which has name in full.

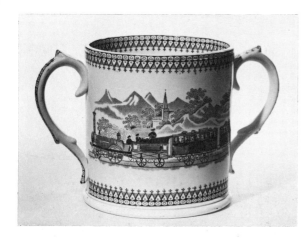

276. *John & Richard Godwin (printed initial mark) of Cobridge, earthenware mug decorated with coloured over railway print (c. 1845–55). 6¼ inches high.*

Godden of Worthing

Several potters produced wares bearing railway prints in the 1830's, 1840's and 1850's. Many bear the makers' names or initials.

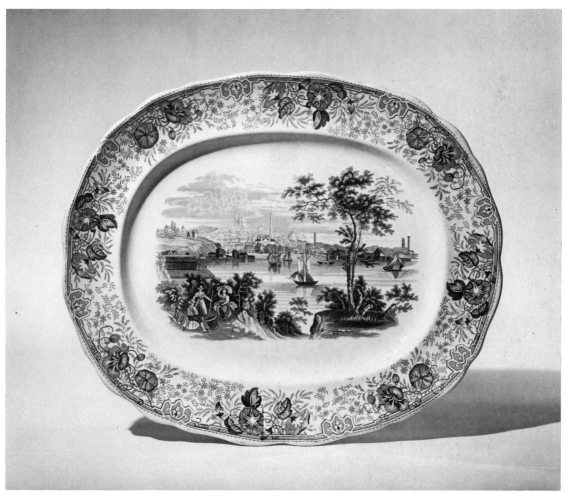

277. *"T Godwin, wharf" (printed mark) earthenware platter made for the American market. Brown transfer print of Baltimore (c. 1830–40). Thomas Godwin potted at Burslem from 1834 to 1854; the word "wharf" relates to his address. Printing in red, brown and green was introduced during the late 1820's (see* British Pottery and Porcelain, *1780–1850).*

Ellouise Baker Larsen Collection, Smithsonian Institution, U.S.A.

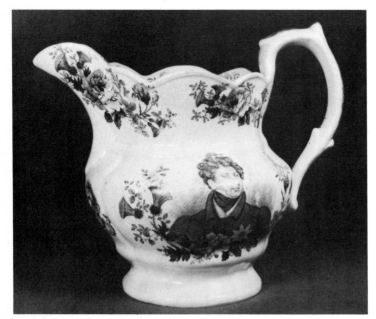

278. Goodwin, Bridgwood & Harris pottery jug, printed motifs—"To the memory of his late Majesty King George IV . . . departed his life June 26th 1830". Printed lion and crown crest mark (below) with initials G.B.H. (c. 1830–1). 7 inches high.

Willett Collection, Brighton Museum

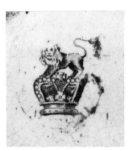

278. a. Crest on jugs above and below.

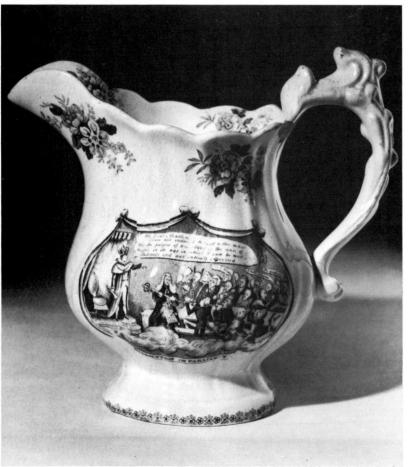

279. Earthenware jug, decorated with printed subjects relating to the Reform Bill of 1832. Printed crown and lion mark, probably used by Goodwins & Harris (of the Crown Works, Lane End, c. 1831–8) for the same basic mark was used by the slightly earlier partnership of Goodwin, Bridgwood & Harris, with their initials G.B.H. (see Plate 278).

Thomas Grainger, a former Chamberlain ceramic artist, established his own factory at Worcester in 1801. With a partner named Wood, he traded as Grainger & Wood, or Grainger, Wood & Co from 1801 to 1812. For the first few years this firm decorated porcelains purchased in the white. Marked examples of this are rare, and similar in general style to Chamberlain Worcester porcelains (see Plate 280).

The factory was rebuilt in 1812 and, having taken a new partner, Thomas Grainger traded as Grainger, Lee & Co; several different marks include this title. Lee retired about 1837 and for two years prior to his death in 1839 Thomas Grainger traded as Grainger & Co.

George Grainger succeeded his father in 1839 and the firm's style and marks were amended to G. Grainger & Co. In 1848 a refined opaque earthenware body was successfully introduced under the name "Semi-Porcelain"; this description, or the initials "S.P.", occurs on several marks of the period. The Grainger porcelains were generally very fine but, as they are usually unmarked, specimens are mistaken for those of better known manufacturers.

During the Victorian era the Grainger firm produced good Parian china, and a class of decorative pierced openwork designs in vases, teawares, and so forth. Good *pâte-sur-pâte* floral designs were also made from about 1880. In 1889 the Royal Worcester Company took over the Grainger concern, but the factory and the use of the Grainger shield mark (no. 1771) was continued until 1902.

Further details, with some designs of animals and basket forms, will be found in G. Godden's *British Pottery and Porcelain, 1780–1850*.

Printed or impressed mark (c. 1870–89). Later version given below.

Printed mark (c. 1889–1902). "England" added below from 1891. The shield marks were not used before 1870, or from 1889 with the words "Royal China Works". The date 1823, given in several books, is an error.
Year letters occur under this mark, from 1891, see below:

A	1891	D	1894	G	1897	J	1900
B	1892	E	1895	H	1898	K	1901
C	1893	F	1896	I	1899	L	1902

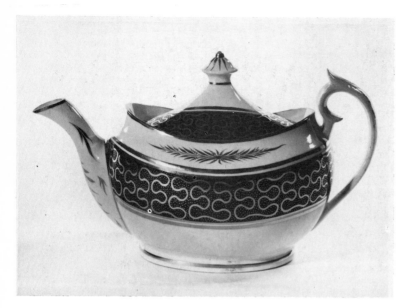

280. *"Grainger, Wood, Worcester War-ranted" (painted mark) porcelain teapot. Pattern no. 321, wide band of underglaze blue with gilt enrichments (c. 1801–12). 6¼ inches high.*
Marked porcelains of this period are ex-tremely rare and unmarked examples often pass as Chamberlains Worcester.

GRAINGER, LEE AND CO, WORCESTER

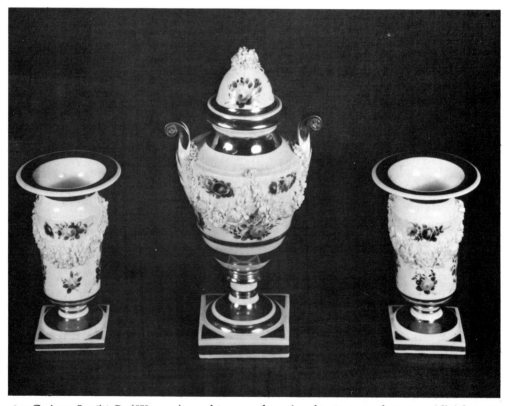

281. *Grainger, Lee & Co (Worcester) porcelain vases of superb quality. Festoons of minute modelled flowers in unglazed china, with gilding and flower painting to rival any factory of the period. Written marks (c. 1812–25). Centre vase 7¼ inches high.*

J. & E. Vandekar, London

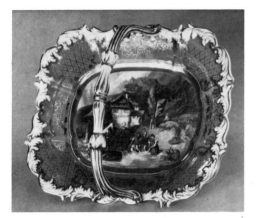

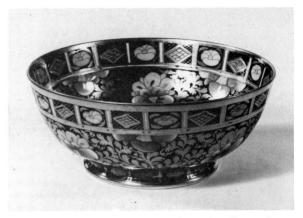

282. "Grainger Lee & Co, Royal China Works, Worcester" (painted mark) porcelain basket, finely painted with a Swiss view. Richly gilt (c. 1825–30). 8 × 7¼ inches.

W. Ramsay Strachan Collection

Other basket forms, from a factory pattern book, are reproduced in British Pottery and Porcelain, 1780–1850.

283. Large Grainger, Lee & Co (painted mark) porcelain punch bowl, decorated with rich "Japan" pattern in blue, red and gold (c. 1812–20). 11½ inches diameter.

Godden of Worthing

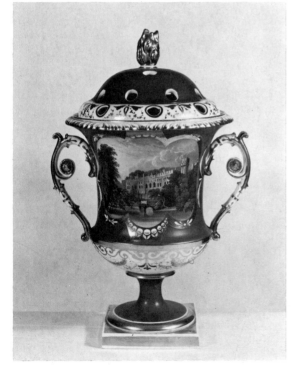

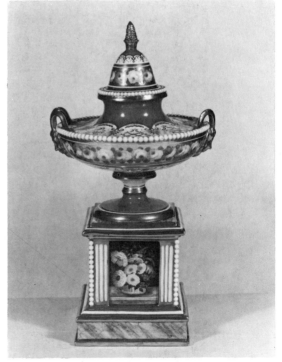

284. "Grainger, Lee & Co" (painted mark) vase with saxon blue ground, richly gilt. Painted panel of Warwick Castle (c. 1815–25). 13 inches high.

Messrs Christie, Manson & Woods Ltd

285. Grainger, Lee & Co (painted mark) vase and cover. Pink ground with flower painting of the finest quality (c. 1815–25). 11½ inches high.

Messrs Christie, Manson & Woods Ltd

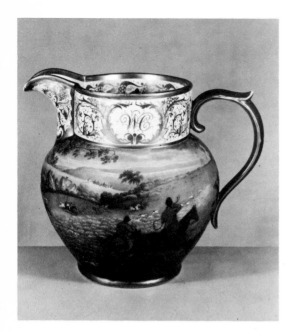

286. Fine quality jug, presented to William Cobbett by the citizens of Coventry. Painted mark "Grainger, Lee & Co. Worcester" (c. 1820).

Messrs Christie, Manson & Woods Ltd

287. Grainger, Lee & Co, Worcester. Porcelain vase with apple-green ground, painted panel of Rochester, Kent. Painted mark (no. 1772). 7 inches high (c. 1812-25). Note the shape, other examples are often unmarked.

Lucile Pillow Collection,
Beaverbrook Art Gallery, Fredericton, Canada

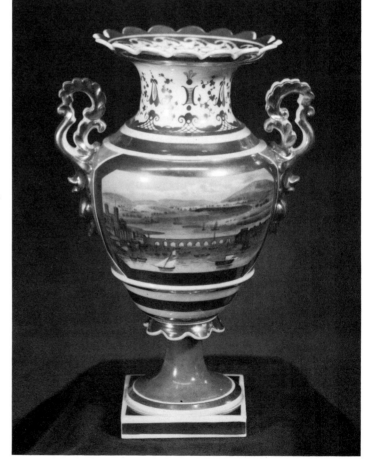

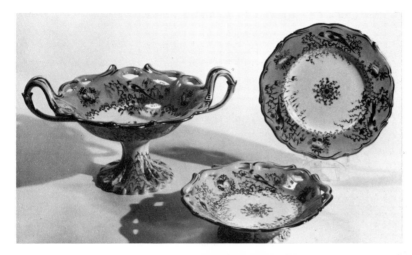

288. *Grainger Worcester dessert service forms of the 1840–50 period. Unmarked (except for retailer's mark), but the pattern, no. 1699x, corresponds with that in the factory pattern book. Centrepiece 8¼ inches high.*

Godden of Worthing

289. *Grainger Worcester dessert service of the 1845–55 period, showing unusual moulded leaf border and floral handles. This pattern occurs in the Grainger pattern book. Unmarked as is most Grainger porcelain of this period.*

Godden of Worthing

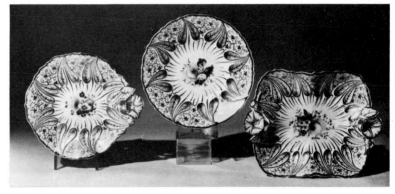

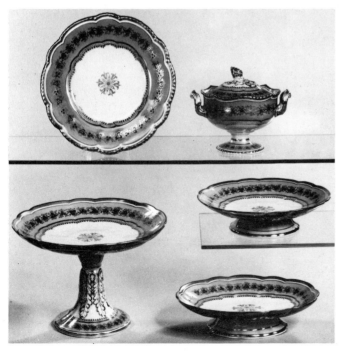

290. *Grainger Worcester part dessert set in "chemical porcelain". Printed mark no. 1766 (c. 1850–60). Pattern no. 574. Plate 9½ inches diameter.*

Godden of Worthing

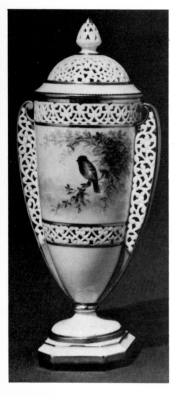

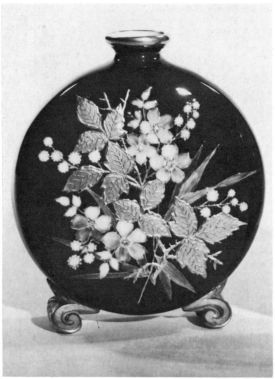

291. (Far left) Grainger Worcester porcelain vase with pierced work. Printed shield mark (no. 1771) (c. 1890). 11$\frac{1}{4}$ inches high.

Godden of Worthing

292. G. Grainger pâte-sur-pâte vase (see page xxvi). Impressed shield mark (c. 1880). 5$\frac{3}{4}$ inches high.

Godden of Worthing

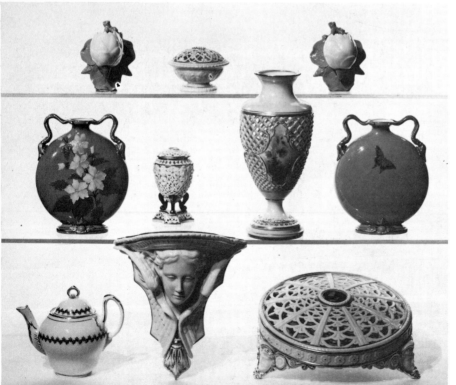

293. A selection of porcelains by George Grainger of Worcester (c. 1865–95). Printed or impressed shield marks (nos. 1770 and 1771). The openwork pieces are typical, as is the floral pattern pâte-sur-pâte vase, middle row (left).

Godden of Worthing

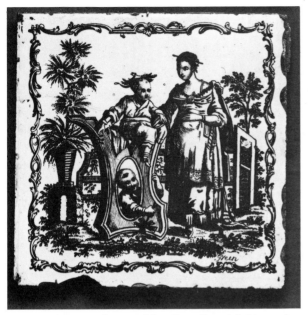

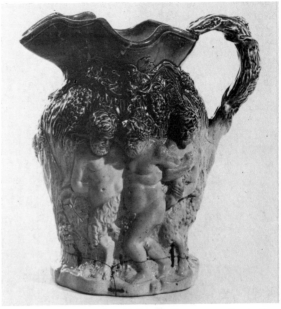

294. *Earthenware tile printed by Guy Green of Liverpool (c. 1770-80). Printed mark "Green". Earlier examples are signed "Sadler" (see Plate 505).*

Victoria & Albert Museum

295. *Stephen Green (moulded marked) stoneware jug made at the Imperial Pottery, Lambeth, London (c. 1830-40). 8½ inches high. Few examples of Green's stonewares are marked. The pottery was sold in 1858. Other potters made this form.*

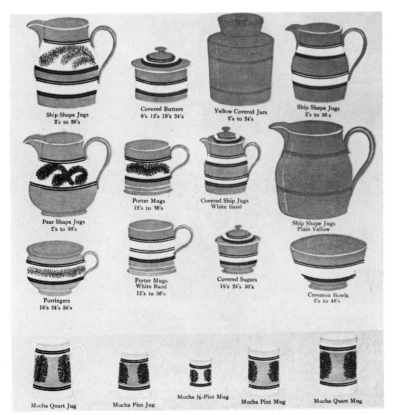

Ship Shape Jugs
2's to 36's

Covered Butters
9's 12's 18's 24's

Yellow Covered Jars
2's to 24's

Ship Shape Jugs
2's to 36's

Pear Shape Jugs
2's to 36's

Porter Mugs
12's to 36's

Covered Ship Jugs
White Band

Ship Shape Jugs
Plain Yellow

Porringers
18's 24's 30's

Porter Mugs
White Band
12's to 36's

Covered Sugars
18's 24's 36's

Common Bowls
2's to 48's

Mocha Quart Jug

Mocha Pint Jug

Mocha ½-Pint Mug

Mocha Pint Mug

Mocha Quart Mug

296. *T. G. Green & Co's Church Gresley (Derbyshire) pottery. Some examples with the tree-like "Mocha" decoration much favoured for beer tankards, etc. (see page xvii). Such utilitarian wares seldom bear a factory mark. The company was founded in 1864 and has continued for over one hundred years.*

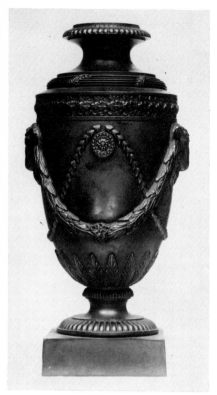

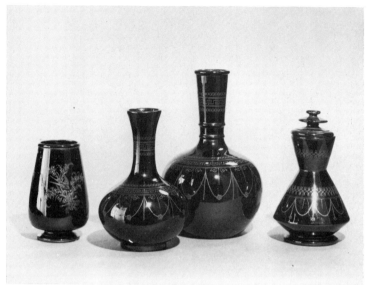

297. *Basalt vase bearing unique impressed mark "S Greenwood". This is a fine quality piece, but the potter is unrecorded (c. 1780–90). 9⅝ inches high.*

British Museum

298. *Black glazed earthenwares, decorated by Guest Brothers' acid engraved process (c. 1877–80). Circular mark—"Guest Brothers. Patent 1877". Centre vase 8½ inches high.*

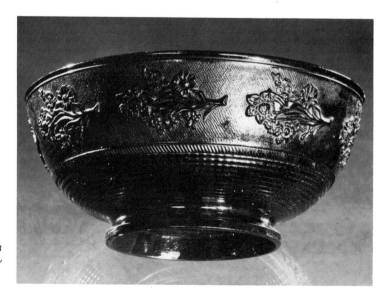

299. *"Hackwood" (impressed mark) bowl in a type of glazed Egyptian black body popular in the 1835–45 period. 6½ inches diameter.*

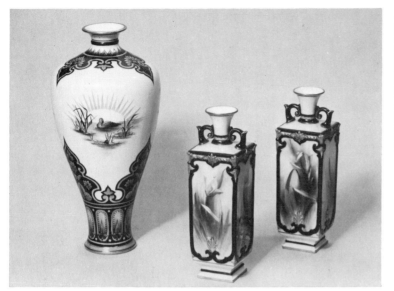

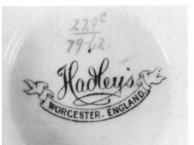

300. a. *Printed mark found on late Hadley Worcester porcelains between August 1902 and July 1905.*

300. *Hadley Worcester porcelain vases, bearing printed name marks (nos. 1871 and 1873, right). For a contemporary account see G. Godden's* Victorian Porcelain. *This Worcester modeller established his own factory in 1896; it was taken over by the Royal Worcester Company in 1905.*

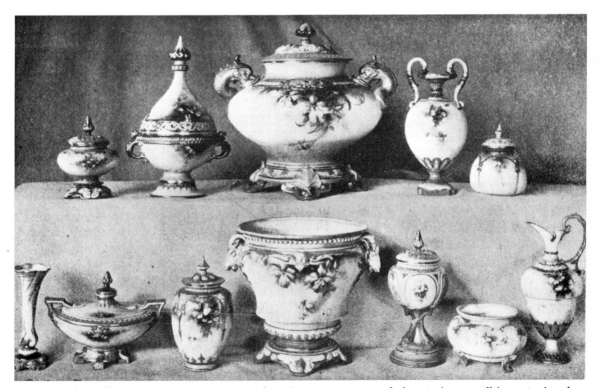

301. *Typical "Hadley Ware" Worcester, reproduced from the Pottery Gazette of 1899. Such ware will bear printed mark no. 1871.*

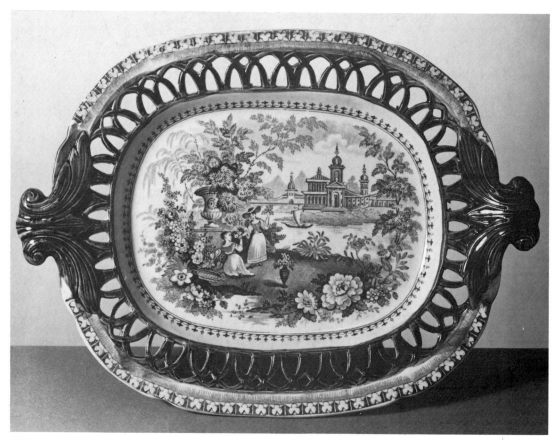

302. "R. Hall" (printed mark) blue printed basket stand, showing the quality and decorative merits of the wares of the lesser potters. Ralph Hall's name occurs in Tunstall directories, etc., from 1822 to 1849. 12 inches long.

Victoria & Albert Museum

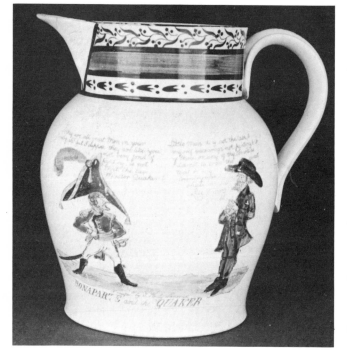

T. HARLEY

303. Bonaparte jug, the printed subject signed "Manufactd by T Harley, Lane End" (c. 1802–8). 6 inches high. Several patterns relating to Napoleonic subjects were produced in the 1800–15 period.

Willett Collection, Brighton Museum

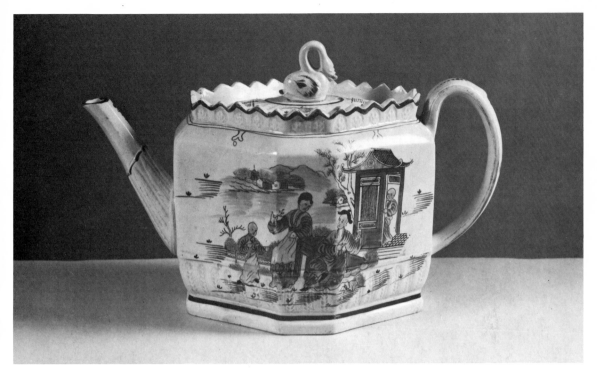

304. *Harley (impressed marked) earthenware teapot decorated with Chinese styled pattern in printed outline, coloured over by hand. Thomas Harley worked at Lane End from c. 1802 to 1808. 6 inches high.*

Victoria & Albert Museum

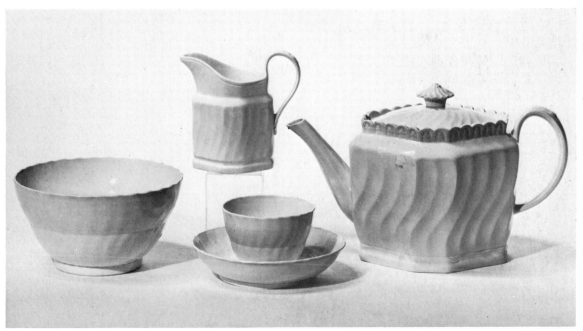

305. *Harley (impressed mark on teapot) teaware shapes of the 1805–15 period. Thomas Harley potted at Lane End from c. 1802 to 1808; marked specimens are rare. Teapot 6¼ inches high.*

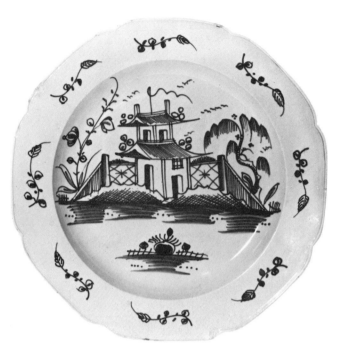

306. *Creamware plate painted with Chinese-type landscape of a type made by several potters. This specimen bears the impressed initials I.H., attributed to J. Heath of Hanley (c. 1770–90). 9½ inches diameter.*

307. *Heath & Son (impressed marked) teapot of so-called "Castleford" type (see page xxiii). Heath & Son of Burslem are listed in a Staffordshire directory of c. 1797. 5½ inches high.*
City Museum & Art Gallery, Stoke-on-Trent

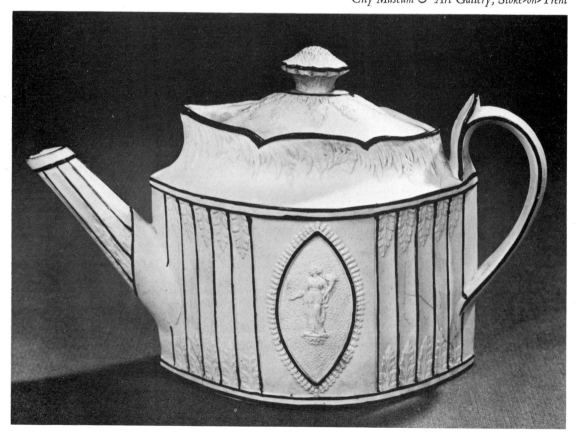

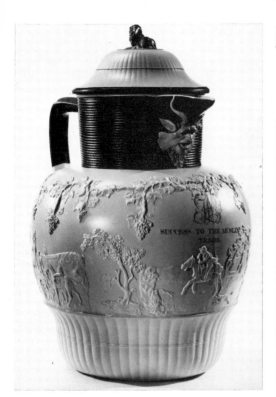

308. *A superb "Herculaneum" presentation jug in stoneware-type body. Impressed name mark (c. 1800). 20 inches high.*

Godden of Worthing

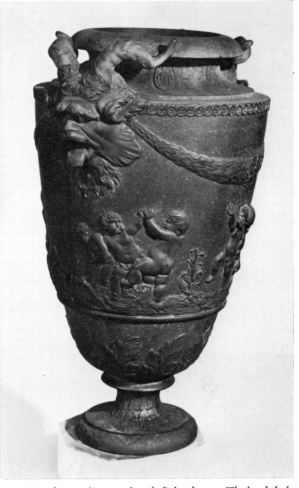

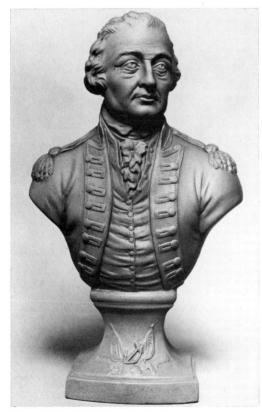

309. *Herculaneum (impressed marked) basalt vase. The basalt body of this Liverpool vase is of a very gritty texture (c. 1810). $11\frac{5}{8}$ inches high.*

Liverpool Museum

310. *A fine quality, impressed marked "Herculaneum" stoneware bust of Admiral Lord Duncan (died 1804) (c. 1800). $8\frac{3}{4}$ inches high.*

Victoria & Albert Museum

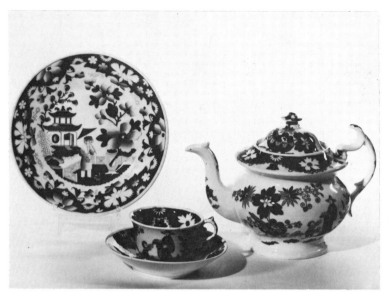

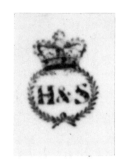

311. *Porcelain teawares by Hilditch & Son of Lane End. The main part of the design is in underglaze blue. Initial mark H & S with a crown over (mark no. 2027, above) (c. 1822–30). Teapot 6½ inches high.*

HILL POTTERY CO

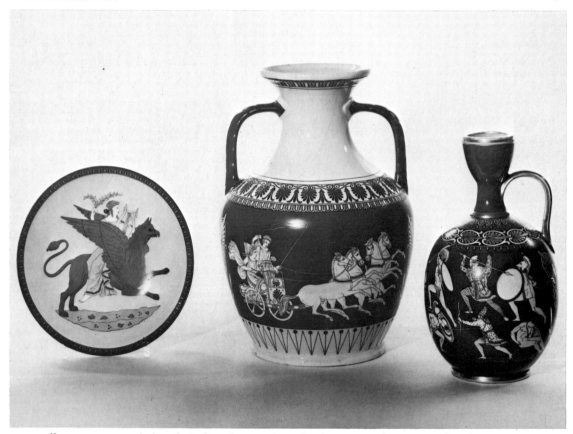

312. *Hill Pottery Company's (Burslem) classical patterned porcelain bearing printed J.S.H. initial marks. The ewer is copied from a design published in February 1856. Hill Pottery Co (c. 1861–7). Vase 10 inches high.*

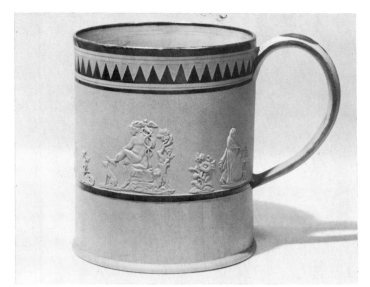

313. *"S Hollins" impressed marked buff bodied stoneware mug of fine quality. The dark parts in this illustration are in a bright silver colour which Hollins used with restraint (c. 1800–10). 5½ inches high.*

Godden of Worthing

314. *S. Hollins (impressed marked) buff stoneware moulded teapot of fine quality, with typical enamel enrichments (c. 1790– 1800).*

Godden of Worthing

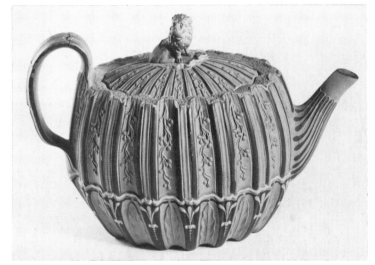

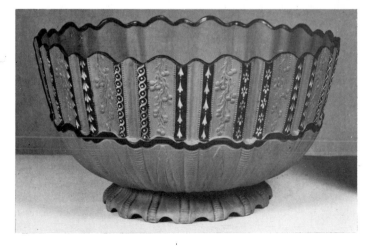

315. *S. Hollins (impressed marked) moulded buff stoneware bowl, decorated with slight enamelled pattern (c. 1790–1800). 5 inches high.*

Victoria & Albert Museum

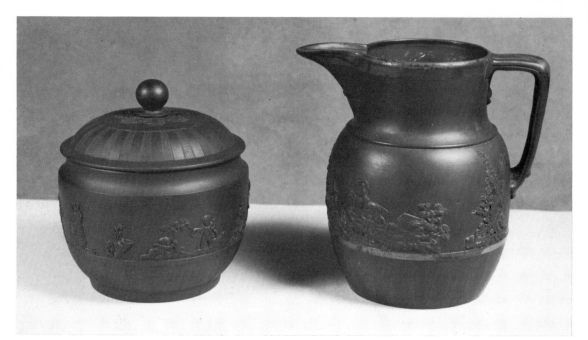

316. *S. Hollins (impressed marked) basalt-type body of a dark brown colour. Note the silvered rim of the jug; this is typical of Hollins, but has often worn away with use (c. 1790–1800). Sugar 4½ inches high.*

Victoria & Albert Museum

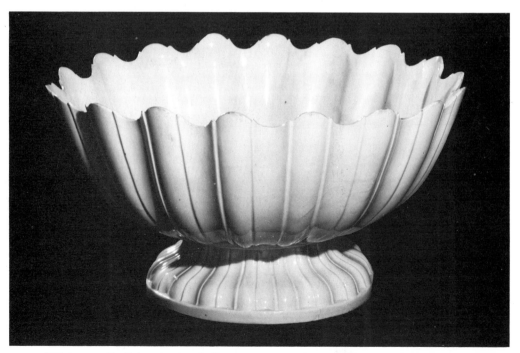

317. *"T & J Hollins" (impressed marked) creamware monteith-type bowl. Bowls with a deeply scalloped edge are called monteiths. Wine glasses were hung by their stems and feet so that the glasses were cooled by water in the bowl (c. 1795–1820). 6 inches high.*

D. M. & P. Manheim

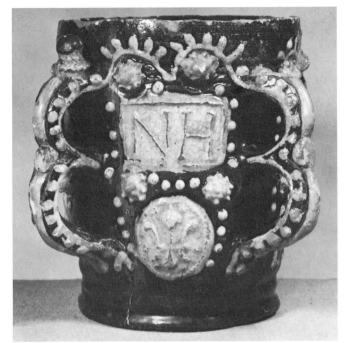

318. *Wrotham slip decorated tyg with the initials NH, attributed to the potter Nicholas Hubble (see page xii) (dated 1654). 6 inches high. For further information on Wrotham pottery, see* The Transactions of the English Ceramic Circle, *vol. 3, part 2.*

Fitzwilliam Museum, Cambridge

319. *Wrotham slip decorated cistern with initials NH and date 1678. These initials are attributed to Nicholas Hubble (see* The Transactions of the English Ceramic Circle, *vol. 3, part 2, and page xii). 13⅜ inches high.*

British Museum

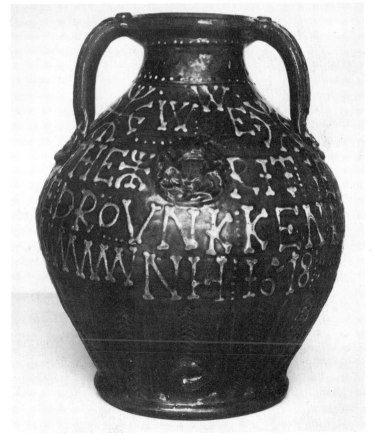

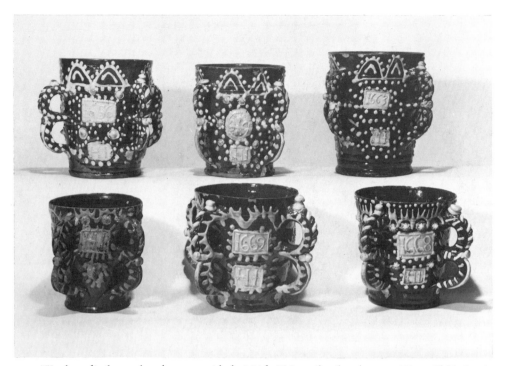

320. *Wrotham slip decorated earthenwares with the initials H.I. attributed to the potter Henry Ifield. See the* Transactions of the English Ceramic Circle, *vol. 3, part 2. Examples dated from (top left) 1656; 1661; 1663; 1668; 1669; 1668. The last example $5\frac{3}{4}$ inches high.*

Fitzwilliam Museum, Cambridge

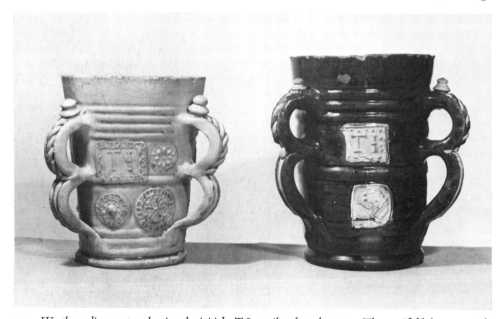

321. *Wrotham slipware tygs bearing the initials T.I. attributed to the potter Thomas Ifield (see page xii). The right-hand tyg is dated 1621, the other 1632. $6\frac{1}{2}$ and $7\frac{1}{4}$ inches high. The name tyg is an old term for multiple-handled beakers of this type.*

Fitzwilliam Museum, Cambridge

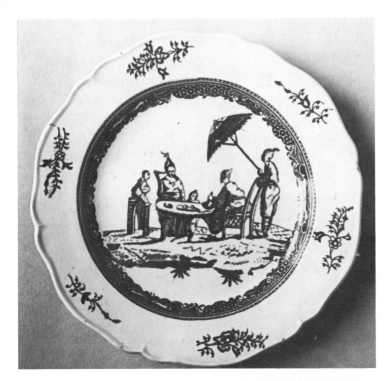

322. "Indeo" (impressed marked) cream-ware plate, decorated with underglaze blue print. Marked examples from the Indeo Pottery, Bovey Tracey, Devonshire, are very rare (c. 1780).

Dr Bernard Watney

323. "Nathaniel Ireson" (signed and dated) delft-type earthenware jug, painted in blue and manganese purple (1748). 14½ inches high.

Fitzwilliam Museum, Cambridge

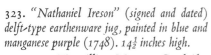

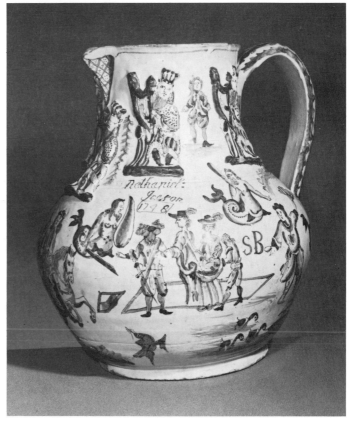

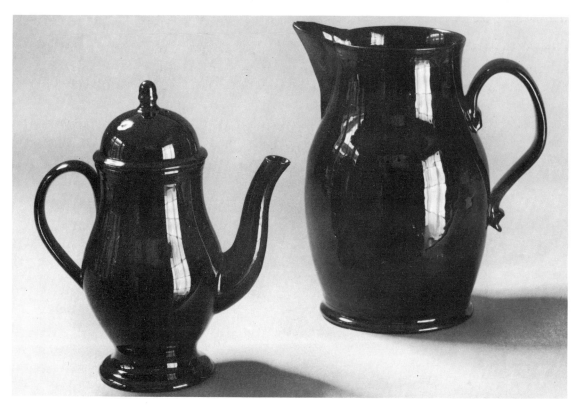

324. *Glossy black glazed red earthenwares of a type traditionally attributed to Jackfield in Shropshire. Such wares were also made in quantity in the Staffordshire Potteries (see page xiv) (c. 1760–80). Coffee pot 9 inches high.*

Godden of Worthing

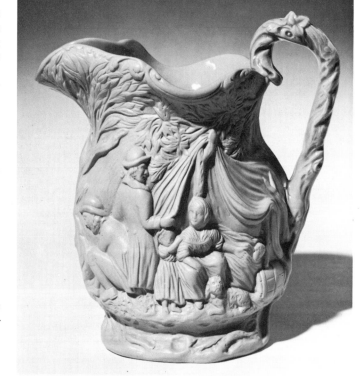

JONES AND WALLEY

325. *The Gipsy jug in stoneware. "Published July 1, 1842 by Jones & Walley" of Cobridge. $6\frac{1}{2}$ inches high. This pattern was produced by other British and American potters in the 1840's.*

George Jones (& Sons)

George Jones was employed by Messrs Mintons until he established his own Trent Pottery in Stoke in 1861. Very fine, colourful "Majolica"-type earthenwares were made in many fancy designs. Porcelain was introduced in 1872. *Pâte-sur-pâte* decorated earthenwares (see Plate 328) was also made by this enterprising firm during the period 1876–86; see *Victorian Porcelain* (1961).

Most specimens are marked with a monogram of the initials G.J., often above a crescent-shaped device. From the latter part of 1873 "& Sons" occurs in the crescent; "England" was added after 1891.

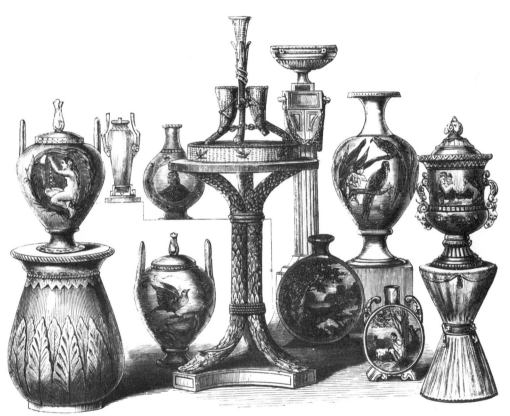

Engraving of George Jones exhibits at the 1873 Vienna Exhibition, reproduced from the Art Journal.

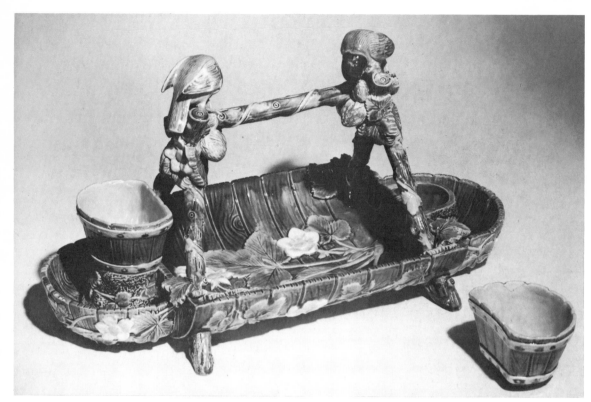

326. *George Jones "Majolica" glazed earthenware strawberry dish, of a design registered in 1875. Impressed G.J. monogram mark (no. 2217). This firm produced many decorated dishes, baskets, etc., in colourful "Majolica" (see page xxv). 14½ inches long.*

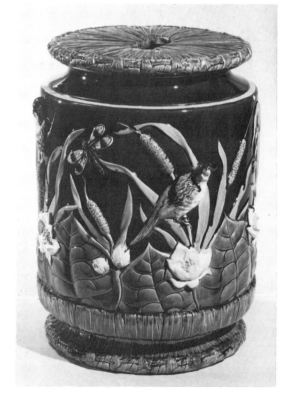

327. *Garden seat in "Majolica" glazed earthenware. Pattern registered by George Jones & Sons of Stoke in May 1874. 19 inches high.*

Godden of Worthing

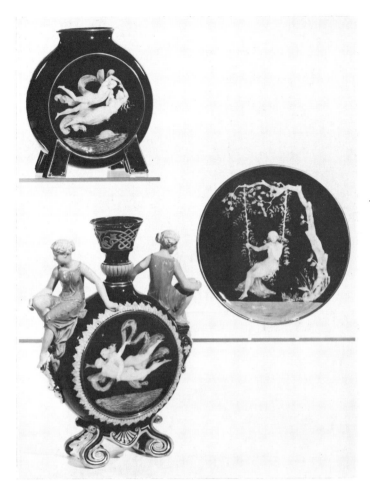

328. *George Jones's pâte-sur-pâte wares (see page xxvi) modelled by F. Schenck (c. 1880–90). Impressed monogram and crescent mark (no. 2218). Large vase 14¼ inches high, model no. 75.*

Godden of Worthing

KEELING AND TOFT, HANLEY 1805–26

329. *Keeling & Toft (impressed marked) basalt wares with figure motifs in relief. Jug 5 inches high (c. 1805–15).*
City Museum & Art Gallery, Stoke-on-Trent

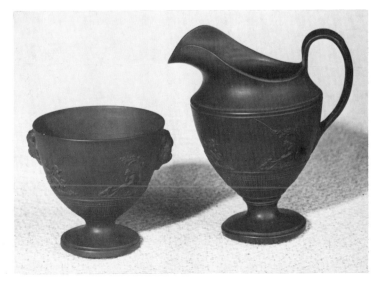

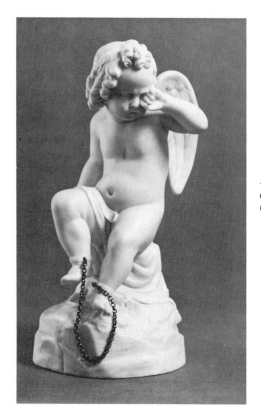

330. "S Keys & Mountford" impressed marked Parian figure. John Mountford is credited with introducing the popular Parian body while employed by Copeland & Garrett. The Stoke partnership of Keys & Mountford dates from 1850 to 1860. $8\frac{3}{4}$ inches high.

J. KISHERE, LONDON c. 1800–43

331. Kishere Pottery, Mortlake (impressed marks nos. 2293A and 2294). Stoneware jug and jar, of a type made at several potteries. Marked specimens are rare (c. 1820–30). Jug 8 inches high.

Victoria & Albert Museum

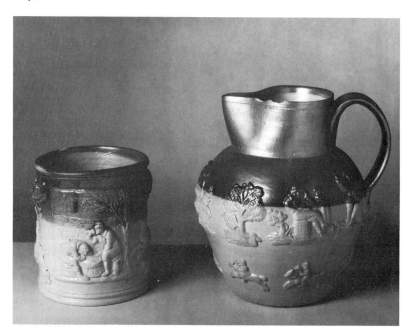

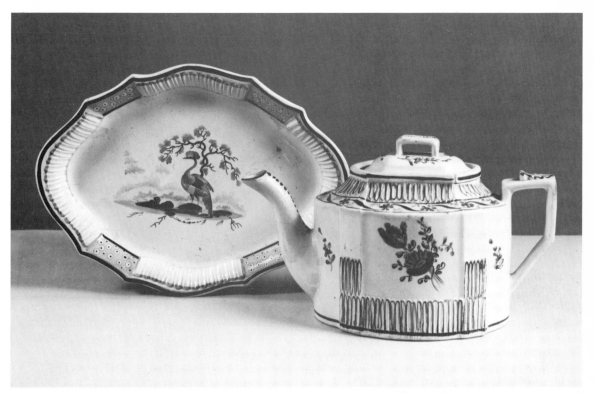

332. *Lakin & Poole (impressed marked) creamware teapot, with sliding cover, and a teapot stand of a different pattern. This Burslem partnership relates to the period* c. 1791-5. *Teapot 4 inches high.*

Victoria & Albert Museum

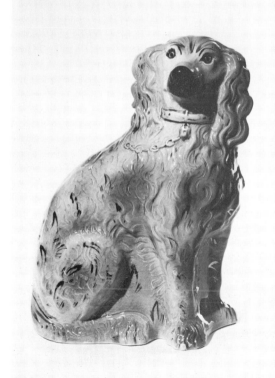

333. *Lancaster & Sons' Staffordshire dog (printed mark) of a type which were seldom marked. Early twentieth century, note glass eyes at this period.* 12¾ *inches high.*

Leeds Pottery

The Leeds Pottery was established in the late 1750's. Although its name is mainly associated with cream-coloured earthenwares, often with pierced openwork borders (Plate 337), the works also made quantities of shiny black earthenware of the so-called "Jackfield" type, glazed and unglazed red earthenware of the Elers type, and white and enamelled salt-glazed stoneware (see pages xiii, xiv). The Leeds creamwares were either undecorated, decorated in underglaze colours, with over-glazed enamels, or printed. Figures, groups, and animals were also made, as were basalts and lustred earthenwares (see Plates 343–5).

In general the early wares are unmarked. From about 1775, the impressed mark "Leeds Pottery" was employed (this has been copied on the many nineteenth- and twentieth-century reproductions). After 1800 the name "Hartley Greens & Co" was added to the "Leeds Pottery" mark; occasionally the firm's mark occurs on its own. The impressed or incised initials "L.P" were also used. The firm became bankrupt in 1820, but the pottery was continued by other potters until 1878.

The Leeds Pottery shapes are well documented as a series of pattern books were issued in 1783, 1785, 1786, 1794, and 1814. Various other drawing and order books have been preserved and are in the Art Library of the Leeds City Art Gallery or in the Victoria & Albert Museum, Print Room; some pages are reproduced in Plate 342.

The reader seeking further information need only consult Donald Towner's *The Leeds Pottery* (1963) for a full review of the history and products of the Leeds factory; the last and most comprehensive pattern book (of 1814) is also reproduced.

Late in the nineteenth and early in the twentieth century typical eighteenth-century Leeds creamwares were produced by James Senior and his son, George, and by John Thomas Morton. These reproductions often bear the original impressed mark "Leeds Pottery", and in general these wares are thicker in potting than the original, the glaze often very thick and much crazed (specimens are reproduced in Plates 346–8).

For a full appreciation of English cream-coloured earthenwares the reader should consult Donald Towner's standard work *Creamware* (1978) and also Peter Walton's *Creamware and other English Pottery at Temple Newsam House* (1976).

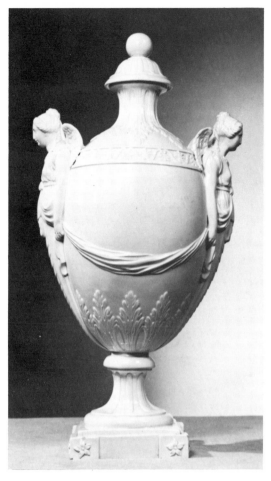

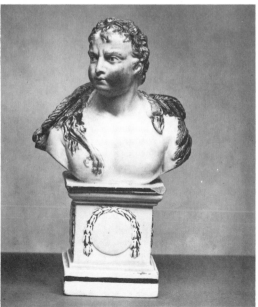

334. *Leeds Pottery creamware vase of classical form,* with rare incised monogram mark of the initials LP for "Leeds Pottery" (c. 1795). 12½ inches high.*
Victoria & Albert Museum

* This is really a candelabrum, metal arms with candle-holders were originally fitted. This form occurs in the Leeds pattern books.

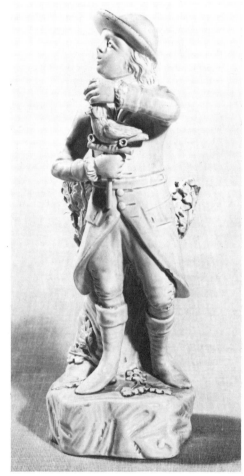

335. *"Leeds Pottery" impressed marked earthenware figure of a falconer (c. 1780–90). 7½ inches high.*
Leeds City Art Gallery and Temple Newsam House

336. *Leeds Pottery bust, emblematic of Air, in coloured and oil gilt creamware. Impressed mark "Leeds Pottery", twice in crossed form (c. 1780). 6½ inches high.*

Schreiber Collection, Victoria & Albert Museum

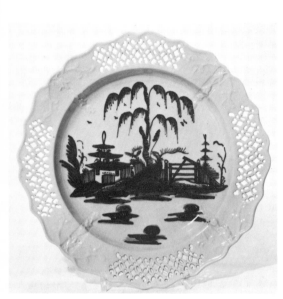

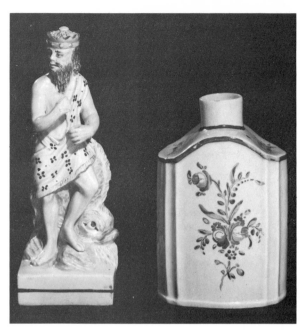

337. *"Leeds Pottery" (impressed marked) creamware plate, with typical pierced border. Chinese styled landscape painted in underglaze blue (c. 1780). 9½ inches diameter.*

338. *"Leeds Pottery" (impressed marked) creamwares. Rare figure of Neptune 7½ inches high. Tea container (cover missing) 5½ inches high. Similar pieces were made by several manufacturers but examples are seldom marked (c. 1790).*

D. M. & P. Manheim

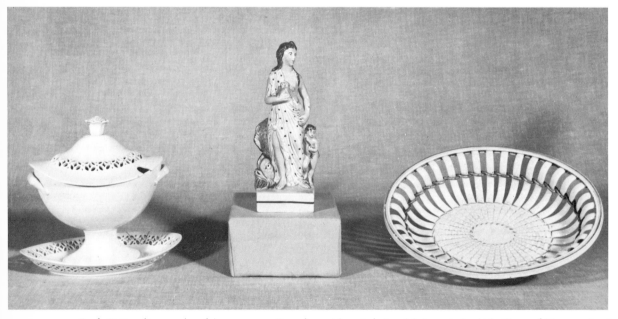

339. *Leeds Pottery (impressed marks) creamwares. Sauce boat with typical pierced design. 7 inches high. Figure of Venus painted in overglaze enamel colours. 7½ inches high. Openwork basket, similar baskets were made at several potteries but are seldom marked. 11 inches long (c. 1790/1800).*

Temple Newsam House, Leeds

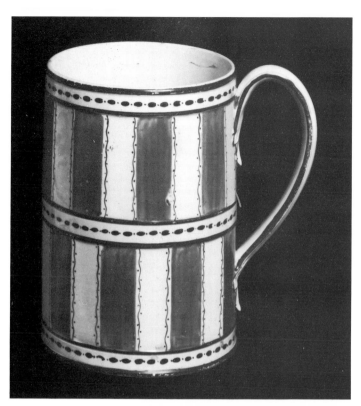

340. *A creamware tankard with rare incised mark "Leeds" (c. 1790). 6 inches high.*

D. M. & P. Manheim

341. *"Leeds Pottery" (impressed marked) earthenware teapot, decorated with green slip which has been turned away to give a geometrical pattern. The "engine turning" process was much used in the Potteries from c. 1770. 6½ inches high.*

Victoria & Albert Museum

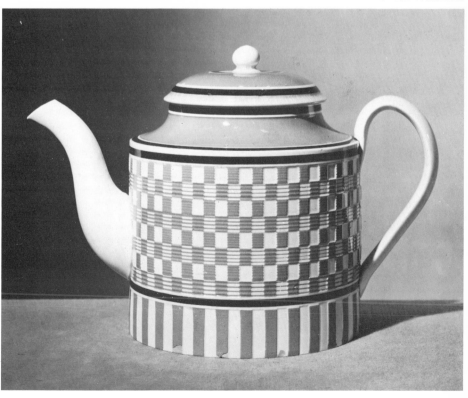

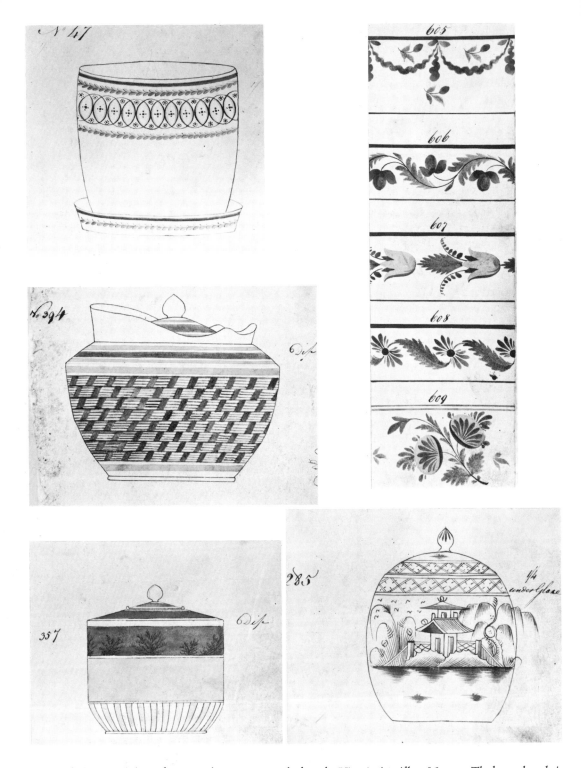

342. *Sample designs and shapes from a Leeds pottery pattern book at the Victoria & Albert Museum. The lower three designs represent teapot bodies (without handles or spouts). Design 357 shows a Mocha motif, see page xvii (c. 1790–1820).*

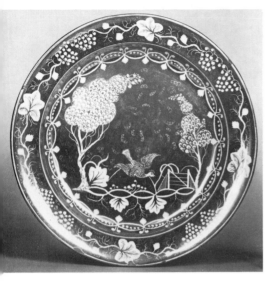

343. (Left) *Leeds Pottery (impressed marked) dish covered with a platinum (silver) lustre. The white design was protected so that these parts resisted the lustre, hence the term "Resist lustre" (c. 1815–20). 14½ inches diameter.*

Fitzwilliam Museum, Cambridge

344. *Leeds Pottery basalt wares with impressed marks—"Hartley Greens & Co/Leeds Pottery" (cup and saucer) and "Leeds Pottery" on creamer and tea kettle (c. 1795–1815). Creamer 5 inches high. Several original moulds for the relief ornamentation of Leeds basalt wares are illustrated in Kidson's* Old Leeds Pottery *(1892).*

Godden of Worthing

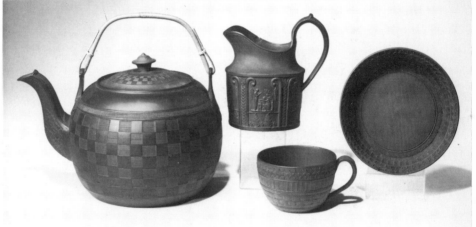

345. *"Leeds Pottery" impressed marked basalt wares (c. 1800–20). The creamer also has the name mark "Hartley Greens & Co". Coffee pot 10 inches high.*

Leeds City Art Gallery and Temple Newsam House

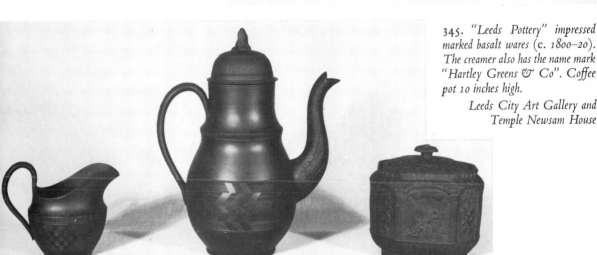

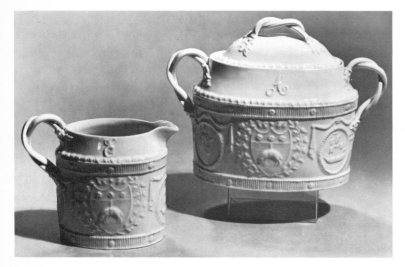

346. Part of a Leeds creamware teaset made to commemorate the royal visit to Leeds in July 1908. Impressed mark "E.A. Royal Visit to Leeds. July 7, 1908. W. L. Hepton. Lord Mayor. Leeds Pottery. J.S." The addition of the initials J.S. (for James Senior) under the standard Leeds Pottery mark is unusual. Creamer 3½ inches high (1908).

347. Leeds-type creamwares reproduced (c. 1888–1916). Impressed mark "Leeds Pottery". Jug 7 inches high. Note the crazed glaze; such wares are rather thicker than original pieces.

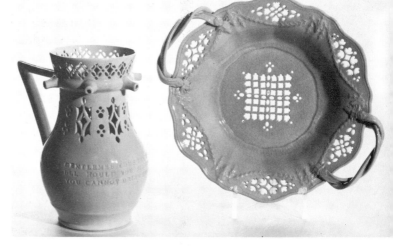

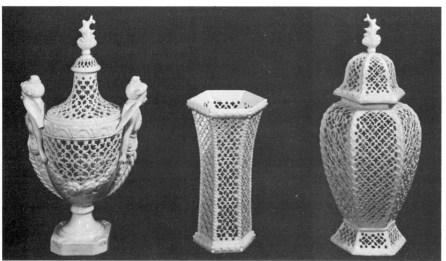

348. Reproductions of Leeds creamware made at Leeds between 1888 and 1916. These examples bear the impressed mark "Leeds Pottery", a form of mark also found on genuine specimens. Centre vase 6¾ inches high.

Leeds City Art Gallery and Temple Newsam House

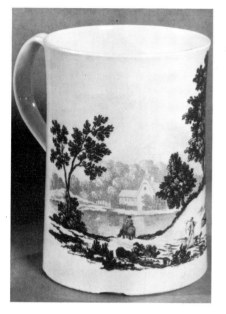

349. *Liverpool porcelain, decorated with very fine black print, which is signed in the foreground "Liverpool". Probably printed by Sadler of Liverpool. A similar example is recorded signed I. (J.) Sadler, Liverpool (c. 1760). 5¾ inches high.*

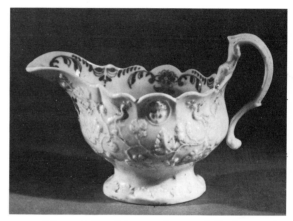

350. *Liverpool Porcelain sauce boat, probably from Seth Pennington's factory, the moulded design including Liver birds (from the Liverpool city crest). Most Liverpool porcelains are unmarked. Note the bubbled glaze, the underglaze blue inner body is of typical dark inky colour (c. 1775–80). 7 inches long.*

Chanctonbury Gallery, Washington, Sussex

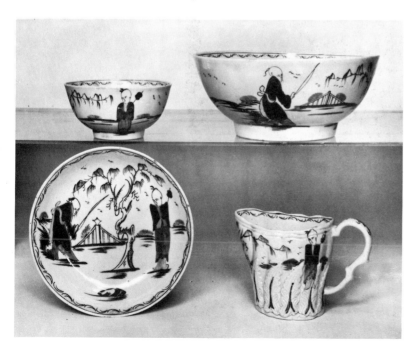

351. *Liverpool porcelains bearing the rare ꟼP mark in underglaze blue (c. 1780).*

Sotheby & Co

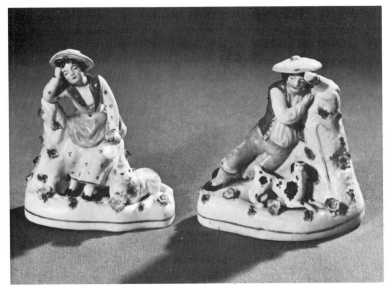

352. *Lloyd (impressed marked) porce-lain figures. John Lloyd produced "toys" at Hanley in the 1840's. Girl 5½ inches high.*

City Museum & Art Gallery,
Stoke-on-Trent

353. *Lloyd, Shelton (impressed marked) Staffordshire earthen-ware dog (c. 1834–52). 5½ inches high. Note: base is missing from similar dogs made after* c. *1850; compare with Plate 333.*

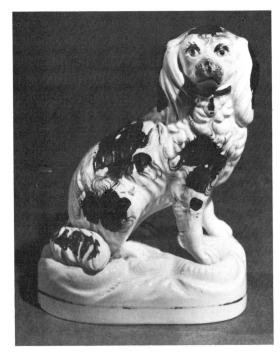

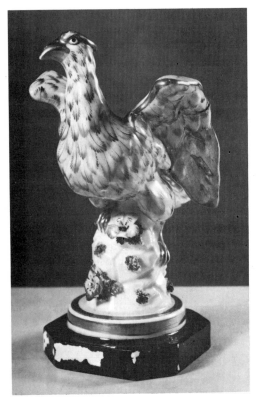

354. *(Left) Lloyd, Shelton (impressed marked) bird. Other animal forms were also made but are very rare (c. 1834–52).*

Victoria & Albert Museum

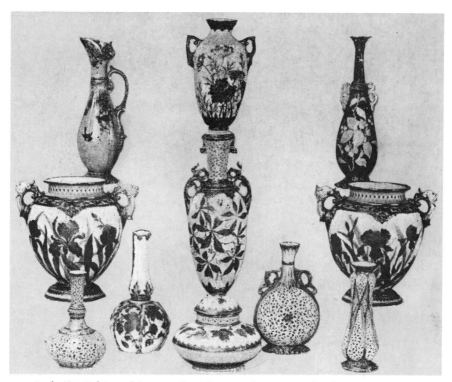

355. *Locke & Co's porcelains, reproduced from an advertisement of early 1899 date. Such wares would have the printed globe mark with name "Locke & Co, Worcester, England".*

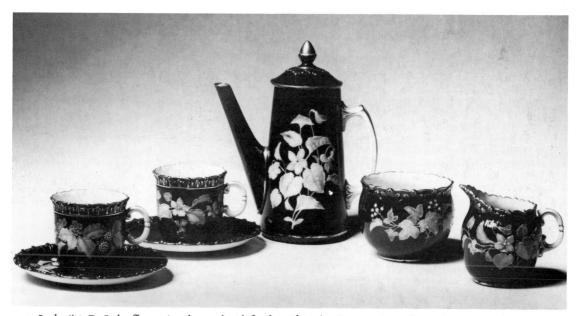

356. *Locke & Co Ltd coffee service, decorated with floral motifs in the pâte-sur-pâte technique (see page xxvi) (c. 1900–4). This Worcester firm produced other floral wares in the pâte-sur-pâte style.*

Godden of Worthing

Longton Hall

William Littler's name is associated with the Longton Hall porcelain works in Staffordshire. Recent research has, however, shown that the works were established by William Jenkinson c. 1749. In October 1751 Jenkinson took as partners William Littler and William Nicklin; they traded as William Littler & Co, as is proved by early newspaper advertisements such as this in *Aris's Birmingham Gazette*, July 1752: "This is to acquaint the public that there is now made by William Littler & Co at Longton Hall, near Newcastle, Staffordshire, a large quantity and great variety of very good and fine ornamental P O R C E L A I N or C H I N A W A R E, in the most fashionable and genteel Taste. . . ." William Jenkinson withdrew from the concern in 1753; subsequent partners were Nathaniel Firmin and Robert Charlesworth.

Typical Longton porcelains are shown in Plates 357–9. Most specimens are rather thickly potted and consequently heavy; leaf motifs were favoured for dishes and plates, sauce boats, etc.; figures and groups were also made. The blue and white decorated examples can be very good and neatly painted. Some Longton Hall porcelain was decorated by Sadler at Liverpool with overglaze printed designs. Many examples of Longton Hall porcelain show a scum-like line at the edge of the glaze on bases, etc. The best known class of Longton Hall porcelain is that decorated with borders, etc., of a rich, streaky underglaze blue; such specimens are with very few exceptions the only ones that bear the accepted factory mark of two crossed "L's" (or "J's") with a short tail of dots (marks nos. 2412–14). Some blue and white and some enamelled examples bear workmen's signs or numbers.

The Longton Hall works closed in 1760. The notice of a closing-down sale held in Salisbury in September 1760 is interesting as it shows the extent of the stock which consisted of "upwards of ninety thousand Pieces . . . Figures and flowers, mounted in chandeliers, Essence Jars, Beakers, Vases and Perfume Pots, magnificent Dessert Services, Sets of Bowls, Mugs, Dishes and Plates ornamented with Columbines and Central Groups, Tea, Coffee and Toilet equipages of elegant patterns superbly furnished. . . ."

For further information and illustrations of unmarked specimens the reader is referred to Dr Bernard Watney's *Longton Hall Porcelain* (1957) and to his contribution to *English Porcelain, 1745–1850* (1965). Recent research has proved that after the closure of the Longton Hall factory William Littler moved to West Pans, near Musselburgh, Scotland—see *Transactions of the English Ceramic Circle*, vol. 5, part 2 (1961). Further information, showing that Littler's Scottish venture probably continued to at least 1777 and that he attempted to manufacture (as well as decorate) pottery and porcelain at West Pans, is contained in a Paper *West Pans Story* published in the *Transactions of the English Ceramic Circle*, vol. 6, part 2 (1966).

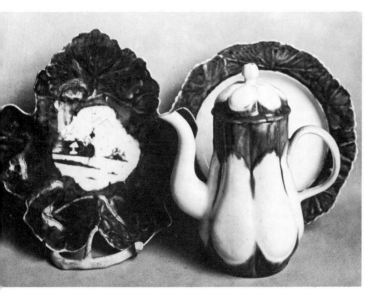

357. *Three typical examples of Longton Hall porcelain, bearing the crossed "L's" mark in underglaze blue (mark no. 2413). The rich streaky blue borders on these specimens are characteristic (c. 1749–60). Coffee pot 8¼ inches high.*

Dr Bernard Watney

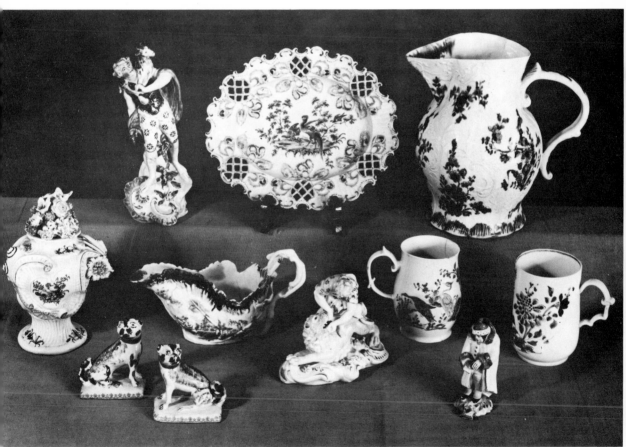

358. *A selection of typical Longton Hall porcelain (c. 1749–60). Dogs only are marked with crossed "L's" in underglaze blue. The handle forms of the two mugs are characteristic of Longton Hall examples. Large jug 9¾ inches high.*

City Museum & Art Gallery, Stoke-on-Trent

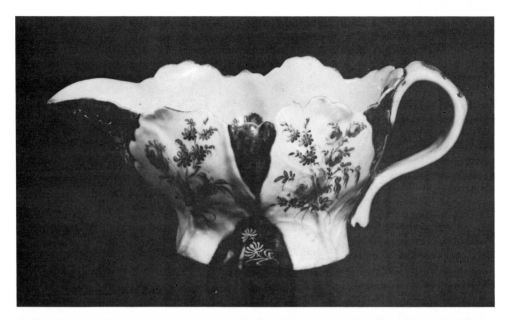

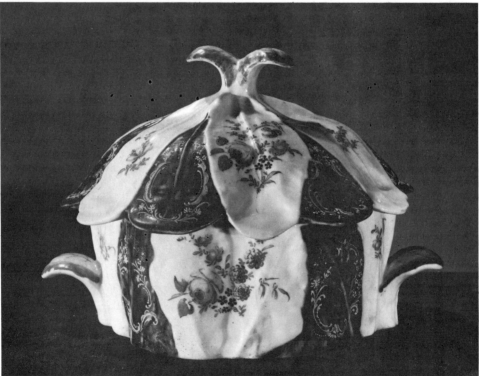

359. *Longton Hall porcelain sauce boat and tureen. The rich streaky underglaze blue is typical, as is also the slight floral sprays in white on the blue ground. The coloured flower painting is by a hand seen on much Longton Hall porcelain. Crossed "L's" mark (no. 2413) (c. 1749–60). Sauce boat 8 inches long.*

D. M. & P. Manheim

In 1757 a small porcelain factory was successfully established at Lowestoft in Suffolk. The porcelain made there is soft paste and contains some 20 per cent of bone ash; it is rather similar to that produced at the Bow factory.

The early productions of the factory, under the management of Robert Browne, were painted in underglaze blue (overglaze enamels were not used before about 1770). These patterns usually show the Chinese influence—anglicized Chinese landscapes, Chinese fishermen, etc. A charming series of pieces were decorated with moulded patterns in relief, enhanced with underglaze blue panels (see Plate 361). Teawares and sauce boats form a large proportion of the Lowestoft output. The blue and white porcelains made before about 1773 often have a workman's number painted on the inside edge of the footrim. The rims of the teapot covers are glazed over, not wiped clear as are Worcester rims.

In 1771 Robert Browne Junr. succeeded his father as manager and within a few years several changes were made: overglaze enamel colours were used, transfer printing in underglaze blue was introduced, and some figures and animals were made in small quantities. Copies were made of Worcester and other porcelains, imitating both the form and the pattern (see Plate 362); the Worcester crescent mark and the Dresden crossedswords mark were copied on blue and white specimens. Other post1773 wares are unmarked. The Lowestoft porcelain appears softer than Worcester and of a more open grain. Slight brownish discoloration sometimes occurs at the edge where the glaze skin has been damaged. As a general rule the enamelled pieces do not bear any mark.

From about 1765 to the closure in or before 1802 the Lowestoft factory made numerous inscribed and dated pieces to commemorate special events. These examples are a great help in tracing the changing styles in form and methods of decoration; a selection is given in a paper by A. J. B. Kiddell, Esq., printed in the *Transactions of the English Ceramic Circle*, no. III, 1931. A series of mugs, inkwells, etc., were made for local sale and bear inscriptions such as "A Trifle from Lowestoft" or have the names of other nearby places (see Plate 363).

In 1902 and 1903 a quantity of moulds, broken fragments, and factory wasters were found on the site; these have proved very useful in identifying the true products of the factory. Many of these pieces are illustrated in W. W. R. Spelman's (otherwise unreliable) *Lowestoft China* (1905). Dr B. Watney's *English Blue and White Porcelain of the 18th Century* (1973) is most helpful on this aspect of the factory's wares. Other helpful sources of information are a Paper by John Howell on the introduction of polychrome decoration at Lowestoft published in the *Transactions of the English Ceramic Circle*, vol. 9, part 3, 1975; a catalogue by Sheenah Smith, *Lowestoft Porcelain in Norwich Castle Museum*, vol. 1, The Blue & White Wares (Norwich, 1975) and G. Godden's *The Illustrated Guide to Lowestoft Porcelain* (Barrie & Jenkins, London, 1969). Good representative collections can be seen at the Castle Museum, Norwich; Christchurch Mansions, Ipswich; Fitzwilliam Museum, Cambridge; Lowestoft Borough Library; and at the Victoria & Albert Museum in London.

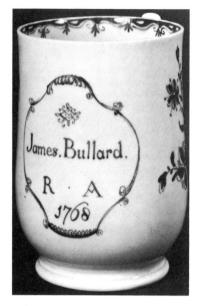

360. *Lowestoft porcelain mug, of early bell shape, painted in underglaze blue (dated 1768). Painter's mark "3" on inside of foot-rim. 5¾ inches high.*

Godden Collection

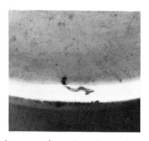

360. a. *Detail of Lowestoft workman's number mark painted on inside of foot-rim.*

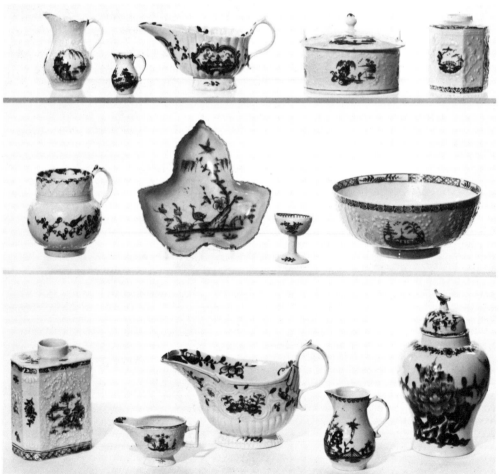

361. *Lowestoft (soft paste) porcelains of the 1760's, painted in underglaze blue. The moulded wares are particularly attractive, all with painter's numbers; in most cases on the inside of the foot-rim (see typical detail above).*

Godden Collection

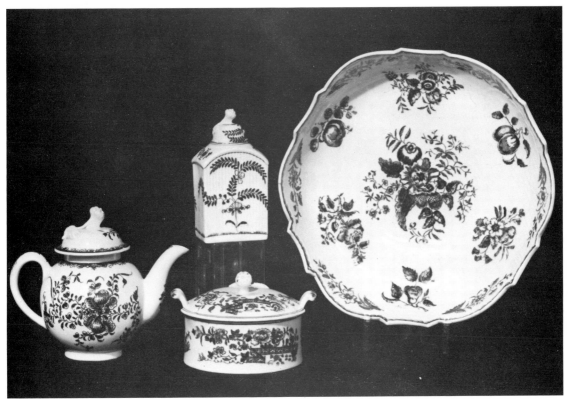

362. *Lowestoft soft paste porcelains decorated in underglaze blue. Teapot with the Worcester crescent mark (c. 1780). Covered butter dish decorated with a Worcester printed pattern (c. 1780). Fluted tea-caddy with the Dresden crossed-swords mark in underglaze blue (c. 1775). Moulded and blue printed salad bowl with a copy of the Worcester filled in crescent mark in blue (c. 1785). 10 inches diameter.*

Godden of Worthing

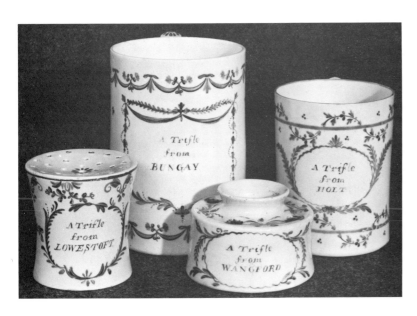

363. *Lowestoft porcelains of the "Trifle" type made for the local visitors' markets (c. 1785–95). Note late type cylindrical mug form. Apart from these "Trifle" pieces the later coloured Lowestoft porcelains do not bear a factory mark.*

Godden Collections

207

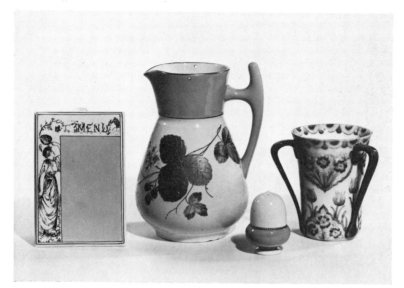

364. *Earthenwares by James Macintyre & Co, of Burslem (c. 1890–1900). Impressed name and monogram marks, nos. 2821 and 2822. Also printed mark no. 2823. Jug 7¼ inches high.*

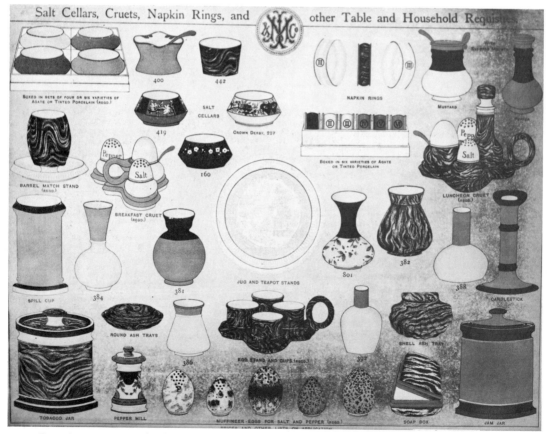

365. *James Macintyre & Co's advertisement of 1888, showing typical wares of the period. The monogram mark can be seen at the top centre.*

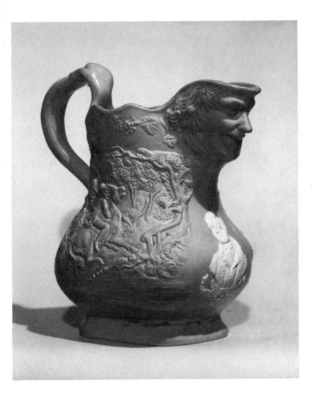

366. *Moulded earthenware jug, impressed mark—*
"Machin & Potts, June 20th 1834". 6¼ inches high.

British Museum

367. *Earthenware "Reform Bill" jug of*
1832. Initial mark M & T, of Machin
& Thomas of Burslem (c. 1831–2).
5 inches high.
Glaisher Collection, Fitzwilliam Museum

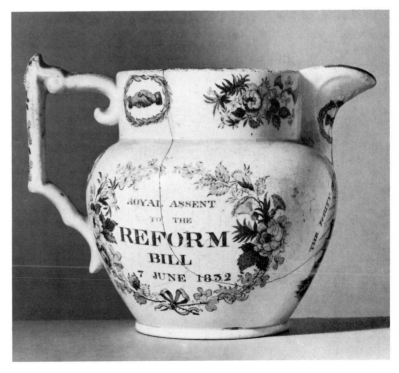

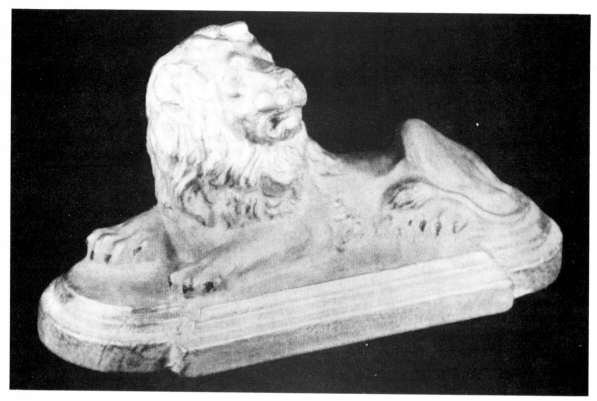

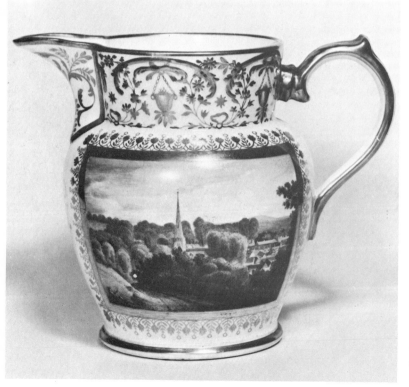

368. *Madeley porcelain lion, bearing the unique mark "T.M.R. Madeley S". The initials are those of the owner of the Madeley Works, Thomas Martin Randall. The S after Madeley relates to the county, Shropshire. This is the only recorded marked specimen of Madeley porcelain (c. 1828–40).*

Present owner unknown
Photo: S. W. Fisher

369. *Porcelain jug, by family tradition made at T. M. Randall's small factory at Madeley, Shropshire (c. 1826). This unmarked example has been included as no marked useful wares have been recorded. There would seem to be no reason to doubt this traditional attribution.*

Hereford Museum & Art Gallery

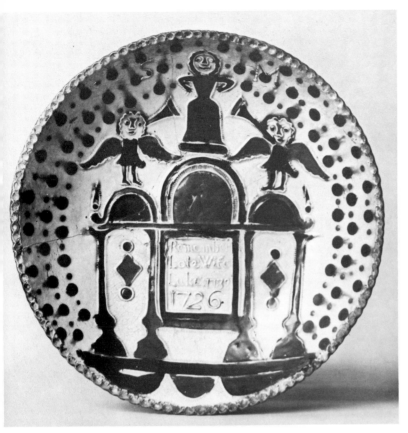

370. *Moulded and slip decorated dish, bearing the initials "SM" (for Samuel Malkin of Burslem). This example is dated 1726. Other dishes by this potter are dated 1712?, 1727, and 1734. Most have the initials S.M. worked into the design (c. 1726). 14 inches diameter.*

Fitzwilliam Museum, Cambridge

See articles by Hugh Tait in Apollo *magazine, January and February 1957.*

MALING, SUNDERLAND *c.* 1762–1815

371. *An attractively primitive earthenware plate, bearing the impressed mark "Maling". William Maling worked the North Hylton Pottery at Sunderland (c. 1800–15). "Maling" marks were later used at Newcastle upon Tyne. 7¼ inches diameter.*

Victoria & Albert Museum

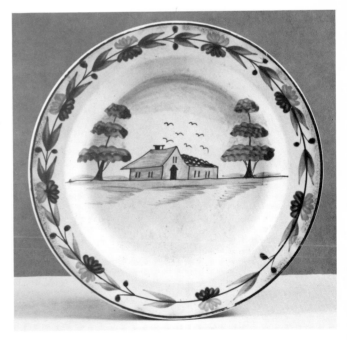

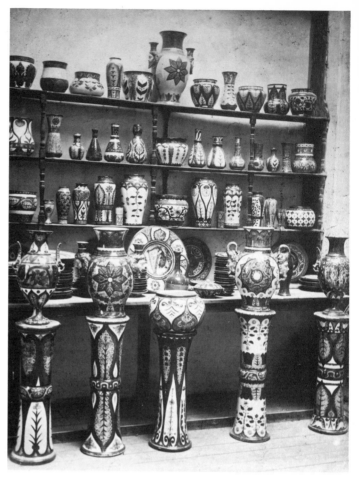

372. *Selection of pottery produced by Carlo Manzoni at his Granville Pottery, Hanley (c. 1895). Reproduced from a contemporary photograph. Such wares should bear the initials C.M. (joined) with the year added.*

J. MARE

373. *"Mare" (impressed marked) earthenware footbath with fine quality blue printed pattern. John Mare potted at Hanley (c. 1800–25). 20 inches long. Pre-1820 footbaths are of this simple form with straight sides, later examples have shaped sides.*

Godden of Worthing

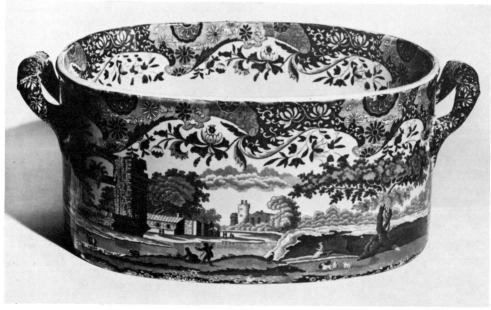

The Martin Brothers (Fulham & Southall)

The Martin Brothers have a claim to be considered the first of the "Studio" Potters. Robert Wallace Martin (1843–1923), Walter Martin (1859–1912), Edwin Bruce Martin (1860–1915), and Charles Martin (d. 1910) worked together in their studio (see Plate 374) as a team, producing salt-glaze stoneware of a unique and varied character.

Robert, usually known as Wallace Martin, was the mainstay of the partnership (he had earlier worked as a stone carver on the Houses of Parliament). He was responsible for the series of grotesque bird models with movable heads, as well as other animal forms. Walter Martin received early training at Doultons' Pottery at Lambeth. He was responsible for "throwing" all the large vases and was also in charge of mixing the clays and of the firing process. The third brother, Edwin, decorated vases, etc., with incised and relief patterns—seaweed, fish, floral motifs, etc. Charles Martin took the responsibility of management and administration off the shoulders of his brothers and was in charge of their retail shop (Plate 378) in Brownlow Street, Holborn.

The Martin Brothers worked from 1873 to 1914. Their wares are marked with their name, place of production (Fulham at first, later London and Southall) and figures signifying the month and year of production—all incised into the soft clay before firing. The various changes in the basic marks are:

RW Martin 84
Fulham

"Fulham" period (c. 1873-4).

RW Martin 9
London

"London" mark (c. 1874-8). Note—no letter prefix to number.

RW Martin 21
Southall
OR *R W MARTIN SOUTHALL.*

"Southall" period (c. 1878).

RW Martin
London & Southall

"London & Southall" marks (c. 1879–82)

RW Martin & Brothers
London & Southall

"& Bros" or "& Brothers" added to name from 1882 onwards.

The reader is referred to Blacker's *The A.B.C. of English Salt-Glaze Stoneware* (1922) and to *Country Life*, 23 March 1961, for full accounts of the Martin brothers. A detailed and well illustrated work of reference is Charles Beard's catalogue of the Nettlefold Collection of Martinware (1936), but this is now very scarce and expensive. All Martinware bears the name or one of the marks reproduced above.

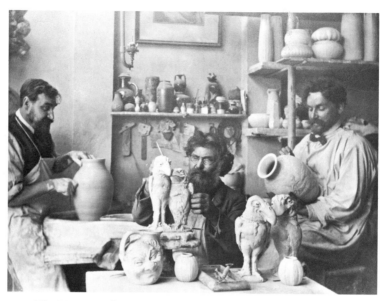

374. *The Martin Brothers at work on their individual specialities* (left to right): *Walter—turning, Wallace (R. W.) Martin—modelling his famous birds, and Edwin who did most of the incised and relief modelled patterns.* Reproduced from an original photograph on glass in the Godden Collection.

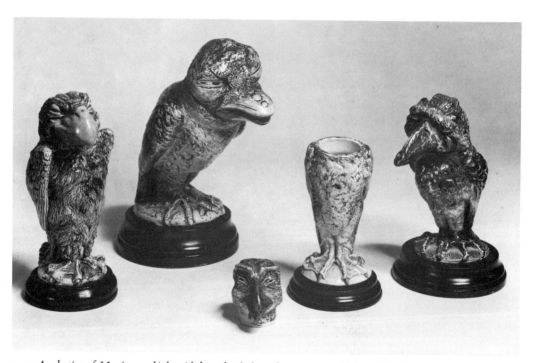

375. *A selection of Martinware birds with loose heads (one shown separated from its body). Incised name and address marks (see page 213) with date of production. Large centre bird 11½ inches high, dated 1887. Similar models were made into the twentieth century.*

Godden of Worthing

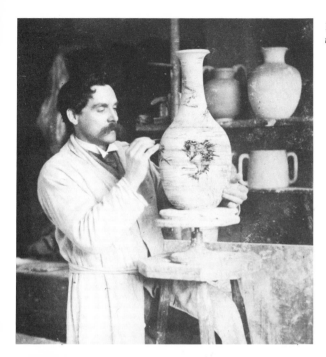

376. *Edwin Martin decorating a typical Martin Bros vase.*

Southall Public Libraries

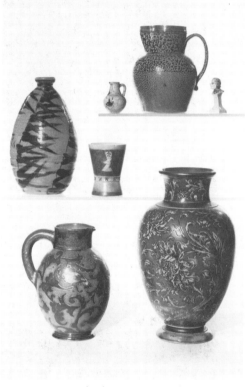

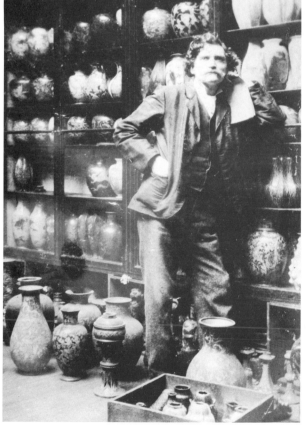

377. *Martin Brothers' stonewares with incised name marks, with place-name (Fulham, Southall or London) and date. Crested beaker dated 1873. Large vase (1893). $13\frac{1}{2}$ inches high.*

Godden of Worthing

378. *Charles Martin in the Martin Brothers' shop in Brownlow Street, Holborn (c. 1900). Showing typical vase forms and styles of decoration.*

Southall Public Libraries

Masons

Miles Mason was the first member of the Mason family to start potting, at Lane Delph, in the Staffordshire Potteries. Good quality attractive porcelain was made by Miles Mason from about 1802 to 1813. Specimens usually bear the impressed mark "M. Mason"; occasionally the full name "Miles Mason" was used and this name may occur with a mock Chinese square seal mark. Marked examples of Miles Mason's porcelains are rarely found today, but are always well potted and bear restrained and tasteful patterns (see Plates 382–3).

Miles Mason's son, Charles James Mason, was the one destined to lasting fame for, in his name, the famous Ironstone patent of July 1813 was taken out. This was for "a process for the improve‑ment of the manufacture of English Porcelain", although the new body was in no sense a porcelain but a heavy, hard, opaque earthenware for which the name Ironstone was especially apt. Typical specimens of Mason Ironstone are boldly decorated and colourful (see Plates 384–5). Early pieces have a crisp compact body and bear self‑explanatory impressed marks in line or circular form. From 1813 to 1848 the Mason firms produced vast quantities of their "Patent Ironstone". The forms are varied and range from miniature pieces to huge vases and fireplaces. This durable Ironstone china was especially suited to the manufacture of colourful dinner and dessert services.

There were various changes in the title of the Mason firm; these changes are reflected in several different marks: "G. M. & C. J. Mason. 1813–29", "C. J. Mason & Co. 1829–44", "C. J. Mason. 1845–48". In 1848 Charles J. Mason became bankrupt and his possessions were sold. Most of the moulds and patterns were purchased by Francis Morley of Shelton. Morley was in partnership with George Ashworth from 1858 to 1862 and the Mason patterns, etc., subsequently came into the hands of Messrs G. L. Ashworth & Bros of Hanley, a firm which today produces Mason‑type wares.

Charles Mason soon re‑established himself at Longton for, in April 1849, he registered at the Patent Office the dish shown in Plate 387. He also exhibited a formidable display of Ironstone wares at the 1851 Exhibition. Charles Mason's name does not occur in rate records after 1852. Standard works on Mason wares are R. Haggar's *The Masons of Lane Delph* (Lund Humphries, London, 1952) and *The Illustrated Guide to Mason's Patent Ironstone China* by G. Godden (Barrie & Jenkins, London, 1971); an enlarged revised version of this out‑of‑print work is to be published by the Antique Collectors' Club of Woodbridge in 1980. The reader is also referred to R. G. Haggar's and E. Adam's joint work *Mason Porcelain and Ironstone 1796–1853* (Faber, London, 1977).

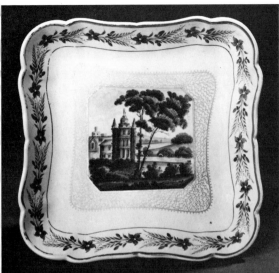

379. *"M Mason" impressed marked porcelain dish of fine quality. Landscape painted in sepia (c. 1802–13). 8 inches square.*

City Museum & Art Gallery, Stoke-on-Trent

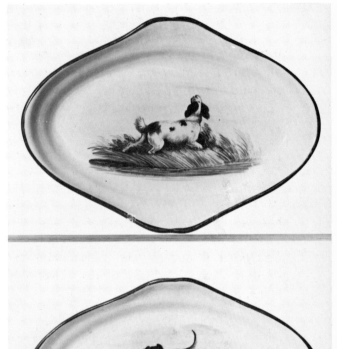

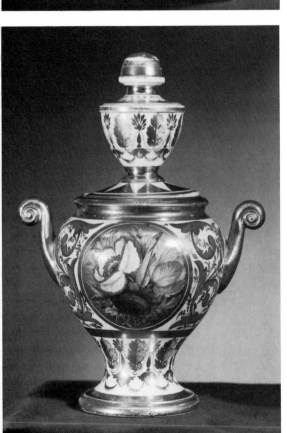

381. *M. Mason (impressed marked) porcelain vase and cover. One of a pair. Floral panels on gold ground. 7 inches high (c. 1802–13). Marked Miles Mason vases are very rare.*

Lucile Pillow Collection,
Beaverbrook Art Gallery, Fredericton, Canada

380. *"M Mason" (impressed marked) porcelain dishes, with very rare animal subjects painted in sepia (c. 1802–13). 10¾ inches long.*

Godden of Worthing

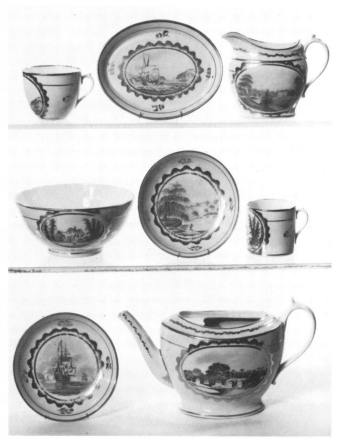

382. *Part of a rare M. Mason (impressed mark on teapot) porcelain tea service, decorated with fine bat printed panels (c. 1802–13). Most Mason teawares are unmarked.*

Godden of Worthing

383. *M. Mason (impressed marked) porcelain tea service (c. 1802–13). Miles Mason of Lane Delph (Fenton) retired in 1813. Teapot 5¼ inches high. Pattern no. 91.*

Godden of Worthing

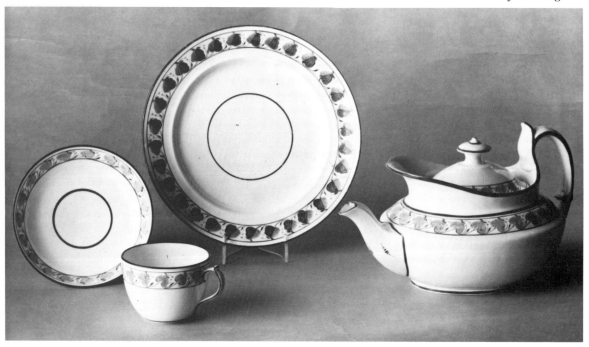

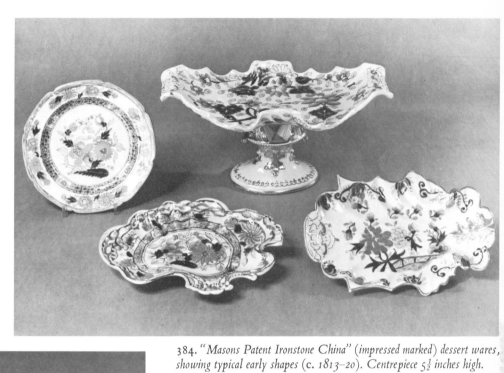

384. *"Masons Patent Ironstone China" (impressed marked) dessert wares, showing typical early shapes (c. 1813–20). Centrepiece 5½ inches high.*

Godden of Worthing

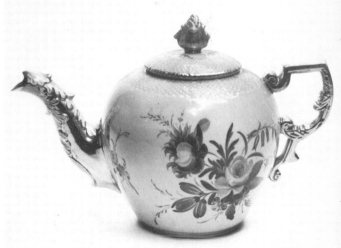

385. *"Masons Patent Ironstone China" (impressed marked) vase and a miniature ewer, with typical colourful "Japan" pattern (c. 1813–25). Vase 15 inches high.*

Godden of Worthing

386. *A fine quality Mason's Ironstone teapot with richly gilt handle, spout, etc. Flowers painted in enamel colours. Impressed mark "Patent Ironstone China" (c. 1813–20). 5¼ inches high.*

Sotheby & Co

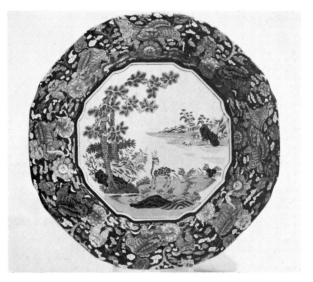

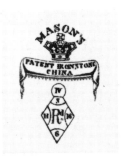

387. *Mason's Ironstone dish of a form registered in 1849. Note late version of standard printed mark below with angular outline to crown. 10¼ inches diameter.*

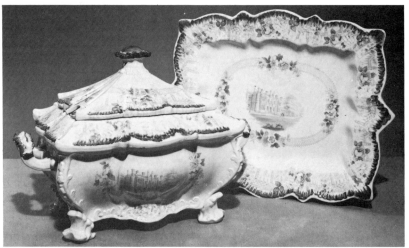

388. *C. J. Mason & Co (printed mark) Ironstone tureen cover and stand. Decorated with printed scenic and floral pattern (c. 1829–45). Tureen 10 inches high.*

Victoria & Albert Museum

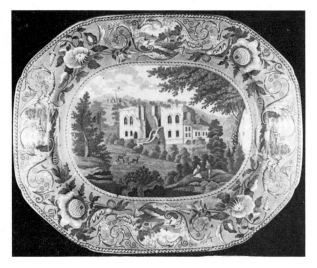

389. (Left) *W. Mason (printed marked) earthenware dish, with underglaze blue print. William Mason (son of Miles Mason) potted at Lane Delph from about 1811 to c. 1815.*

Present owner unknown

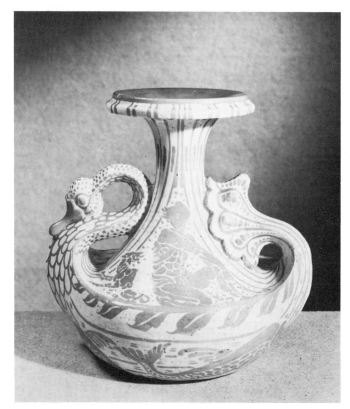

390. *Maw & Co (impressed mark) of Broseley earthenware vase, decorated with lustre pattern designed by Walter Crane, monogram mark on base, see companion mark book (c. 1889). 9 inches high. A good selection of Maw earthenware can be seen in the Shrewsbury Museum.*

Victoria & Albert Museum

E. MAYER, HANLEY c. 1780–1804

391. *E. Mayer impressed marked moulded canewares of good quality. Elijah Mayer potted at Hanley from c. 1773 to 1805. Uncoloured teapot 4½ inches high.*

Victoria & Albert Museum

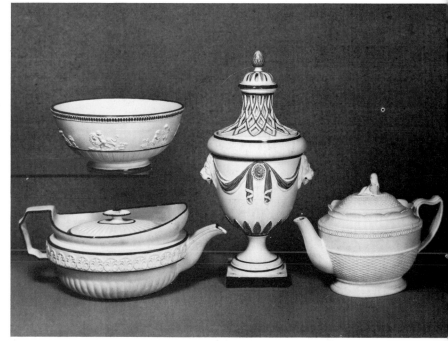

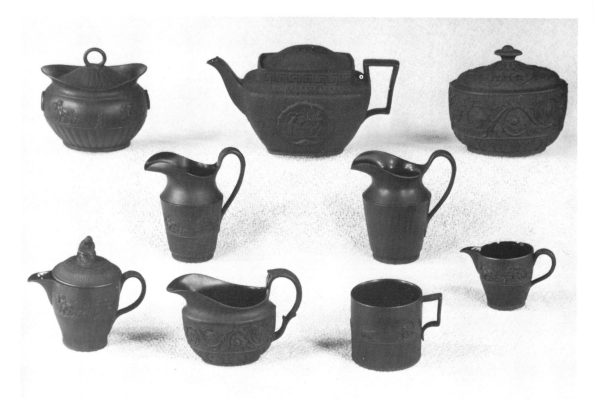

392. *E. Mayer (impressed mark) basalt wares, a representative selection from the Hanley Museum. The teapot (knob missing) commemorates Nelson's victory at Trafalgar in 1805. Height of covered sugar at left 4¾ inches (c. 1800–20).*

City Museum & Art Gallery, Stoke-on-Trent

MAYER AND NEWBOLD, LANE END 1817–33

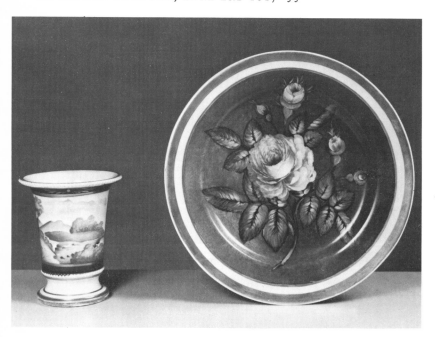

393. *Mayer & Newbold porcelains. The spill vase with initial mark painted in red—M & N. The plate with names written in full. All marked porcelains by this Lane End firm are rare (c. 1817–30). Vase 8⅝ inches high.*

Victoria & Albert Museum

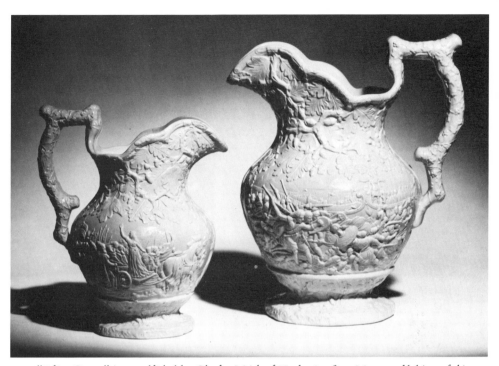

394. *"Julius Caesar" jugs, published by Charles Meigh of Hanley in 1839. Many moulded jugs of this type were produced in the 1830's and 1840's.*

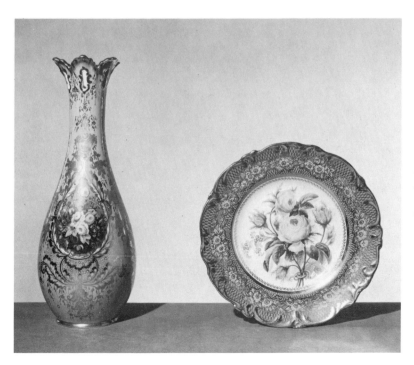

395. *Charles Meigh & Son's decorated earthenwares. The plate has the Royal Arms mark with the name in full. The vase has the standard impressed mark "Opaque/ Porcelain" in oval form (c. 1851) (1851 Exhibition?).*

Victoria & Albert Museum

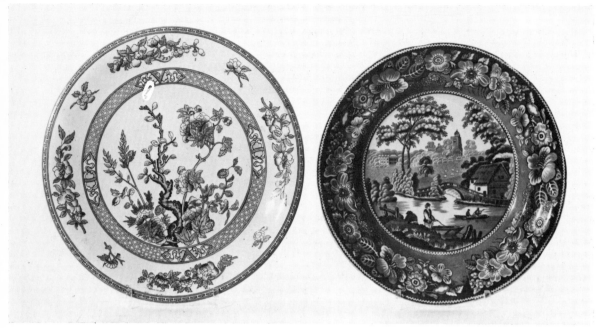

396. J. Meir & Son's earthenware plates. The "Indian Tree" pattern plate has the impressed mark Meir & Son and printed initial mark "J M & S". The blue printed plate has a printed mark with name in full. This Tunstall potter worked c. 1841–97.

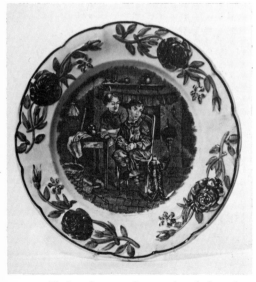

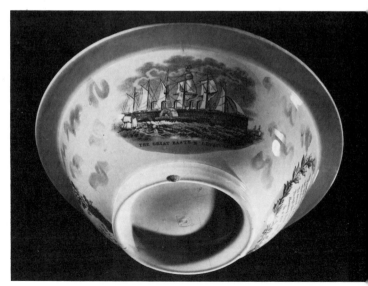

397. Middlesbrough pottery (impressed marked) earthenware plate with relief moulded border coloured over and printed centre (c. 1834–44). Many similar inexpensive plates were produced at this Yorkshire pottery.

398. Middlesbrough pottery bowl, showing impressed mark—"London" and an anchor. The printed panel shows the Great Eastern Leviathan launched in 1858. 11 inches diameter.

In 1793, at Stoke-on-Trent, Thomas Minton (1765–1836) founded the world-famous firm that still bears his name. He had earlier been apprenticed to Thomas Turner as an engraver at the Caughley porcelain works. This training stood Thomas Minton in good stead, for his early productions were unmarked earthenwares decorated with printed patterns in underglaze blue. Production was not started until May 1796.

The exact date when Thomas Minton began the manufacture of porcelain is open to some doubt, but the probable year was 1798. The earliest examples from about 1798 to 1805 bear only the painted pattern number, often prefixed by the letter "N" or "No", and these wares are often mistaken for the products of other firms. The existence of several of the early factory pattern books, however, enable the accurate identification of Minton pieces (see Plate 399).

The first factory marked examples would seem to date from about 1805 (see Plate 401). The finest pieces were decorated by former Derby artists—Thomas Steel, Joseph Bancroft, and George Hancock. Their floral painting occurs on tea services, dessert services, and fine, richly gilt punch bowls with flower painted panels. These early 1805–16 porcelains have a painted crossed "L" mark, often with the pattern number written below (mark no. 2684) (see Plate 401a). The standard shapes are often similar to those employed at the Spode factory, but pieces shown in Plates 399–402 have been checked against the pattern books and these standard shapes should be studied. Porcelain was not made between 1817 and 1823.

The Minton porcelains of the 1820's and 1830's are normally unmarked. It is only the existence of factory pattern and design books that show the fine quality ornamental as well as useful wares produced at this period. These fine Minton porcelains have in the past been attributed to the Coalport, Derby, Rockingham, Swansea, and Worcester factories in error.

Sample pages from the Minton design books of the 1820's, 1830's, and 1840's are reproduced in Plates 403–5, but these are only a few of the hundreds of forms produced by Mintons at this period and decorated in a variety of styles. One of the most popular forms of decoration was the application of richly coloured modelled flowers. These floral encrusted pieces are normally called Coalbrook-dale or Coalport, but the Minton records show that most pieces are in fact Minton (see page xxiv). A selection of Minton floral encrusted porcelain is shown in Colour Plate VIII; all these forms match the design books. These pieces are normally unmarked, but some pieces bear a mock Dresden crossed-swords mark in underglaze blue.

Messrs Minton also produced a wide range of fine quality figures and groups, some of which are glazed and finely enamelled. Others are in the bisque—that is, unglazed and undecorated. The enamelled examples have in the past been called Coalport or Derby; the bisque examples Derby, Rockingham, or even Swansea. The bisque figures are in a white rather chalky body, quite different from the later creamy coloured Parian body with its slight gloss. Minton figures from the factory design book are shown in Plate 403, finished examples in Plates 406–7. The figures are normally unmarked; some rare examples of the 1840's bear the incised ermine-like mark (no. 2700).

The detailed study of the Minton records show clearly that their early products have been sadly neglected by ceramic historians and collectors. Forthcoming books on the pre- and post-1850 periods are in preparation and will shed much light on the unidentified Minton wares.

A series of moulded jugs, mugs, etc., in a hard, coloured earthenware was begun in the late 1820's and continued into the 1840's. These wares are marked with a moulded (or applied) scroll device with the initial "M" in the bottom right-hand corner with the model number above (see Plates 408, 408a).

Thomas Minton died in 1836; he was succeeded by his son, Herbert Minton (1793–1858), who joined in partnership with John Boyle and traded under the title Minton & Boyle. Various printed trade marks of this period (1836–41) incorporate the initials "M. & B.". From 1841 the marks include the initial "M. & Co" but from 1845 to 1868 some earthenwares have the initials "M. & H" denoting the partnership between Herbert Minton and Michael Hollins.

The Minton porcelains, from the 1840's onwards, became more and more ornate, but were always of the finest quality. Good figure subject painting was carried out by John Simpson from 1837 to 1847, when he moved to London and became an enamel painter and miniaturist. Simpson was succeeded by Christian Henk and Thomas Allen, both of whom excelled in the French style of figure painting, on vases and other wares, in imitation of the fashionable eighteenth-century Sèvres porcelains (see Plate 416). Anton Boullemier, a French artist employed from 1872, excelled in charming figure compositions.

As the name of Copelands, Mintons' rivals, was associated with the Parian body (which Mintons also produced in quantity) so Mintons' name was associated with the so-called Majolica body which they introduced in 1850. This was basically an earthenware body coated with an opaque white glaze, but subsequently all Victorian earthenwares decorated with semi-translucent glazes were termed Majolica. They were produced by most manufacturers of the period, but none were of such fine quality as the examples made by Mintons.

Throughout the Victorian era Mintons employed the finest ceramic artists, many of whom were attracted from the Continent by the world-wide prestige enjoyed by the firm in the nineteenth century. Information on many of these artists will be found in G. Godden's *Victorian Porcelain*. Apart from the French Art Director, Leon Arnoux, the foreign artist who was to gain further international fame for Mintons, was the Sèvres-trained M. L. Solon, whose forte was the style of decoration known as *pâte-sur-pâte*, in which thin layers of china clay are built up over a coloured ground to give a charming cameo-like effect (see Plate 422). This painstaking technique produced what is today the highest priced range of Victorian ceramics. All Solon's pieces are signed but, as with other successful ventures, there were several imitations both in England and on the Continent. Further information on *pâte-sur-pâte* will be found in *Victorian Porcelain*.

All Minton wares after 1862 were marked either with overglaze printed marks (as chronologically listed in the companion *Encyclopaedia of Marks*) or with impressed name marks—MINTON (1862–73), and MINTONS from 1873 onwards. In addition to these marks nearly all Minton wares from 1842 to the present day will be found to bear impressed year cyphers, the key to which is contained in *The Encyclopaedia of British Pottery and Porcelain Marks*. The standard book on these superb wares is G. Godden's *Minton Porcelain of the First Period* (Barrie & Jenkins, London, 1968 and 1979).

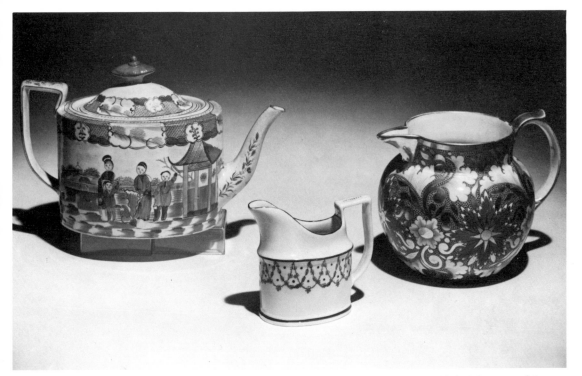

399. *Early Minton porcelains, un-marked except for painted pattern numbers—teapot no. 105, milk jug no. 18, jug no. 178, which match the original pattern books. Other pieces of these forms or patterns can be identified from these examples (c. 1800–10). Jug 5¼ inches high.*

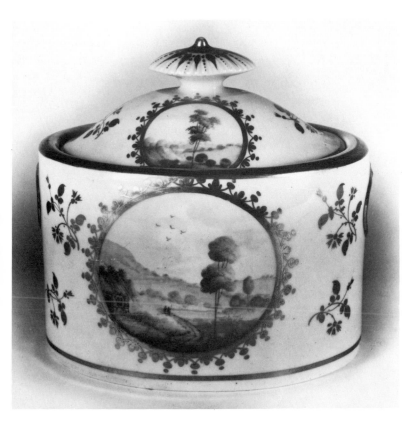

400. *Early Minton porcelain sugar basin and cover. Painted pattern no. 58, which matches the original pattern book. The Pinxton factory issued a similar design without the number "58", but with the titles of the scenes written under the base (c. 1800–5).*

Sotheby & Co

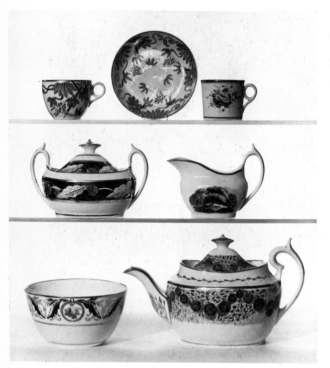

401. *Minton porcelain teawares of various patterns, showing standard shapes of the 1810–20 period. Painted crossed "L" mark with "M" and pattern number below. Pattern (top row, left to right) 85, 767, (middle row) 670, 119, (bottom row) 791, 540. Teapot 6¼ inches high.*

401. a. *Basic Minton crossed "L's" mark. The pattern number was often added below (c. 1805–16).*

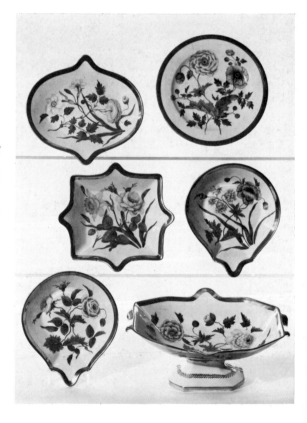

402. *Early Minton porcelain dessert service, showing typical shapes, painted with flowers in the finest manner. Painted mark no. 2684, pattern no. 786 (c. 1810). Centrepiece 12½ inches long.*

Godden of Worthing

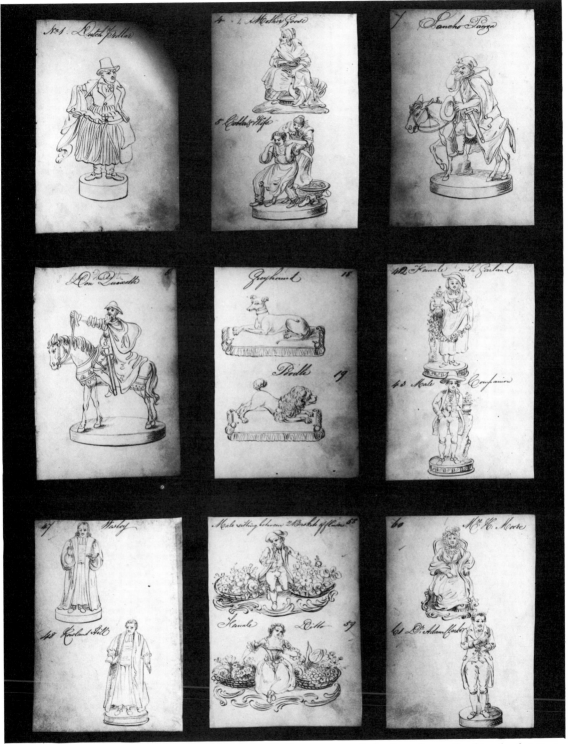

403. *Sample pages from Minton's first figure design book. The figures are unmarked and are often attributed to other factories in error. Nos. 1, 4, 5, 7 and 8 are of small size, finely enamelled and gilt and of narrow section. Nos. 47, 48, 60, 61 are normally in white biscuit (unglazed china).*

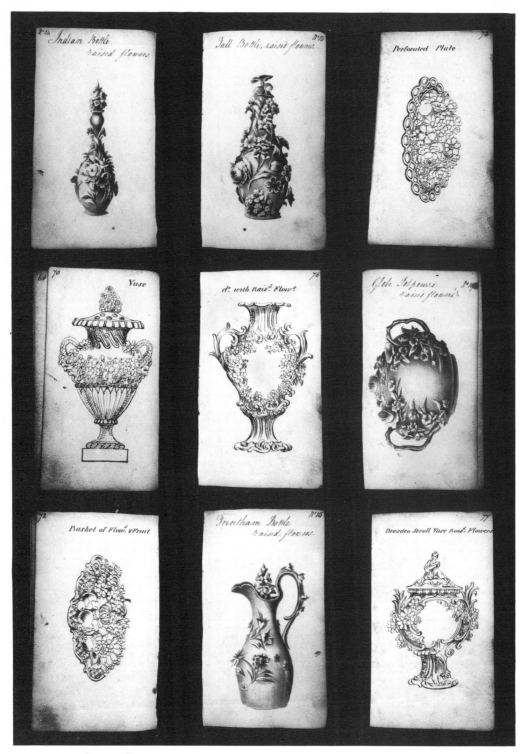

404. *Sample pages from Minton's first ornamental ware design book, showing floral encrusted porcelains of a type often attributed to the Coalport factory. These Minton wares often bear the Dresden crossed-swords mark in blue (see also Colour Plate VIII).*

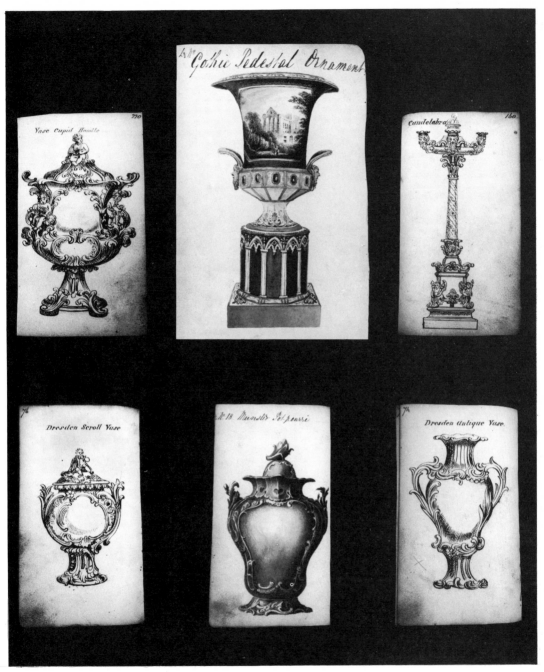

405. *Six Minton designs, examples of over two hundred and fifty vases, etc., drawn in the first (pre-1841) pattern book. Such fine porcelains are unmarked and pass as Coalport, Derby, Rockingham, etc., as the full range and quality of Minton's early porcelain has not as yet been realized. Basic vase forms were finely painted with landscapes, flowers, feathers and figure subjects. The gilding is superb.*

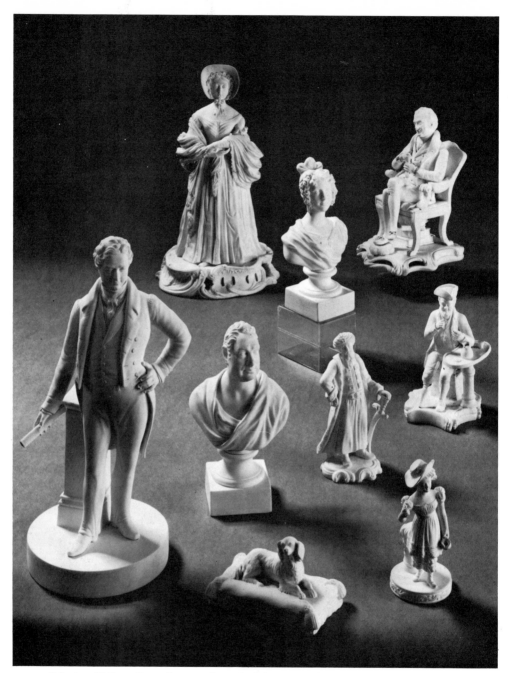

406. *Selection of Minton bisque figures, each matching drawings in the factory pattern books. Such Minton figures are normally unmarked and are mistaken for the products of other factories—Derby, Rockingham, etc. Large figure of Sir Robert Peel (model no. 77) is 11 inches high (c. 1830–47).*

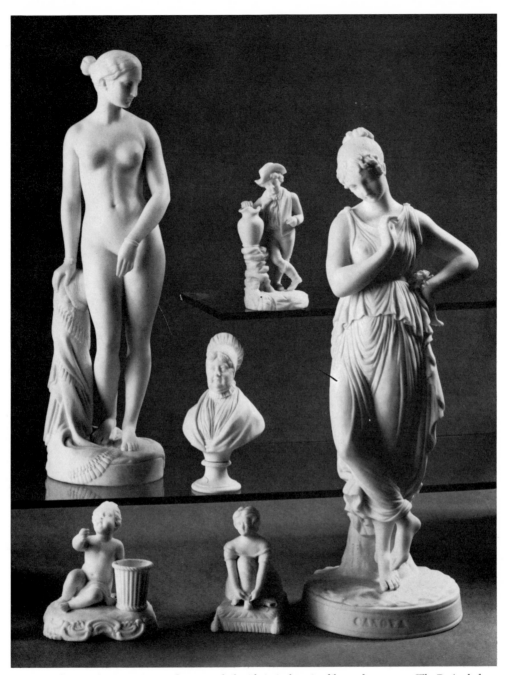

407. *Selection of Minton Parian figures marked with incised ermine-like mark, no. 2700. The Parian body with its slightly creamy tint and very slight glaze or gloss replaced the early matt white, chalky bisque body in about 1847. Earlier models were reissued in the new Parian body and new models introduced in quantity. Canova's Dancing Girl dated 1849 is 15¼ inches high.*

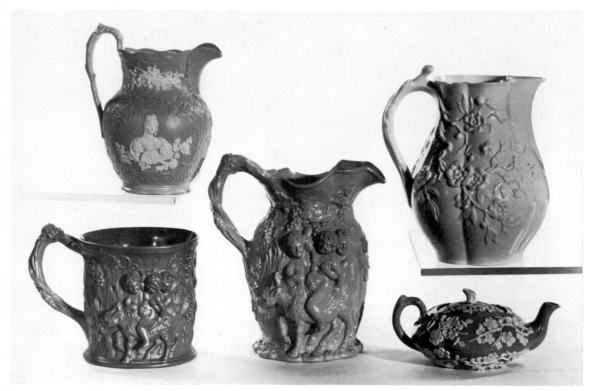

408. *Minton moulded stonewares, bearing the scroll relief mark no. 2690 with "M" under the design number (see detail below). The portrait jug (showing William IV and Queen Adelaide) is design no. 13 (c. 1830–1). Centre jug 6 inches high. Most of these forms were made in several sizes.*

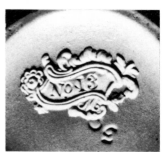

408. a. *Detail of base of 1830–1 Queen Adelaide jug (see above). This relief moulded mark occurs on many coloured earthenware and Parian objects of the 1830–50 period. The model number "no. 13" within the scroll varies. Impressed numbers relate to the size.*

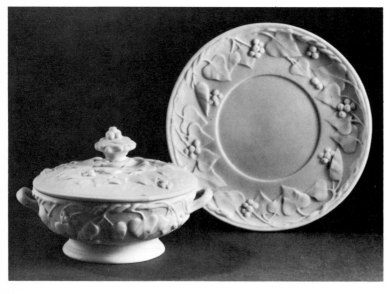

409. *Minton moulded Parian butter dish, cover and stand. Form registered in 1852, model no. 520. The matt white Parian body was used for utilitarian wares as well as figures and groups.*

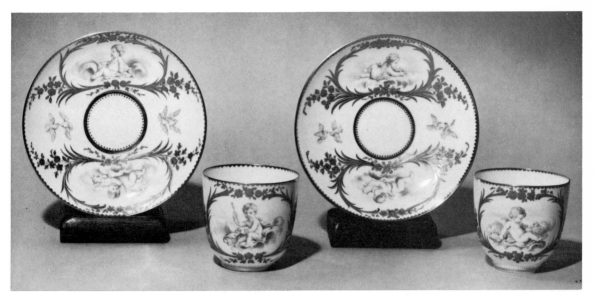

410. *Pair Minton porcelain cups and saucers painted by Thomas Kirkby (c. 1850). Several of Kirkby original designs are preserved. "Ermine" mark no. 2703.*

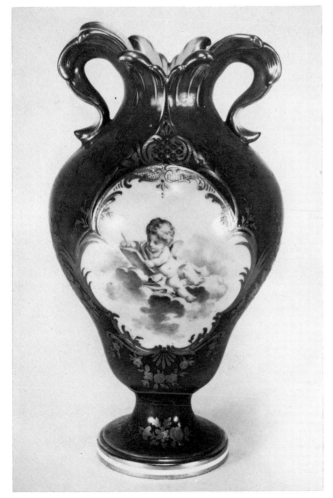

411. *Minton porcelain vase in the Sèvres manner, painted in pink camaieu, on a turquoise ground. Model no. 99 "Sèvres Eard. vase". "Ermine" mark no. 2703. 8¼ inches high.*

Sotheby & Co

Much fine Minton porcelain of the 1850's bears only the small ermine-like device, mark no. 2703.

235

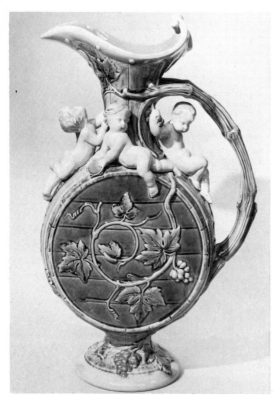

412. Minton "Palissy"-type earthenware ewer with coloured glazes. A model shown at the 1862 Exhibition. Impressed name mark "Minton" with year cypher for 1869. 13 inches high.

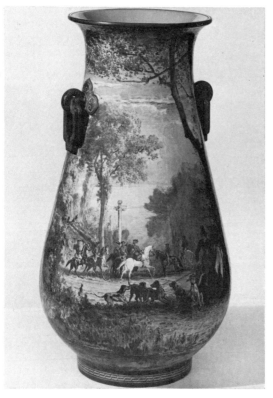

413. A very colourful Minton earthenware dish painted by W. S. Coleman, a famous artist who worked for Mintons from 1869 to 1873; 1869 (impressed year cypher and name mark). 16½ inches diameter. See Victorian Porcelain, Chapter 5.

414. Minton Majolica vase, one of a pair, painted by Edouard Rischgitz (worked 1864–70). Impressed name mark, year cypher for 1865. 20½ inches high.

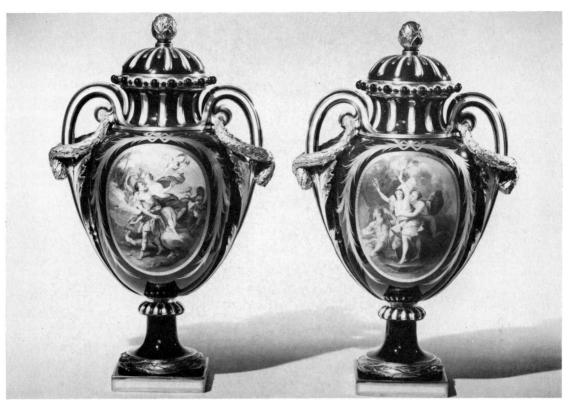

415. *Pair of Minton blue-ground vases in the Sèvres style, with hand-painted figure panels in the manner of C. Henk. Printed mark no. 2705 (c. 1860–70). 17½ inches high.*

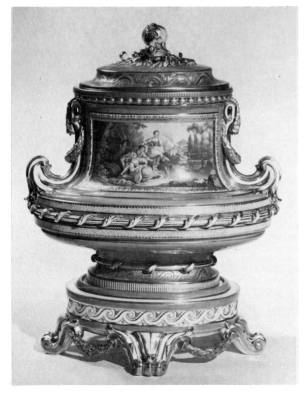

416. *Minton porcelain covered vase and stand (one of a set of three) in the Sèvres style. Turquoise blue ground with the finest quality gilding. Hand-painted figure subject panels in the French style. 16 inches high. Mintons excelled in the reproduction of Sèvres-type wares during the 1860's and 1870's. These wares bear clear Minton name marks; the original marks were not forged.*

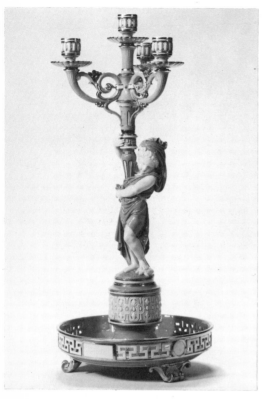

417. *Minton candelabra—centrepiece in celadon and white glaze Parian (c. 1876). Impressed name mark. 24 inches high. Many attractive designs occur in celadon and white in the 1870's.*

Godden of Worthing

418. *Minton's inlaid "Henri Deux" ware. By Charles Toft. Examples bear this artist's signature and are sometimes dated. All examples in this style are rare. The central vase was included in the 1878 Paris Exhibition. 22 inches high.*

City Museum & Art Gallery, Stoke-on-Trent

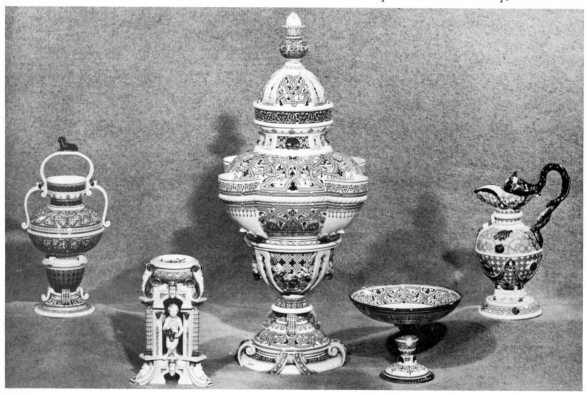

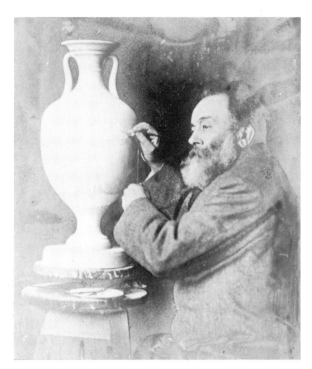

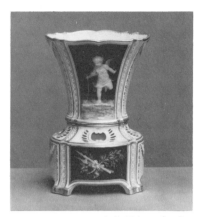

419. *M. L. Solon at work on a pâte-sur-pâte vase (see page* xxvi*), a contemporary photograph from the Wenger collection.*

420. *Minton vase (of a Sèvres form), decorated with pâte-sur-pâte panels, by M. L. Solon. Year cypher for 1898.* $6\frac{7}{8}$ *inches high.*
Victoria & Albert Museum

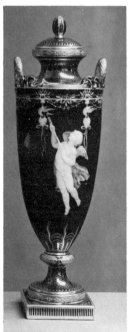

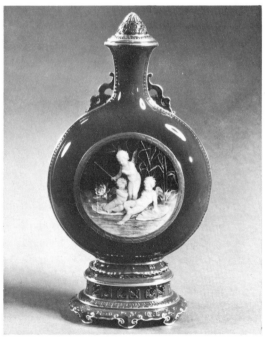

421. *Minton vase, decorated by M. L. Solon in his pâte-sur-pâte technique (see* Victorian Porcelain*), 1898.* $13\frac{1}{2}$ *inches high.*
Victoria & Albert Museum

422. *Minton vase with pâte-sur-pâte panel by L. Birks, one of several apprentices trained by M. L. Solon. Gold printed mark no. 2713, impressed "Mintons" name mark and year cypher for 1886.* $13\frac{1}{2}$ *inches high. For a full account of the expensive pâte-sur-pâte technique see* Victorian Porcelain, *Chapter 8.*

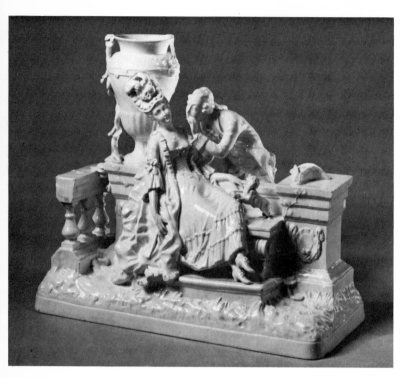

423. *Minton porcelain group, one of many decorative groups. One of Minton's registered designs bearing the diamond shape mark, see* Encyclopaedia of British Pottery and Porcelain Marks, *pages 526–7. Impressed name mark (c. 1876). 14½ inches long.*

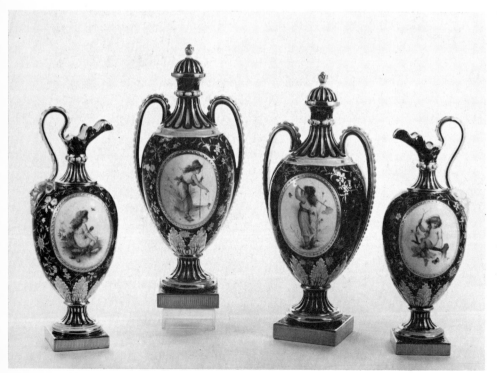

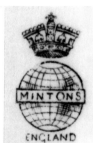

424. a. *Minton printed mark no. 2713. Without crown above (c. 1863–72). With crown, without "England" below (c. 1873–91). With "England" below (c. 1892–1912).*

424. *Set of Minton porcelain vases and ewers. The figure panels painted by A. Boullemier (signed) after designs by W. S. Coleman (c. 1885). Printed mark no. 2713 (see right). 12½ and 11 inches high.*

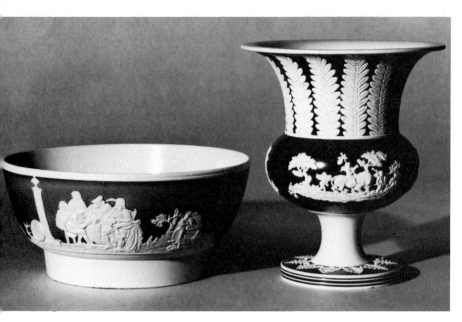

425. Stonewares of Turner-type, bearing the impressed mark of J. Mist of 82 Fleet Street, London. This name mark relates to the London selling agent, not to the manufacturer (c. 1810–15). Vase 7¾ inches high.

Godden of Worthing

MOORE BROS, LONGTON 1872–1905

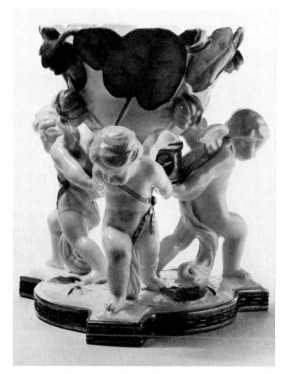

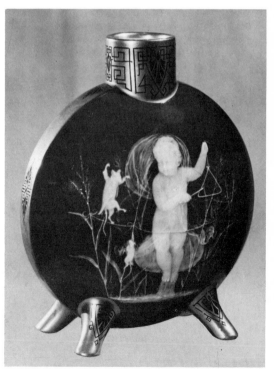

426. "Moore" (impressed marked) porcelain centrepiece of typical form—with cupids and lily leaves. This design was registered in 1873. 8 inches high.

Godden of Worthing

427. Moore Brothers (impressed name mark) vase, decorated in the cameo-like pâte-sur-pâte style (c. 1878–82). H. Sanders did this type of work for the Moore firm.

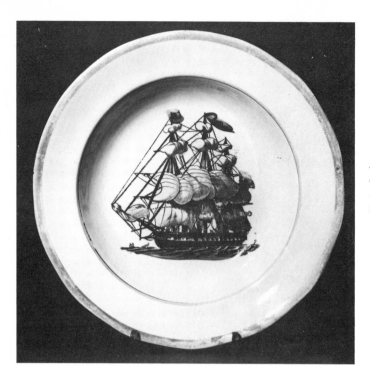

428. *Moore & Co (impressed marked) earthenware plate, made at the Wear Pottery, Sunderland (c. 1845–55). This firm continued to 1874. Most late wares are unmarked.*

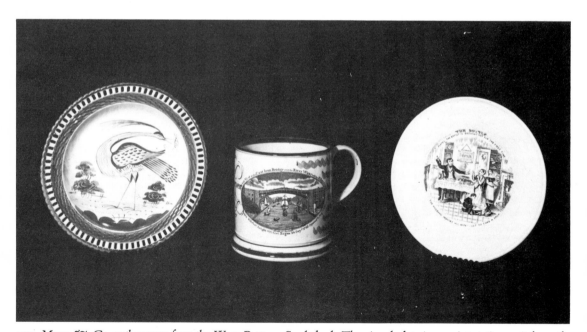

429. *Moore & Co earthenwares from the Wear Pottery, Sunderland. The pierced plate is very interesting as it bears the impressed mark "Moore & Co". Similar plates were made at Swansea (see Plate 564). The mug has a printed view of the Wear-mouth Bridge and incorporates the name "Moore & Co". 4¾ inches high. The printed plate has a moulded rim and is one of a series entitled "The Bottle". Printed and impressed marks (c. 1810–15, c. 1830, and c. 1850).*

Sunderland Museum

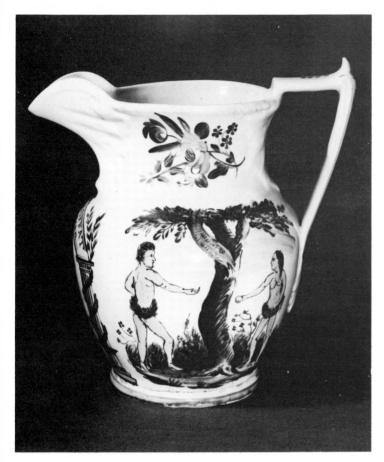

430. *Porcelain jug inscribed and dated "Musselburgh . . . 1827". Probably made at Musselburgh, Prestonpans or Portobello. Scottish ceramics rarely bear factory marks. 8½ inches high.*

Royal Scottish Museum, Edinburgh

J. MYATT, STAFFORDSHIRE POTTERY LATE EIGHTEENTH CENTURY

431. *"Myatt" (impressed marked) glazed redware (see page xiii) teapot, with applied relief motifs. Joseph Myatt was potting at Longton in the 1790's. 4⅜ inches high.*

Victoria & Albert Museum

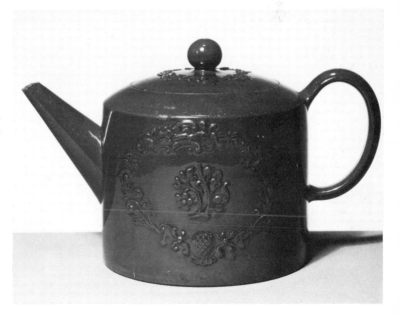

Nantgarw

The Nantgarw works in Wales were established on an experimental basis late in 1813 by William Billingsley (formerly of Derby and Pinxton) and Samuel Walker. W. W. Young was taken as a partner in 1814 and in this year the partners applied to the Board of Trade for Government aid. L. W. Dillwyn of the near-by Swansea works was asked to report on the Nantgarw project; he observed: "I found much reason for considering that the body was too nearly allied to glass to bear the necessary heat, and observed that nine-tenths of the articles were either shivered or more or less injured in shape by the firing. . . ." Nevertheless, it was apparent that the faults were capable of being rectified, and it was agreed in September 1814 that the Nantgarw concern be removed to the larger, better equipped, Swansea factory.

In about 1817 this arrangement was terminated, Billingsley and Walker returned to Nantgarw, where they continued to produce a delicate soft-paste porcelain until 1820, when the moulds, etc., were purchased by John Rose of the Coalport factory.

The Nantgarw porcelain, when correctly fired, was wonderfully translucent and mellow, but in gaining these properties the percentage of spoilt wares was very great, as the glassy body could not be fully controlled in the firing. The porcelain was in great demand by the London decorators, as it was the nearest English approach to the popular Sèvres china. Apart from the London decorated examples, finely painted tea, dessert, and dinner services and numerous other useful as well as ornamental objects were made and decorated at the Nantgarw works. The place-name mark "Nantgarw" occurs on some specimens, both impressed and printed. Reproductions have been made in the nineteenth and twentieth century, but once he has examined a true specimen and felt and seen the characteristic warm translucent body, the collector should not be deceived by later copies, with their harder body and wooden painting.

A wide range of specimens will be found in W. H. John's *Nantgarw Porcelain* (1948) and in E. M. Nance's *The Pottery and Porcelain of Swansea and Nantgarw* (1942).

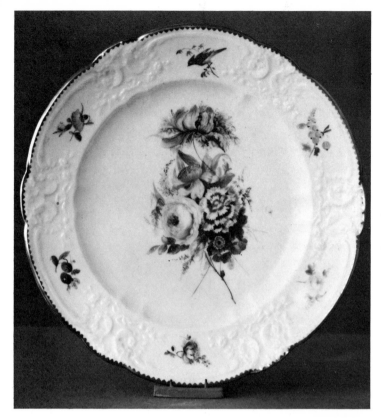

432. "Nant-garw, C W" (impressed marked plate). A typical and attractive specimen from this Welsh factory (c. 1813–22). 10 inches diameter. This moulded border was later used at Coalport and other factories.

Victoria & Albert Museum

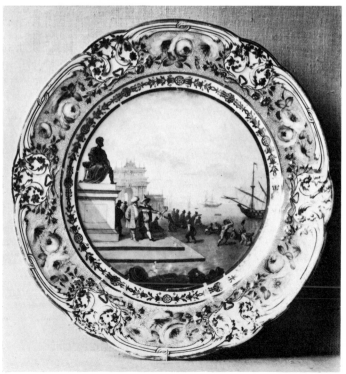

433. "Nant-garw, C W" (impressed marked) plate of superb quality. Nantgarw plates, etc., with ornate decoration are believed to have been sold in the white to London decorators and retailers, who finished them to order or to their own taste (c. 1820). 10 inches diameter.

Allen Collection, Victoria & Albert Museum

James Neale (& Co)

James Neale had been selling agent in London for Humphrey Palmer's Wedgwood-type earthenwares. On Palmer's failure in 1776, James Neale took over and continued the Church Works at Hanley.

Very good creamware basalt and jasper objects were made, the early examples of which are often marked "N", "NEALE" or "I. NEALE". From c. 1778 the mark was amended to "NEALE & CO", and this was continued through several partnerships to about 1795, although the title "Neale & Wilson" was sometimes used during the period 1784–95. The mark "Neale & Bailey" was also used c. 1790–1814, but this style was probably confined to goods sold at the retail shop in London as Robert Wilson took over and continued the Church Works in 1795.

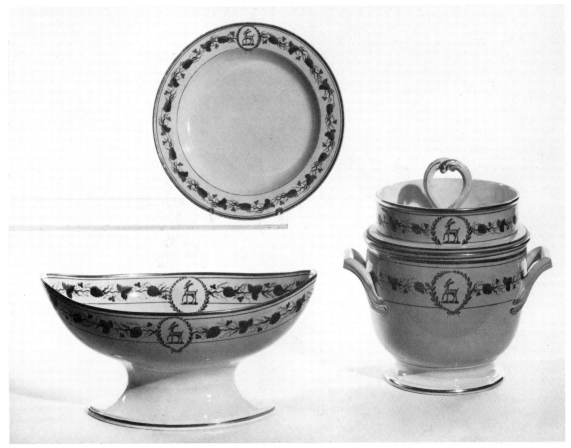

434. *Neale & Co creamware dessert service of simple Wedgwood-type pattern. Impressed marks nos. 2845, 2846, and the crown with "C" under with the addition of the name "Neale" (c. 1778–86). Fruit cooler 10¼ inches high.*

Godden of Worthing

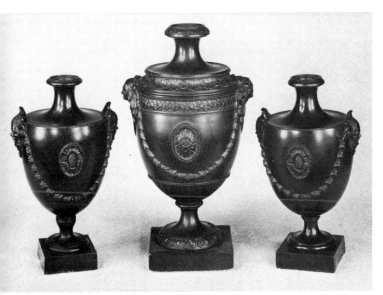

435. *J. Neale, Hanley (circular impressed marks). Basalt vases in the Wedgwood manner. The other side of these vases is decorated with figure subjects in oval panels (c. 1776–8). 12½ and 10 inches high.*

City Museum & Art Gallery, Stoke-on-Trent

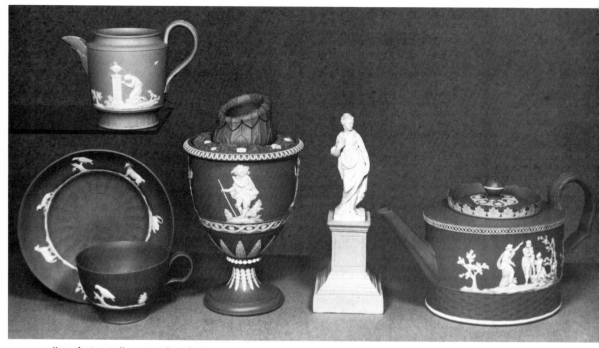

436. "Neale & Co" impressed marked jasper wares (see page xx) of fine quality. This form of mark was used by this Hanley firm from c. 1778 to at least 1788. Rare figure 7 inches high.

Victoria & Albert Museum

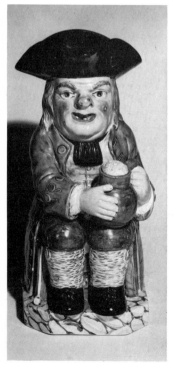

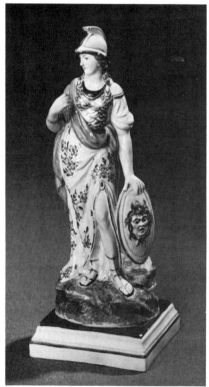

437. (Far left) Neale & Co (impressed marked) earthenware "Toby" jug (c. 1785). 10¼ inches high. "Toby" jugs were made by many potters, including Ralph Woods. Early examples have pleasing semi-translucent coloured glazes. After about 1790 the enamel colours are heavy and opaque.

Godden of Worthing

438. Neale & Co (impressed marked) earthenware figure of Minerva (c. 1778–86). 8 inches high.

City Museum & Art Gallery,
Stoke-on-Trent

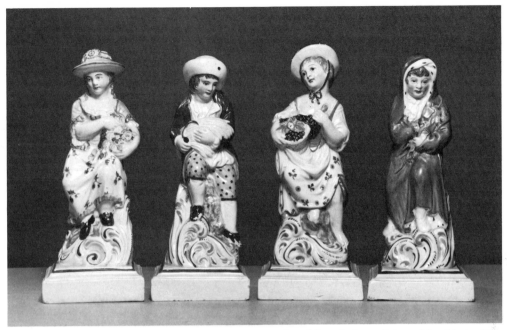

439. *The four seasons in cream-coloured earthenware. Impressed mark "Neale & Co" (c. 1780). 5¼ inches high.*
Fitzwilliam Museum, Cambridge

NEWCASTLE POTTERY, NORTHUMBERLAND EARLY NINETEENTH CENTURY

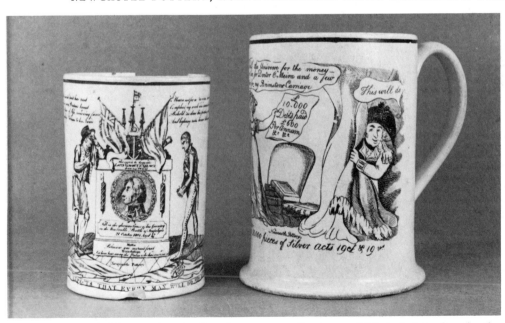

440. *Two rare marked "Newcastle Pottery" earthenware mugs. One laments Nelson's death in 1805, the other*
shows the Duke of York and Mrs Clarke "Burning the Books of Curious Arts . . ." (c. 1809).
Willett Collection, Brighton Museum

New Hall Company (Tunstall & Shelton, Staffordshire)

About 1781 Messrs Hollins, Warburton & Co purchased the patent rights of Richard Champion of Bristol to produce true or hard-paste porcelain from Cornish materials. Champion wrote in September 1781: "I have now entered into an agreement with ten Potters. . . ." The foremost working partners in the Staffordshire concern were Samuel Hollins, Anthony Keeling, Jacob Warburton, William Clowes, Charles Bagnall, and John Turner. At first production was tried at Tunstall, but by 1782, when Champion left for London, the production of porcelain was successfully established at "New Hall", Shelton. At various periods some of the partners left and others, notably John Daniel, joined the concern which in the nineteenth century traded as Hollins, Warburton, Daniel & Co.

The early porcelains were of hard paste and typical patterns comprised floral sprays (Plate 441) or mock Chinese figures in landscape. It must be noted that the traditional New Hall floral patterns were made by most contemporary potters and many examples are attributed to New Hall in error. The New Hall shapes (Plates 441-4) and hard porcelain should be studied. The early wares often bear pattern numbers, prefixed by "N" or "No" painted in a bold free manner (see Plate 441), never small and neat; in teasets only the larger pieces would be marked, not the cups and saucers. The highest number recorded on the early hard-paste porcelains is 940. A workman's mark reproduced as no. 4403 on page 745 of the companion *Encyclopaedia of British Pottery and Porcelain Marks* helps to identify much New Hall porcelain. Underglaze blue printing was practised at New Hall and a rare mark of a crowned lion rampant found on these pieces is now attributed to this factory (Plate 674).

A new type of bone china was introduced about 1812; this was softer than the earlier variety and comparable to that used by Chamberlain at Worcester and several of the leading Staffordshire firms. The shapes (Plate 444) also followed those then in vogue. Bat printed scenes, figure, floral, and fruit patterns were employed and some fine dessert sets were made (Plate 443). Most of these wares were unmarked and examples pass for Worcester or other popular wares. The printed mark of the words "New Hall" within a double circle was sparingly used, and the pattern numbers on the later bone china wares would seem to range from 1040 to about 2200. The New Hall factory in the main produced only useful wares, mainly tea services; some attractive jugs were also made. The works were offered for sale in 1831, but the business would seem to have continued, probably on a reduced scale, until 1835. In 1841 the premises were described as "all the places in bad repair . . . I do not consider it tenable in its present state. The ovens also are too large for the Hovels and all the sagger Houses are small and inconvenient."

The standard book is *New Hall and its Imitators* by D. Holgate (Faber, London, 1971); Mr G. E. A. Gray's contribution to *English Porcelain 1745-1850* (1965) is also most helpful, but much research remains to be done on the question of New Hall porcelain and the many contemporary potters who were producing very similar wares, and in this regard the recent book *Godden's Guide to English Porcelain* (Granada, London, 1978) will prove helpful.

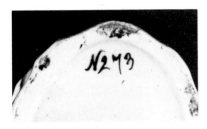

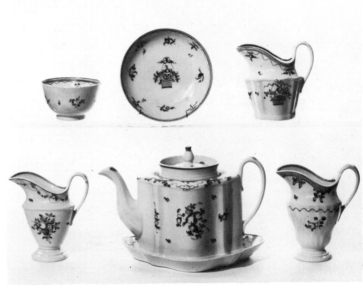

441. *New Hall porcelain teawares of typical shapes and painted patterns. Painted pattern numbers—"No 173", "N 241", "195", etc. See typical example (above). The teapot is pattern no. 195; another example of this form and decoration is dated 1798. Teapot 9½ inches long. The stand is separate (c. 1790–1800).*

Godden of Worthing

442. *New Hall porcelain teaset, decorated in gold only (c. 1790–1800). Pattern no. 52 painted on main pieces. Teapot 6 inches high.*

Godden of Worthing

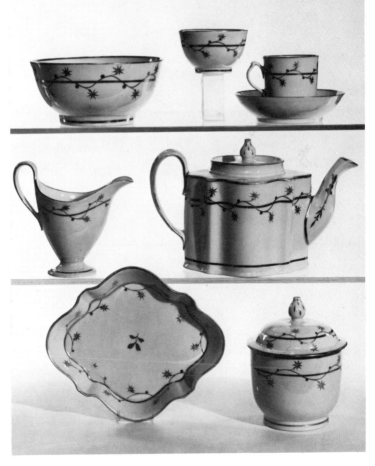

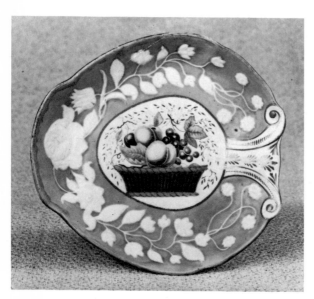

443. *New Hall dish from a dessert service, with relief moulded floral border. Printed mark—"New Hall" within double circle* (c. 1810). *7¾ inches long.*

City Museum & Art Gallery, Stoke-on-Trent

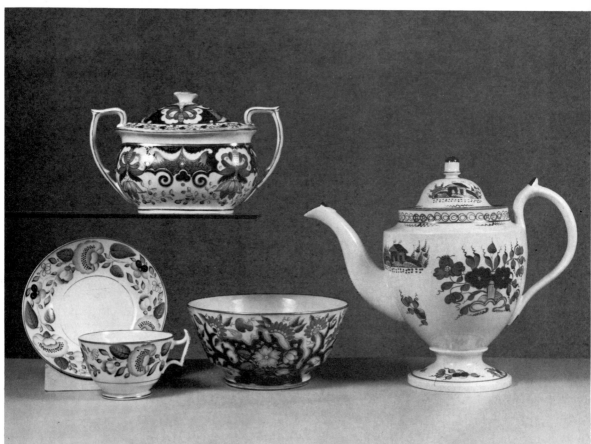

444. *New Hall porcelains, bearing the printed name within a double-lined circle (mark no. 2875). The coffee pot is rare, the other items were parts of tea services* (c. 1812–20). *Coffee pot 8¾ inches high.*

Victoria & Albert Museum

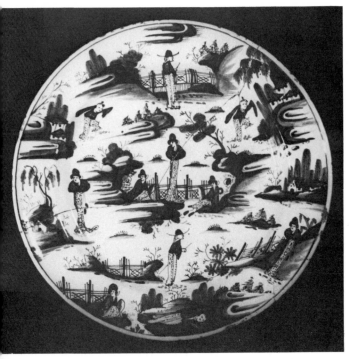

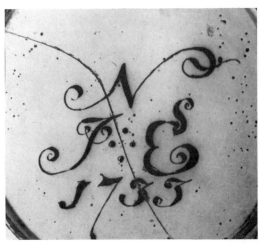

445 & a. Bristol delft-type earthenware (see page xi) dish, painted in polychrome by John Niglett. Signed (?) with initials and dated 1733 (see detail of reverse). 14¼ inches diameter.

Bristol City Art Gallery

W. NORTHEN, LONDON c. 1847-92

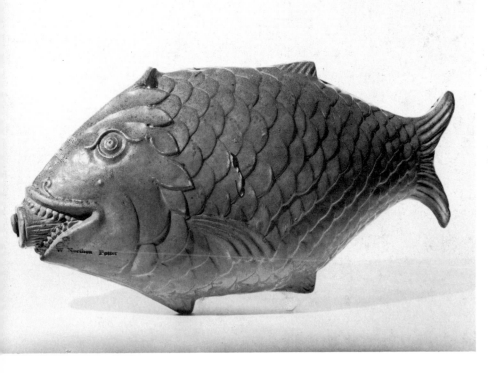

446. A stone hot-water (?) bottle made by W. Northen of Vauxhall, Lambeth (impressed mark), for the Dolphin Hotel, Shoreham, Sussex (impressed name). Northen potted from c. 1847 to c. 1892. 15½ inches long.

Marlipins Museum, Shoreham, Sussex

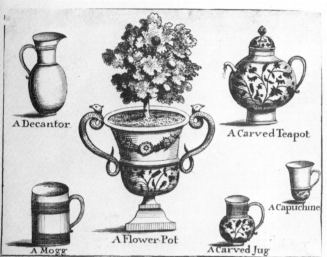

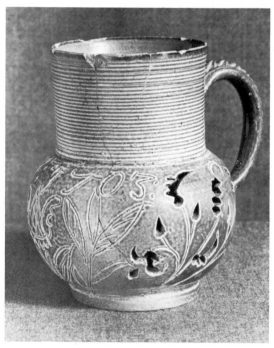

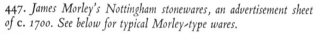

Such as have Occasion for these Sorts of Pots commonly called Stone-Ware, or for such as are of any other Shape not here Represented may be furnished w.th them by the Maker James Morley at y̆ Pot-House i̇ Nottingham

447. *James Morley's Nottingham stonewares, an advertisement sheet of c. 1700. See below for typical Morley-type wares.*

Bodleian Library, Oxford

448. *Nottingham stoneware (see page xii) mug with incised inscription "Nottm. 1703". Compare with James Morley's Advertisement "A Carved Jug". 3⅞ inches high*

Victoria & Albert Museum

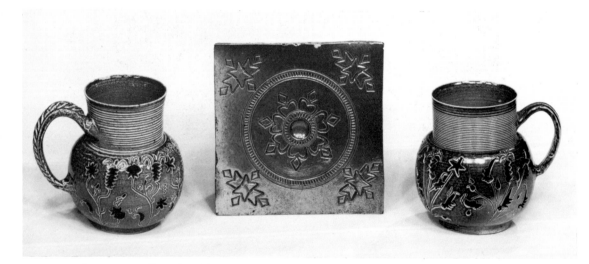

449. *Nottingham stoneware "carved jugs" similar to one depicted in James Morley's advertisement (c. 1700). Approximately 4 inches high. The tile was originally in Charles Morley's house; this Nottingham potter was entered in the list of burgesses in 1723. 5¼ inches square.*

E. N. Stretton, Esq.

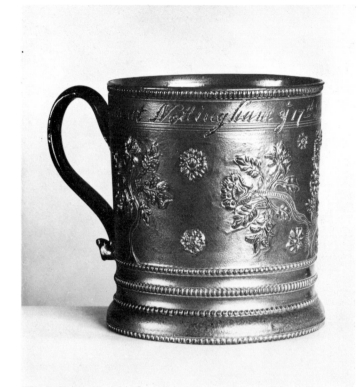

450. *Nottingham stoneware mug with incised inscription—"Made at Nottingham ye 17th day of August. A.D. 1771".*

Victoria & Albert Museum

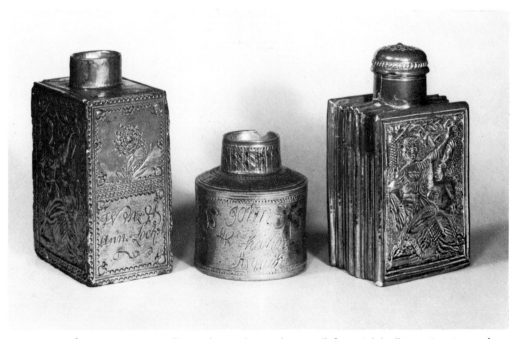

451. *Nottingham stoneware tea-caddies with incised potters' names* (left to right): *"Wm & Ann Lockett, Janr ye 6. 1755", "John Asquith, maker, 1756", and a moulded caddy by William Lockett dated 1764. Other Nottingham wares sometimes have the place-name added.*

Nottingham Museum

255

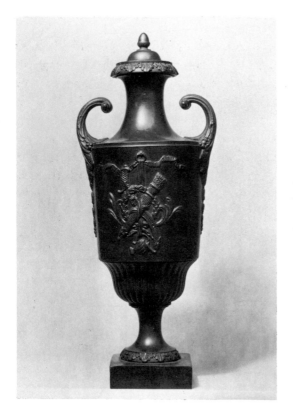

452. *Basalt vase with impressed mark "Made by H Palmer, Hanley, Staffordse". Figure panel on front signed "Voyez Sculpt 1769". 12 inches high.* See Transactions of the English Ceramic Circle, *vol. 5, part 1.*

British Museum

PEARSON AND CO, WHITTINGHAM MOOR c. 1805+

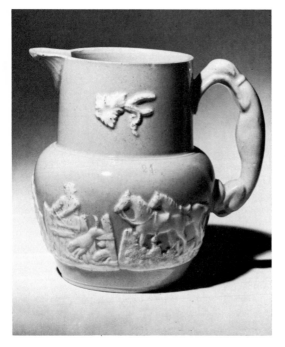

453. *Stoneware jug impressed marked—Pearson & Co, Whittington Moor Potteries, near Chesterfield (dated 1890). Similar jugs were also made at earlier periods. 6½ inches high.*

The Pinxton porcelain works in Derbyshire were established by John Coke and William Billingsley (the latter from the Derby factory) in 1796. In April 1799 the partnership was dissolved, Billingsley going to Mansfield where he started a decorating establishment. Coke continued the Pinxton works until *c.* 1803 when John Cutts took over and continued until the closure in or about 1813.

Typical Pinxton porcelain is similar to puce-marked Derby porcelain of the 1790–1800 period; the body is often very translucent, the glaze is warm and friendly, the shapes are restrained and tasteful. Attractive landscape painting and pleasant floral patterns were employed. Marked specimens are rare, impressed letters occur and the written pattern number is sometimes prefixed by the cursive letter "P" (see Plate 454a). A painted crescent and star mark or an arrow-like device were occasionally used, as was the word "Pinxton", but this is extremely rare. The shapes are a good guide to Pinxton porcelain, the very narrow teapot is rather similar to Barr Worcester but of a warmer, more refined porcelain.

Recent research and discoveries are recorded in *The Connoisseur* magazine of January and February 1963 and the late C. L. Exley's *The Pinxton China Factory* (1963).

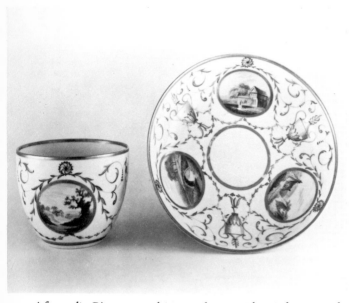

454. *A fine quality* Pinxton *porcelain cup and saucer with typical scenic panels and attractive tracery in sepia. Pattern number mark, see detail (right).*

I. M. Booth Collection

454. a. *Base of scenic panelled cup showing typical form of painted pattern number with letter "P" prefix.*

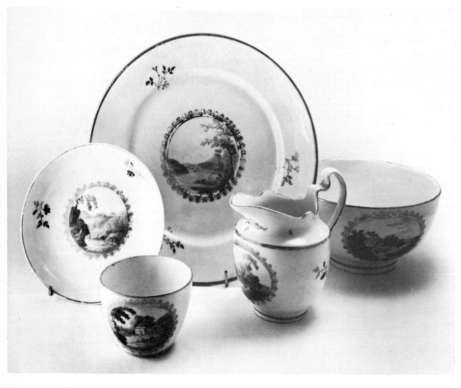

455. Pinxton *porcelain teawares, painted with panels of local views. The creamer shape is typical of this factory. The Pinxton gilding is normally partly worn on useful wares (c. 1795–1800).*

I. M. Booth Collection

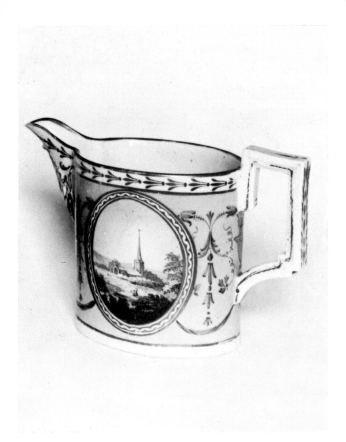

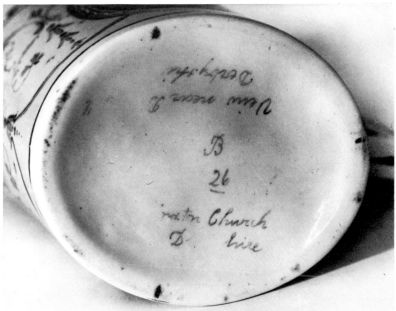

456. *Pinxton porcelain creamer of fine quality, typical form and decoration, showing views of Pinxton and Breadsall churches (see right for detail of base). This piece may have been made or decorated at Mansfield (see Plate 52).*

Mr & Mrs R. Coke-Steel Collection

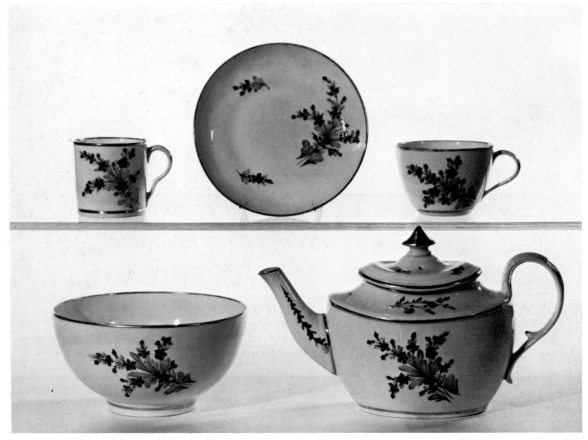

457. *Pinxton porcelain teawares in a soft Derby-like porcelain. The coffee-can handle should be noted as it identifies unmarked Pinxton coffee cans and matching teawares (c. 1796-1800). Teapot 6 inches high.*

Godden of Worthing

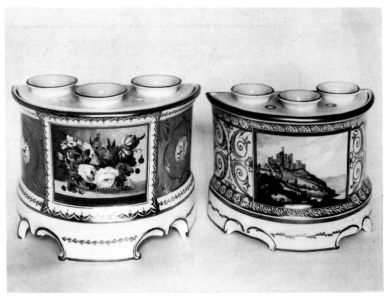

458. *Two very rare Pinxton crocus pots with loose tops. The form of moulded base appears to be peculiar to Pinxton (c. 1796-1800). 7 inches and 7½ inches high. Both one of pairs.*
Mr & Mrs R. Coke-Steel Collection (floral pot)
Mrs & Mrs I. M. Booth Collection (scenic pot)

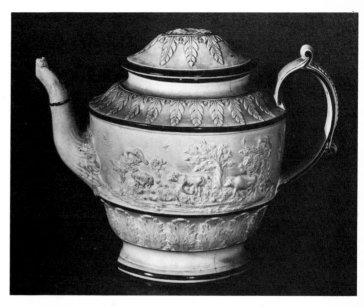

459. *"B. Plant, 1814" (incised mark) moulded stoneware teapot of fine quality. 8 inches high. This is probably a unique marked example by Benjamin Plant of Lane End, Longton (c. 1780–1820).*

R. H. & S. L. Plant Ltd

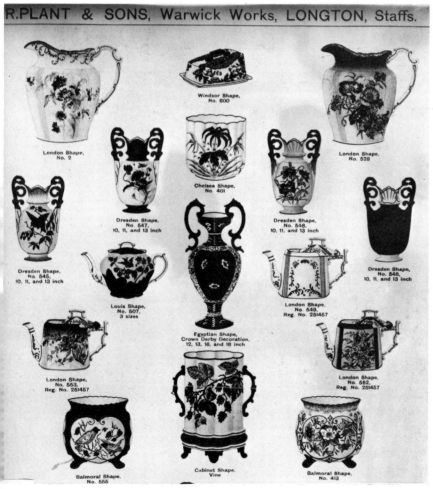

460. *R. Plant & Sons advertisement of 1895, showing typical forms and patterns of the period. This firm potted at Longton from 1895 to 1901.*

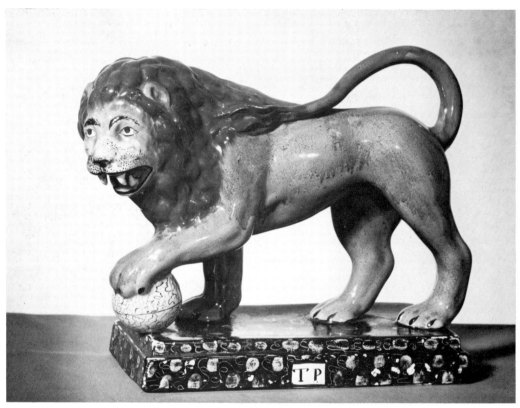

461. *Thomas Plant earthenware lion, signed with initial. Many other potters made similar lion models but specimens are seldom marked* (c. 1825–50). *8 inches high.*

R. H. & S. L. Plant Ltd

Plymouth porcelain, like that of Bristol, is hard paste (see page xvii). The works were established by William Cookworthy in or slightly before 1768. A small mug in the British Museum is painted in underglaze blue with the Arms of the City of Plymouth and is dated 14 March 1768; this specimen proves that the works were able to produce marketable ware by that date. Within three days, on 17 March 1768, a patent was taken out by William Cookworthy "for making a Kind of Porcelain Newly Invented".

The early wares were, in the main, painted in underglaze blue with floral or Chinese-type patterns; in addition there were enamelled wares often painted with floral patterns or with exotic birds in landscape. Figures and groups and rare animal and bird models were also made.

The standard mark was the chemical sign for tin—the joined numerals 2 and 4 (mark no. 3071). The "T" or "To" mark used by the much-travelled modeller known as Tebo also occurs on Plymouth porcelain (see page 320). The Plymouth works ceased production in 1770 when William Cookworthy transferred the works to Bristol, but the Plymouth tin mark may well have been continued at Bristol until about 1772. For further information see F. Severne Mackenna's *Cookworthy's Plymouth and Bristol Porcelain* (1946).

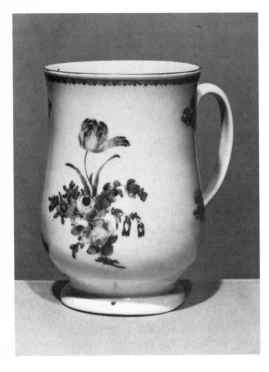

462. Plymouth (hard paste) porcelain tankard, bearing the painted mark of a "2" and "4" joined (mark no. 3071). The flower painting and simple gilt border are typical of Plymouth porcelains (c. 1768–70). 6 inches high.

Albert Amor Ltd

463. Plymouth (hard paste) porcelains (c. 1768–70), bearing the tin mark—"2" and "4" joined. The mortar and inkwell are painted in the typical inky underglaze blue colour. The sauce boat is inscribed in red —"Mr Wm Cookworthy's Factory. Plymouth. 1770".

Plymouth Museum & Art Gallery

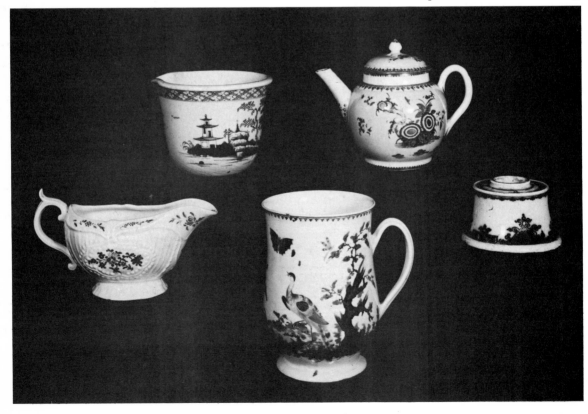

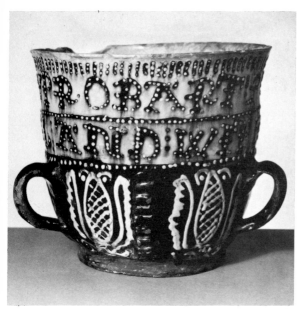

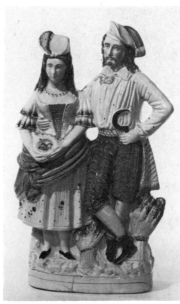

464. (Far left) *Staffordshire slip decorated Posset cup, inscribed "Robart Pool mad this cup and with a guid Poset fil" (late seventeenth, early eighteenth century). 8 inches high.*

Victoria & Albert Museum

465. *Poole & Unwin earthenware cottage ornament of a type normally unmarked. This firm potted at the Cornhill Works, Longton, from c. 1871 to 1876. Initial mark. 15 inches high.*

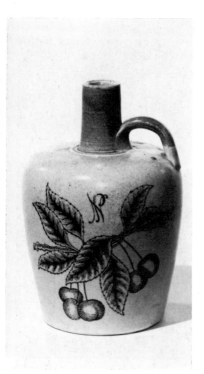

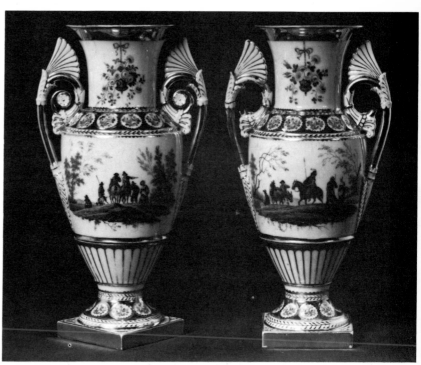

466. *Port Dundas Pottery Co, Glasgow (impressed marked), stoneware bottle, decorated with a printing process introduced c. 1874. 7 inches high.*

467. *Paris porcelain vases decorated in London by John Powell of Wimpole Street. Each with long inscription (see mark no. 3130A) (c. 1816–17). 10⅛ inches high.*

Godden of Worthing

Pratt Wares

The name Pratt is associated with a range of attractive relief moulded earthenware—jugs, teapots, figures, etc., in which the relief motifs are picked out in colours. Plates 468–9 show very rare jugs of this type marked P R A T T. Most specimens are unmarked and many were undoubtedly made by other potters, both in Staffordshire, the Northern factories, and in Scotland (see page xxii). These illustrated marked specimens were probably made by William Pratt of Lane Delph *c.* 1780–99.

William Pratt's son, Felix, established his own works in 1810 and in 1818 formed a partnership with his brother Richard. The resulting firm of F. & R. Pratt (& Co) (Ltd) of Fenton continued into the twentieth century. The early wares were mainly unmarked, but from 1840 when "& Co" was added to the firm's style several different printed marks have been used, all including the name or initials of the firm. Tasteful Etruscan-pattern vases and other earthenwares were made from about 1845 onwards (Plate 470).

Messrs. F. & R. Pratt's name is mainly associated with a system of multicolour printing extensively used on decorative pot lids, dessert services, jugs, teawares, etc. This type of ware (Colour Plate X) was shown at the 1851 Exhibition and was the main concern of the firm for many years, but most specimens are unmarked. The name or initials of Jesse Austin, the designer, appear on several of the best multicolour printed patterns. From about 1850 to 1900 few examples of Pratt's earthenwares bear a factory mark. For further information on this aspect of F. & R. Pratt & Co's wares, see G. Godden's *Antique China and Glass under £5* (1966), H. G. Clarke's *Underglaze Colour Picture Prints on Staffordshire Pottery* or *The Pictorial Pot Lid Book* (1970), and *The Price Guide to Pot Lids and other Underglaze Colour Prints on Pottery* by A. Ball (1970). Mr Ball is Hon. Sec. of the Pot Lid Circle which publishes informative "newsletters" and holds meetings in various parts of the country. Mr Ball's address is 15 Arden Road, Nuneaton, Warwickshire.

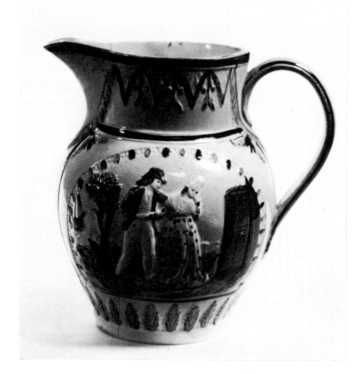

468. *Moulded earthenware jug, bearing the rare impressed mark "Pratt" (c. 1790–1800). 6 inches high.*

British Museum

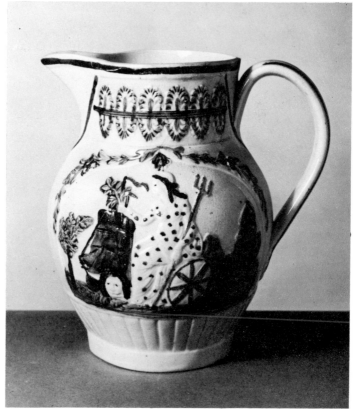

469. *"Pratt" (impressed marked) moulded earthenware jug of a type also made by many other potters in Staffordshire, Yorkshire, etc. This is a very rare marked specimen (c. 1790–5). 5 inches high.*

Victoria & Albert Museum

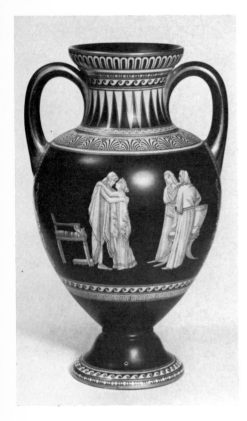

470. *Pratt earthenware vase with classical figure pattern. Printed mark with title in full—"F & R Pratt & Co. Fenton" with crown and wording "Manufacturers to H R H Prince Albert". This mark was used on the best quality pieces during the 1850's. 10 inches high.*

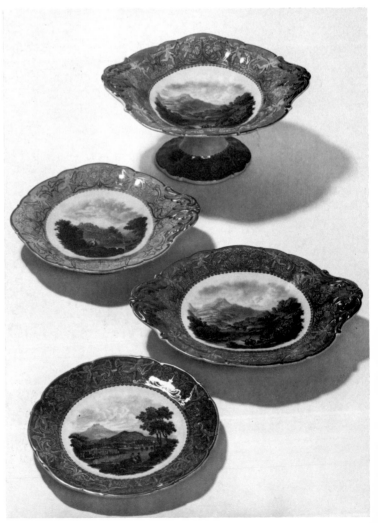

471. *F. & R. Pratt earthenware dessert service, unmarked, but the original drawings for the multi-coloured printed landscape panels were in the factory pattern book. These drawings are by Jesse Austin (c. 1850–60). Comport 6½ inches high.*

Godden of Worthing

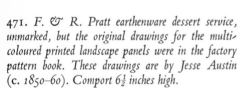

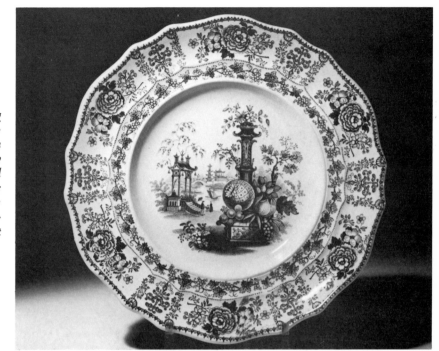

472. Transfer printed plate, bearing the initial mark of Read, Clementson & Anderson of Shelton (c. 1836). This is one of the few examples where the short-lived duration of a partnership enables pottery to be dated to the year by means of a mark. Many Staffordshire firms were of very short duration.

GEORGE RICHARDSON, WROTHAM c. 1642–77

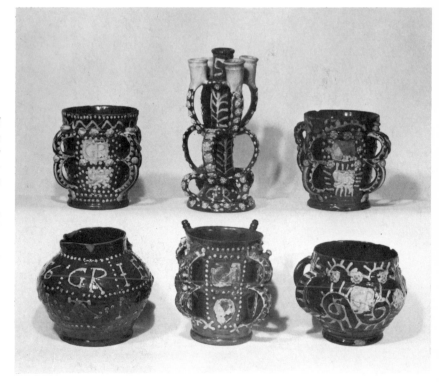

473. Wrotham slip decorated earthenwares (see page xii) with the initials G.R. attributed to the potter George Richardson (see Transactions of the English Ceramic Circle, vol. 3, part 2). Dated from (top left to right) 1654, 1656, 1659, 1656, 164?, 1675. Candlestick 10¼ inches high.

Fitzwilliam Museum, Cambridge

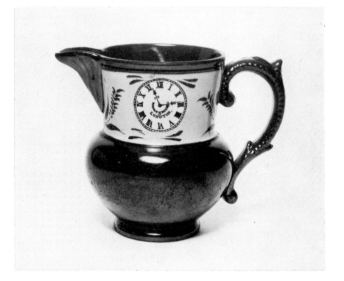

474. Copper lustre jug, marked "Riddle & Bryan, Longton" on clock-face (c. 1835–40). 4¼ inches high. Marked *lustre ware is extremely rare.*

RIDGWAY AND ROBEY, c. 1839

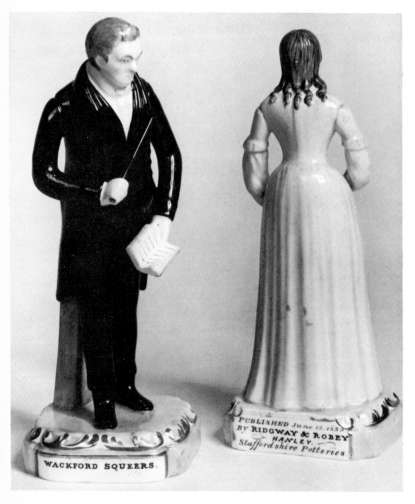

WACKFORD SQUEERS.

PUBLISHED June 15, 1839
BY RIDGWAY & ROBEY
HANLEY.
Staffordshire Potteries

475. Ridgway & Robey character figures in porcelain, from a very rare series published in June 1839. Printed mark on back of base. 8½ and 8 inches high.

The Ridgway family of Shelton potters produced many fine earthenwares and porcelains during the nineteenth century. Their history is rather involved. About 1792 Job and George Ridgway potted at the Bell works at Shelton; from *c.* 1793 to *c.* 1799 the partnership traded as Ridgway, Smith & Ridgway, but from 1799 to 1802 the firm again became that of Job & George Ridgway. In 1802 the two brothers split up and Job built the Cauldon Place works at Shelton; Job's two sons, John and William, then joined the company and succeeded their uncle at the Bell works.

Both the Bell works and the Cauldon Place works produced fine quality earthenwares (with very good blue printed designs), stone china, and porcelains. Their dinner services are noteworthy for their general excellence and durability. Many of the Bell works services bear marks incorporating the title "J. & W. Ridgway" or "J. & W.R." or "J.W.R.". Such examples predate 1830, for in this year the two brothers separated.

William Ridgway continued at the Bell works to 1848, using the style "William Ridgway & Co" or "William Ridgway Son & Co" (*c.* 1838–48). In 1830 John Ridgway joined his father at the Cauldon Place works. His earthenwares, stone china, and porcelain were of the highest quality. He was appointed potter to Queen Victoria and his standard printed mark comprises the Royal Arms with the initials "J.R." placed very small below the central arms motif. In 1840 "& Co" was added. The firm of John Ridgway & Co continued until 1855 when it was succeeded by Ridgway, Bates & Co. The firm of Brown-Westhead, Moore & Co acquired the works in 1862 and were in turn taken over by Cauldon Ltd in 1905.

Recently discovered pattern books of the John & William Ridgway period (1814–30) and those subsequently used by John Ridgway at Cauldon Place and by William Ridgway at the Bell works, indicate that most wares before about 1840 were unmarked. Further research will show that a fine range of Rockingham, Spode, and Worcester *type* wares were made by Ridgways. Sample designs from the early Ridgway pattern books are reproduced in Plates 480, 481a, 483. Unmarked porcelains identified as early Ridgway by means of the original pattern books are shown in Plates 477–9, 481, 484. The standard work on Ridgway wares is G. Godden's *The Illustrated Guide to Ridgway Porcelains* (Barrie & Jenkins, London, 1972).

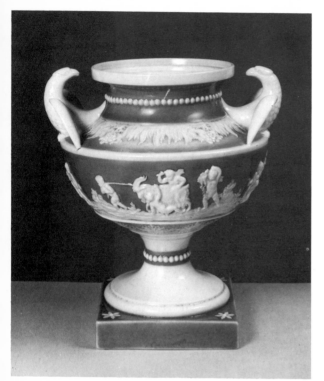

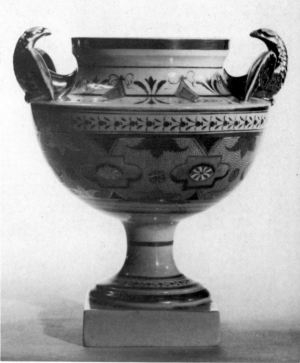

476. *Two early Ridgway porcelain sauce tureens (covers missing) from dessert services. Very rare impressed mark "Ridgway &*
Sons" (c. 1808–13). 6½ inches high. Example on left.

Victoria & Albert Museum

J. AND W. RIDGWAY, c. 1814–30

477. *Fine quality Ridgway porcelain sauce tureen from a dessert set. Painted pattern number—562—which matches the design in the factory pattern book. This typical shape should be noted as it will identify other unmarked Ridgway specimens (c. 1810–15). 6 inches high.*

Godden of Worthing

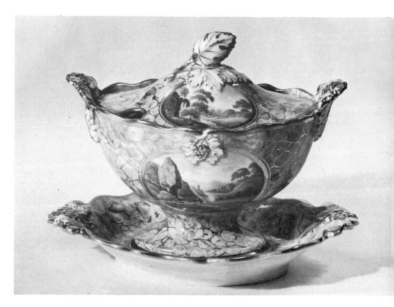

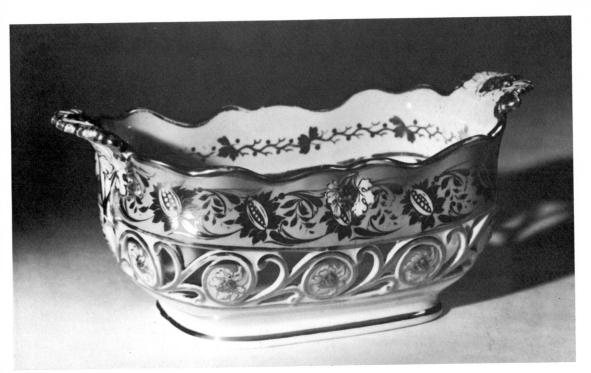

478. Early J. & W. Ridgway fruit basket of a type found in fine quality dessert services. Painted pattern no. 710 which matches this design in the original pattern book (c. 1814–20). 9¾ inches long.

Miss M. A. Beasley Collection

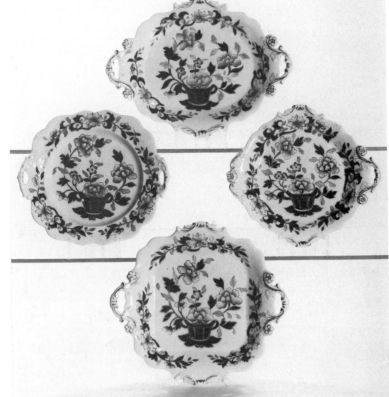

479. Part of a porcelain dessert service by John & William Ridgway, showing typical dish forms with Ridgway's two-handled plate (left). Dark portions of the pattern are in underglaze blue. Pattern no. 1119 matching the original pattern book (c. 1814–20). Top dish 11½ by 8½ inches.

Godden of Worthing

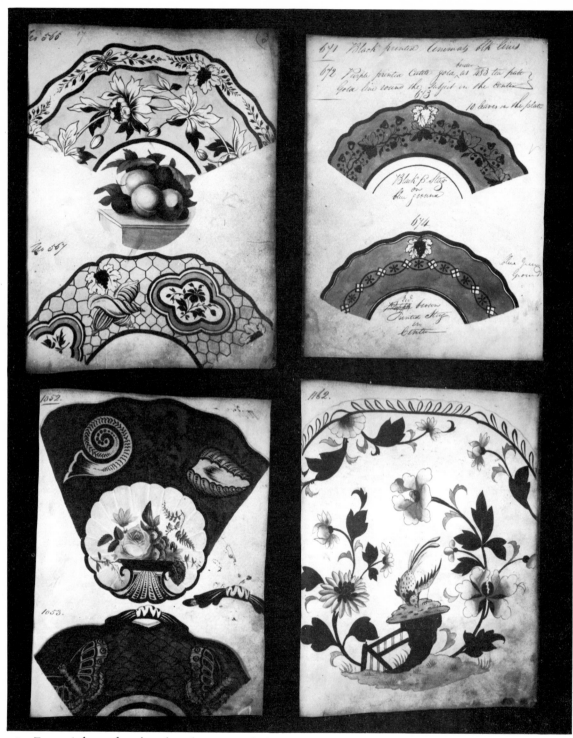

480. Four typical pages from the early Ridgway pattern books, the survival of which enables the unmarked Ridgway wares—both earthenware and porcelain—to be identified. The early plates with relief modelled grapes in the border are shown in patterns 566/7 and 673/4. Many of the plates (forming part of fine dessert services) have printed centres, as noted in patterns 671/4. Other patterns 1052/3, etc., are finely painted and gilt. Note the handled plate shown in pattern 1053.

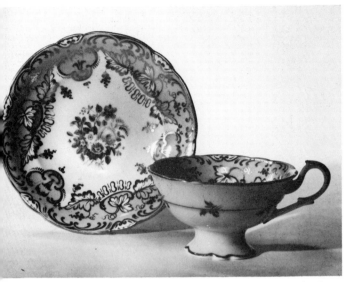

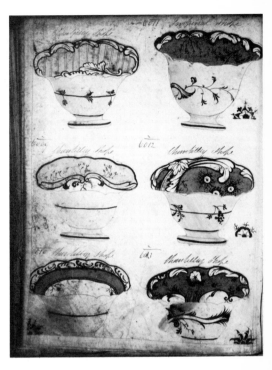

481 & a. *Ridgway cup and saucer of a type often attributed to the Rockingham factory in error. Pattern no. 2/7196 which agrees with the Ridgway pattern book, a sample page of which is reproduced* (right).

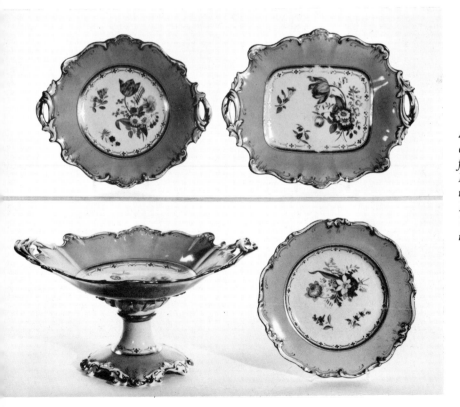

482. *John Ridgway porcelain dessert service, showing typical forms of the 1835–40 period. Printed Royal Arms mark no. 3258 with initials J.R. under. John Ridgway separated from his brother William in 1830. Comport 7¾ inches high.*

Godden of Worthing

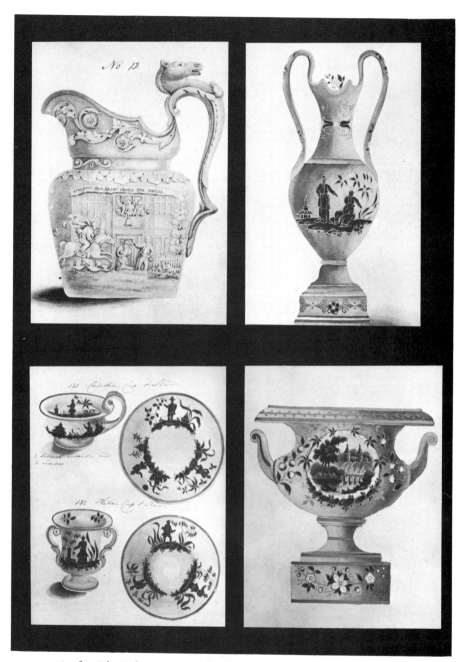

483. In 1830 John Ridgway separated from his brother William, who continued the Church and the Bell Works at Shelton (Hanley) formerly worked by the partnership. The pottery produced by William Ridgway from 1830 to 1854 is often unmarked, except for moulded stoneware jugs (Plate 485). The above four pages from William Ridgway's first pattern book show the attractive earthenwares made. The body is often tinted a delicate light blue, the enamel colours are often raised in slight relief.

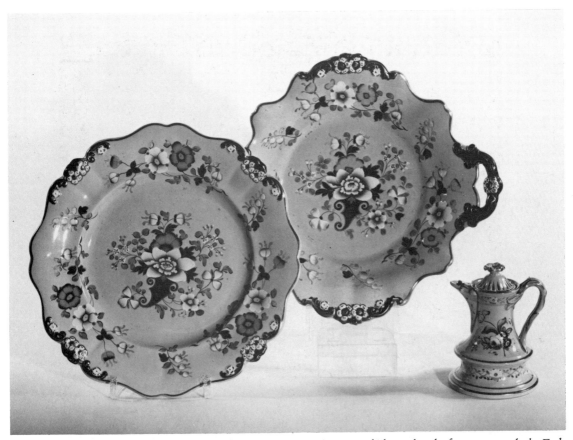

484. *Plate and dish from a William Ridgway dessert service. Pattern no. 57 which matches the factory pattern book. Early William Ridgway wares are unmarked. This plate and dish form should be noted as they will identify other unmarked dessert sets. Toy coffee pot, pattern no. 195, 4¼ inches high.*

Godden of Worthing

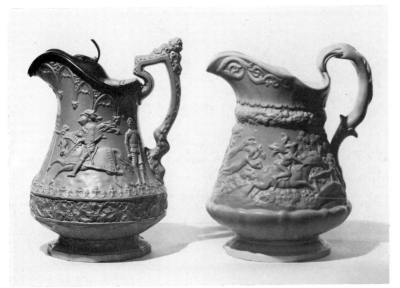

485. *William Ridgway's moulded stoneware jugs. (Left) Impressed mark "Published by W. Ridgway, Son & Co. Hanley. September 1st 1840". (Right) Impressed mark "Published by W. Ridgway & Co. Hanley. October 1st 1835". 9¼ inches high.*

These moulded jugs were made in various sizes. The impressed "Published by . . ." marks give the date that the design was registered. The firm of "W. Ridgway, Son & Co" was separate from the parent firm; its period was 1838–48.

277

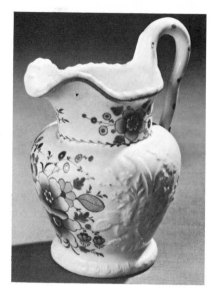

486. *Porcelain jug with moulded name mark "Riley" and date 1823. Many similar jugs are unmarked but are of this period.* 4½ *inches high.*

City Museum & Art Gallery, Stoke-on-Trent

RING AND CO (RING AND CARTER), BRISTOL *c.* 1789–1813

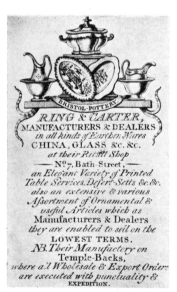

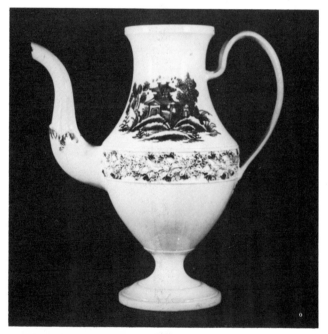

487. *Bristol earthenwares shown on Ring & Carter trade card of c. 1793–1813. The oval dish with Chinese-type scene was painted in underglaze blue, similar patterns were produced by other potters of the period.*

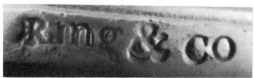

488. *Ring & Co (impressed marked) Bristol creamware coffee pot, Chinese type scene painted in underglaze blue, similar to oval dish shown in trade card (left). Marked examples are very rare (c. 1789–1800).*

Bristol City Art Gallery

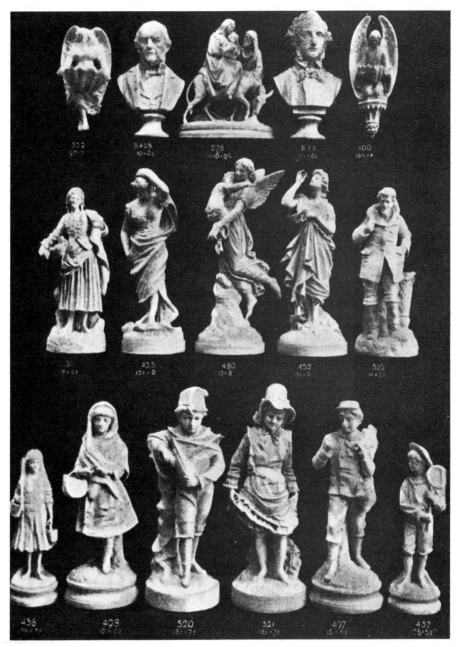

489. *Robinson & Leadbeater's advertisement of 1896, showing typical Parian figures, etc., most of which were unmarked. Rare examples bear the initials R & L within an oval. Messrs Robinson & Leadbeater of Stoke specialized in the production of inexpensive moulded Parian figures and ornaments of which they made a vast quantity from 1864 (see page xxv).*

The Rockingham or Swinton Works

The earthenware works at Swinton in Yorkshire was established about 1745, but the early wares are unmarked and cannot be identified with certainty.

In 1778 Thomas Bingley took over the concern and traded as Thomas Bingley & Co (the other partners being John (and William from 1786) Brameld and a Mr Sharpe). In 1785 an important link was forged with the Leeds factory when the principal partners were John & Joshua Green and William Hartley (partners also in the Leeds concern). At this period the Swinton firm traded under the title Green, Bingley & Co, later to become Greens, Hartley & Co. The pattern books were similar to those issued by the Leeds Pottery; price lists of 1796 record the main wares as ". . . all sorts of Earthenware, Cream Coloured or Queen's, Nankin Blue, Tortoise Shell, Fine Egyptian Black, Brown China &c. &c. All the above sorts enamelled, printed or ornamented with gold or silver."

In 1806 the Leeds partnership was dissolved, and John and William Brameld continued as Brameld & Co, using as a mark the impressed word "BRAMELD" (usually with various small crosses or numerals after). William Brameld died in 1813 and he was then succeeded by his brother Thomas, who was later assisted by his younger brothers, John Wager and George Frederic. The Rockingham trade had prospered and expanded by the early 1820's and it was largely due to their export trade, in particular that with Russia, that the firm faced serious monetary difficulties by 1825, due to the fact that they could not get payment for goods supplied; this resulted in the firm becoming insolvent in 1825. After creditors meetings early in 1826 and after the Pottery had been advertised, Earl Fitzwilliam, of the Rockingham estate, guaranteed a large sum of money to enable the Bramelds to continue and give employment to their former employees. From this period the Earl's crest—a griffin—and the name Rockingham were used as marks on the Brameld or "Rockingham" wares.

At this period too, porcelain, as opposed to the former earthenwares, was introduced. A cup in the Rotherham Museum is the earliest documented specimen; it is marked "Rockingham China Works, Swinton 1826". It is the porcelain ware that most collectors today associated with the name Rockingham.

Rockingham porcelain is remarkably soft and mellow. Apart from useful wares, figures, animal models, ornate vases and baskets were also made, as were some charming figures, groups and busts in unglazed white (bisque) porcelain (Plate 493). From *c.* 1826 the Griffin crest of Earl Fitzwilliam was used as a mark. At first this was printed in red but, from 1830, it occurs in puce with the addition of the words "Brameld. Royal Rockingham Works" and/or "Manufacturer to the King".

So expensively decorated were the finer wares and so soft the porcelain (with resulting costly failure in the firing) that the concern, with its rather incompetent management, could not compete with the strong competition from the more commercial Staffordshire and Worcester firms, and in 1842 the Rockingham works were closed. Recent research by Mr A. A. Eaglestone and Mr T. A. Lockett has led to the discovery of some factory records and notices of the sale of remaining stock in May 1842. These point to the fact that earthenware as well as porcelain was made up to the closure in 1842. The closing down sale notices are most interesting as they list articles of both china (porcelain) and earthenware:

The valuable *Stock of China* which embraces Dinner and Dessert Services, Breakfast, Tea and Coffee equipages; 250 dozens of China plates and Dishes; 300 dozens of tea and Breakfast cups and saucers, milk jugs, slop and sugar bowls, Cream ewers, Water ewers, Jugs etc. A variety of scent Jars, Vases and other decorative articles including some beautifully finished Cabinet specimens.

The Earthenware which is very extensive comprehends a general assortment of Table Ware including 750 dozens in various patterns of Dishes, Plates, Drainers, Vegetable Dishes, Sauce Tureens, Cheese Trays, Salad Bowls, Bakers &c; 190 sets Chamber Services, Slop Jars, Water Jugs; 400 dozens of Tea Plates; Breakfast cups and Saucers in great variety; 70 dozens of Tea Plates; 100 dozens of White Bowls; 150 dozens of Pints and Mugs; 180 dozens of Jelly cans, Preserve Jars, Potting Pots; 80 dozens of Sauce Boats, Mustards; 18 dozens of Dahlia Stands, Eye Baths; 18 dozens of Feeding Boats; 17 dozens of Mortars and Pestles, and Paint Slabs, Jugs, Basins &c and every article for domestic purposes.

From the 1830's Brameld & Co had a London retail establishment, first in Vauxhall Bridge Road and later at "The Griffin" in Piccadilly, at the top of the Haymarket, although other retailers also stocked their goods, particularly the very popular Rockingham teapots (Plate 490).

The collector must be warned that reproductions exist both in hard Continental porcelain and in English bone china; these copies bear a printed Griffin mark. The collector of Rockingham will also be offered as Rockingham nineteenth-century, porcelain that has never been near the factory. Before the new collector becomes acquainted with the Rockingham body and known documented shapes, he should reject all specimens bearing a painted pattern number higher than 2/100, as recent research suggests that true Rockingham pattern numbers range up to 1559 with a subsequent series running from 2/1 to at least 2/78. Therefore, wares with such numbers as 4567 or 4/1234 are not Rockingham nor are the fine Rockingham-type wares bearing the diamond-shaped Patent Office registration mark. The collector will also be offered as Rockingham decorative porcelain cottages and poodles or other animals with added china strips representing fur; it should be noted that no marked Rockingham cottages or furred animals have been recorded and their attribution is based on tradition rather than fact.

These notes have largely been based on the researches of Messrs. A. A. Eaglestone and T. A. Lockett, as published in their joint work, *The Rockingham Pottery* (1964, revised edition 1973). This reference book is an invaluable guide for all Rockingham collectors, as it corrects earlier books and publishes for the first time much contemporary information on the Pottery, its owners, and their products. Dr D. G. Rice's recent book, *Ornamental Rockingham Porcelain*, is a mine of information on this section of the factory's output, as is the same author's work *The Illustrated Guide to Rockingham Porcelain* (Barrie & Jenkins, London, 1971). The latest book on these wares is *The Rockingham Works* by Dr Alwyn and Angela Cox (Sheffield City Museum, 1974).

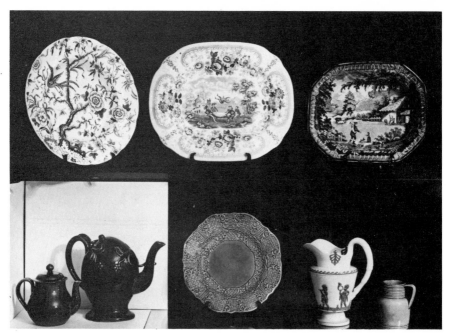

490. Early "Rockingham" earthenwares, mostly marked with the impressed mark "Brameld" (c. 1806–25).

Rotherham Museum

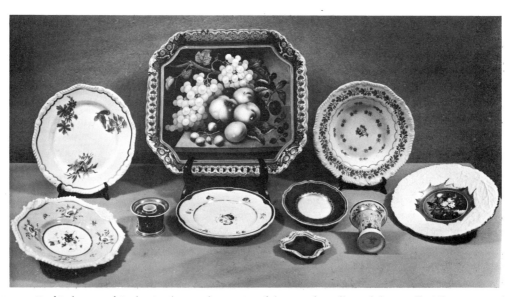

491. Rockingham porcelains bearing the pre-1830 version of the printed Griffin mark (no. 3358). This was printed in red at this period, later in purple or puce. The large tray is signed "T Steel Pinx" (c. 1826–30).

Rotherham Museum

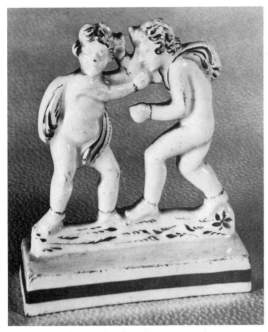

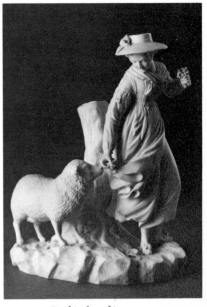

492. *Rare Rockingham porcelain group of boy boxers. Very narrow with flat back; other flat-back groups of this kind were also made by Minton (see Plate 403). 4.7 inches high, 1.2 inches deep. Printed Griffin mark no. 3358 in red (c. 1826–30).*

Rotherham Museum

493. *Rockingham bisque group, one of several very attractive models (c. 1825). Impressed Griffin mark above the words "Rockingham Works/Brameld". Incised "No 4". 6½ inches high.*

Godden of Worthing

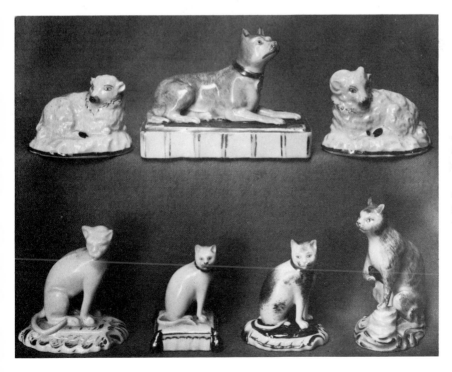

494. *A selection of marked Rockingham porcelain animal models. Sheep model no. 108. Dog no. 87. Cats no. 77. The cat on the right is of Bow porcelain not Rockingham (c. 1826–30). Dog 2⅝ inches high.*

Sotheby & Co

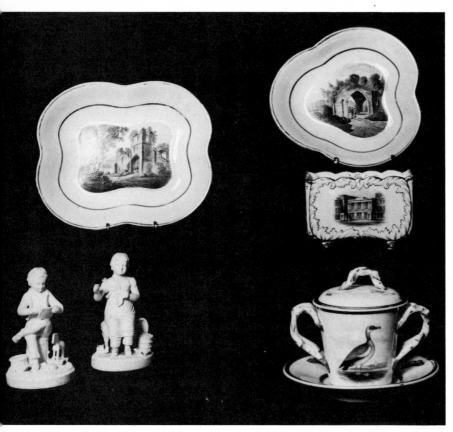

495. Rockingham wares—earthen-ware · dishes with impressed "Brameld" mark (c. 1806–25). Porcelain letter-rack, printed Griffin in puce (c. 1830), mark no. 3359. Two biscuit (unglazed) figures. Impressed Griffin mark no. 3358 (c. 1825–30). 5 inches high. Rare porcelain covered cup and stand with early version of the Griffin mark, printed in red, mark no. 3358 (c. 1825–30).

G. N. Dawnay, Cardiff

496. Sample Rockingham teawares, bearing the post-1830 printed Griffin mark "...to the King". Pattern no. 1139. These teapot and sucrier forms, with crown knob, were much favoured (c. 1830–40). Teapot 6¾ inches high.

Sotheby & Co

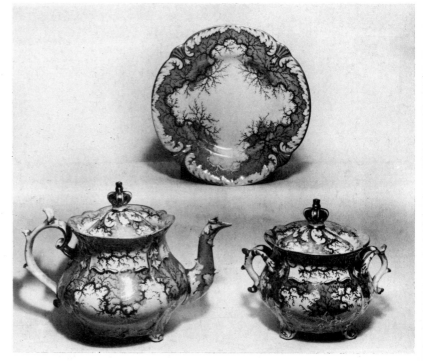

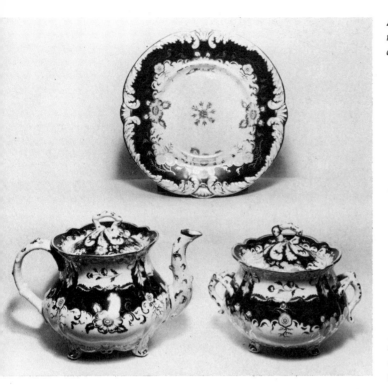

497. Rockingham porcelain teawares of pattern no. 893. Printed mark no. 3359—"To the King" and therefore post-1830. Teapot 6¼ inches high.

Sotheby & Co

498. Rockingham wares, bearing the late version of the printed Griffin mark (no. 3359), with the wording "Manufacturers to the King" (c. 1830-7).

Rotherham Museum

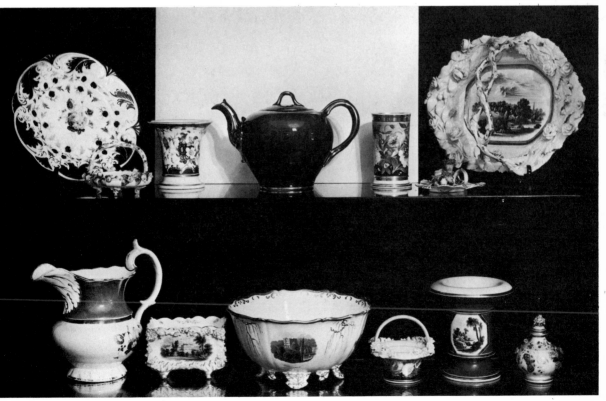

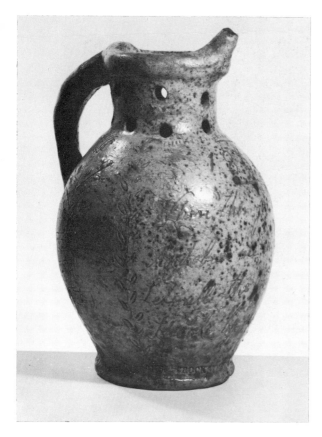

499. *"Rogers & Sons, Crock Strett Pottery" (impressed marked) earthenware puzzle-jug made at Donyatt, Somerset (dated 1864). $8\frac{7}{8}$ inches high. Many West Country wares appear to be of earlier date than that proved by dated specimens.*

Fitzwilliam Museum, Cambridge

JOHN AND GEORGE ROGERS, LONGPORT *c.* 1784–1814

500. *Rogers (impressed marked) creamware sauce tureen of a form much used (c. 1805–15). John & George Rogers potted at Dale Hall, Longport (c. 1784–1814). Many fine quality creamwares bear the simple name mark. 6 inches high. Fine quality underglaze blue printed patterns were a feature of Rogers' output which was exported to many countries.*

Victoria & Albert Museum

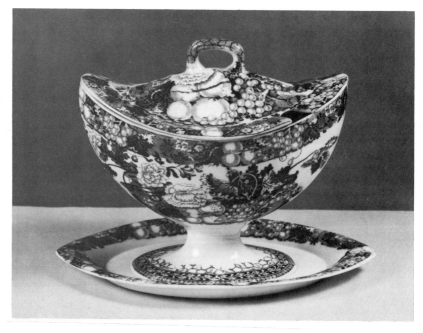

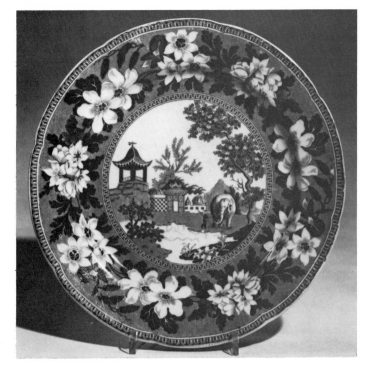

501. *Blue printed earthenware plate by John &*
George Rogers of Longport. The Elephant pattern
is mentioned in an advertisement of 1818. A writer
in 1843 noted that Rogers "were noted for the
excellence of their table-ware" (c. 1815–25).
9¾ inches diameter.

502. *"Rogers" (impressed marked)*
earthenware tureen, decorated with a
fine underglaze blue print, of a type
for which English potters were
famous (c. 1805–15). 11 inches
high. Such tureens were originally
part of large dinner services.

Godden of Worthing

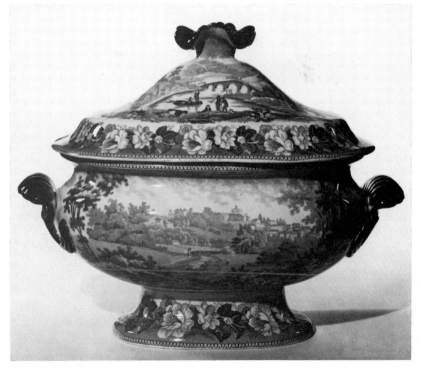

287

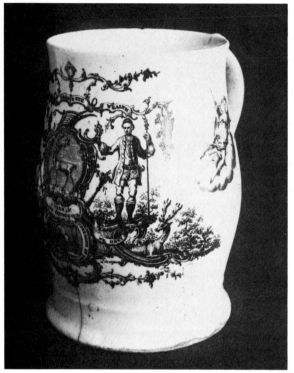

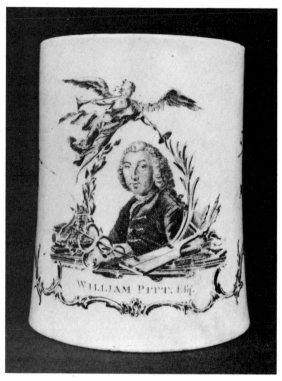

503. *Longton Hall porcelain mug printed by Sadler of Liverpool, with the arms of the Order of Foresters. Print signed "Sadler, Liverpool" (c. 1760). 4 inches high.*

Victoria & Albert Museum

504. *Liverpool porcelain mug, the printed pattern signed "J Sadler, Sculpt" (c. 1760). 5½ inches high.*

Willett Collection, Brighton Museum

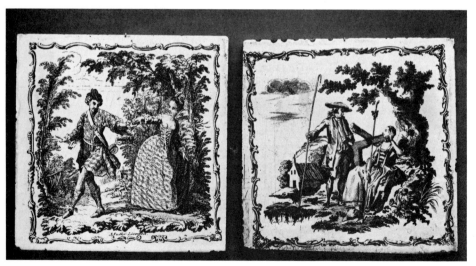

505. *Earthenware tiles printed by John Sadler at Liverpool (c. 1756–70). Signature marks "J Sadler, Liverpool" and "Sadler, Liverpool". Many other examples are unsigned. Green continued to c. 1799.*

Victoria & Albert Museum

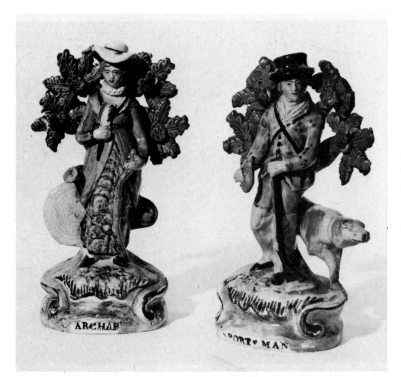

506. *"Salt" (moulded scroll mark) earthenware figures. Ralph Salt potted at Hanley from c. 1820. Many other unmarked figures of this type were made by other potters. 6¾ inches high.*

Godden of Worthing

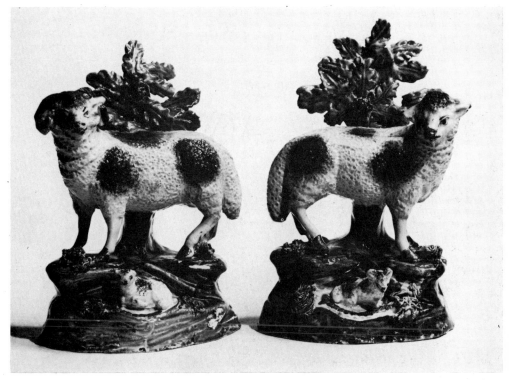

507. *"Salt" (moulded scroll mark) earthenware sheep and ram figures of the 1825 period. 6 inches high.*
Godden of Worthing

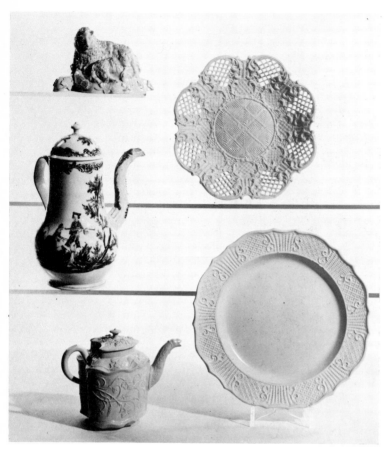

508. A selection of salt-glazed wares (see page xiv). Such eighteenth-century Staffordshire wares do not bear factory marks. The enamelled coffee pot is of a very rare form (c. 1750–70). Teapot 5 inches high.

Godden of Worthing

509. A selection of typical Staffordshire salt-glazed stoneware (c. 1740–80). The coffee pot is decorated with a bright blue which is associated with, and named after, Littler of the Longton Hall factory. The double-handled cup is decorated in the manner known as scratch blue (see page xv). Teapot 8¾ inches high.

City Museum & Art Gallery,
Stoke-on-Trent

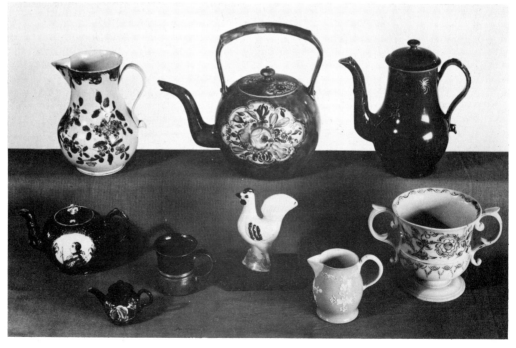

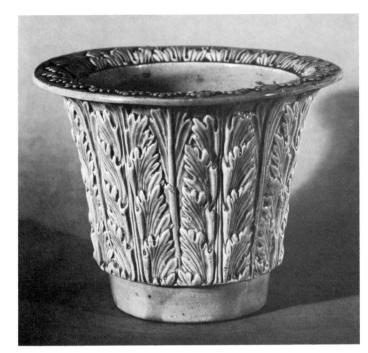

510. *Portobello green glazed earthenware flower pot by Messrs Scott Bros. Late eighteenth century. Impressed mark "Scott/PB". 4.4 inches high. The initial P.B. may be taken to denote Portobello, and differentiates between this pottery and that made by Scott Brothers of Southwick, Sunderland (see below).*

British Museum

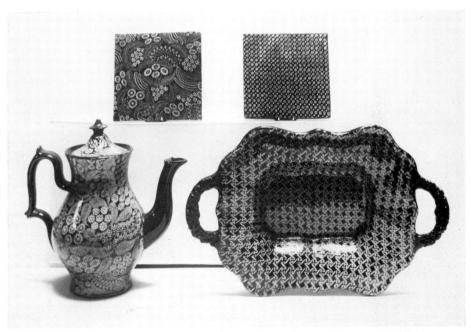

511. *Sunderland pottery from the Scott Brothers' Southwick Pottery. These pieces were given to the Sunderland Museum by members of the Scott family after the pottery closed. The dish has the impressed mark "Scott Brothers" (c. 1845). 11 inches long. Similar wares are attributed to the Portobello factory in Scotland (see companion mark book also British Pottery and Porcelain, 1780–1850).*

Sunderland Museum

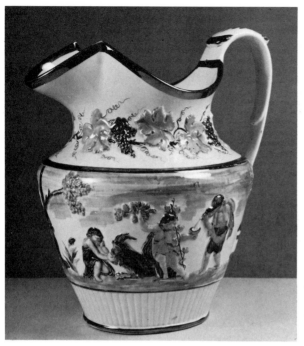

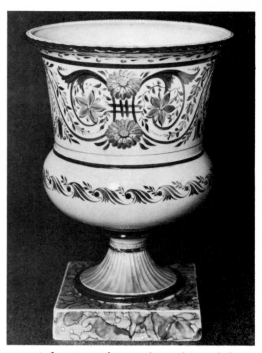

512. *Sewell (impressed marked) earthenware jug of fine quality, decorated in colours and in "purple" lustre. Sewell and later Sewell & Donkin worked the St Anthony's Pottery at Newcastle upon Tyne from c. 1780. This is a very fine example of c. 1815. 9¼ inches high.*

Victoria & Albert Museum

513. *A fine Newcastle vase, decorated in pink lustre. Impressed mark Sewell (c. 1804–28). 8⅞ inches high.*

Laing Art Gallery, Newcastle upon Tyne

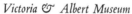

SHORTHOSE AND CO, SHORTHOSE AND HEATH, HANLEY *c.* 1795–1823

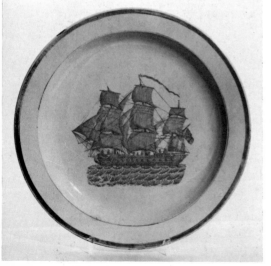

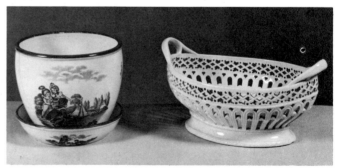

515. *Shorthose & Co (impressed and painted marks) creamwares, showing the high quality of some of the smaller firms' wares. This Hanley Company is of the period c. 1820–3, and is subsequent to the Shorthose & Heath partnership. Pot and Stand 3⅞ inches high.*

Victoria & Albert Museum

514. *"Shorthose & Heath" (impressed mark) creamware plate, decorated with light brown print. This firm potted at Hanley from c. 1795 to 1815.*

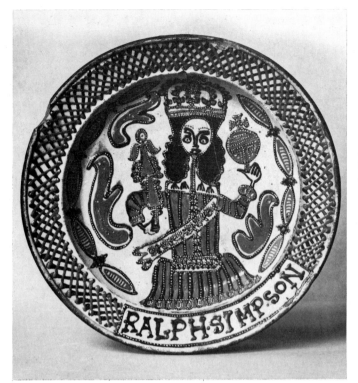

516. *"Ralph Simpson" slip decorated earthenware dish of Toft type (see page xii) (c. 1680–90). 17 inches diameter.*

Fitzwilliam Museum, Cambridge

517. *Slip decorated earthenware dish by Ralph Simpson (1651–1724), similar dishes were made by other potters and depict various subjects (see page xii) (c. 1700). 16¾ inches diameter.*

Victoria & Albert Museum

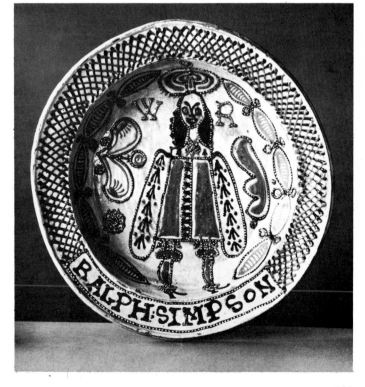

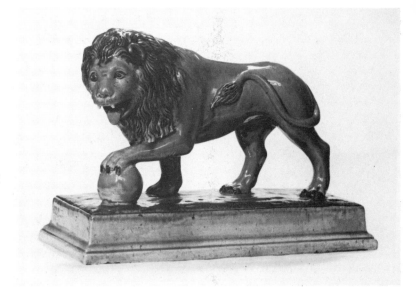

518. *George Skey (impressed marked) earthenware lion, made at the Wilnecote Works, Tamworth (c. 1862–90). 14 inches long.*
Godden of Worthing

SLIP DECORATED STAFFORDSHIRE POTTERY (SEE PAGE XII)

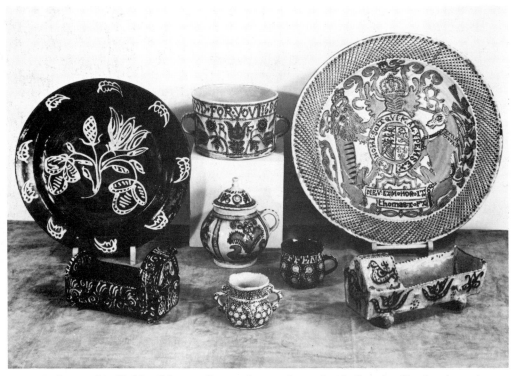

519. *A selection of Staffordshire "slip wares", or earthenware decorated with slip—clay diluted to the consistency of cream, trailed over the ware, in much the same way that one would decorate an iced cake (see page xii) (c. 1680–1720. Diameter of "Toft" dish 20¾ inches.*

City Museum & Art Gallery, Stoke-on-Trent

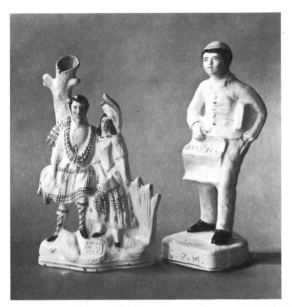

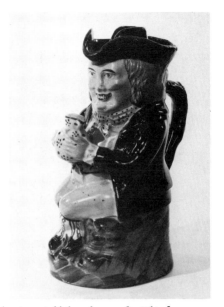

520–1. *Sampson Smith earthenware figures and a Toby jug, bearing moulded mark no. 3584. This firm produced vast quantities of "Staffordshire earthenware" figures, but very few bear a factory mark (c. 1870–80). Toby jug 9¾ inches high.*

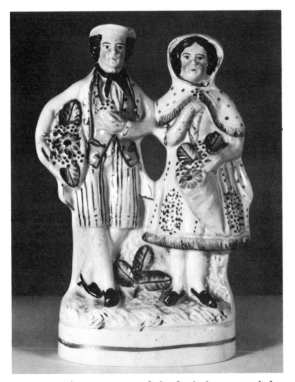

522. *Earthenware group of the flat-back type. Relief mark on base—"Sampson Smith, 1851, Longton". 8¾ inches high.*

Victoria & Albert Museum

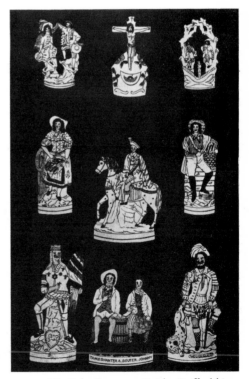

523. *Typical Sampson Smith Staffordshire earthenware figures, from an early twentieth-century catalogue, showing late nineteenth-century models.*

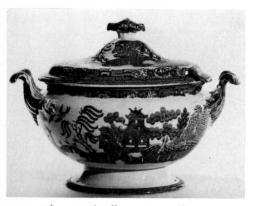

524. Blue printed willow pattern earthen-ware tureen by William Smith & Co of the Stafford Pottery, Stockton-on-Tees, Yorkshire. Impressed mark "W S & Co's /Queens Ware/Stockton" (c. 1825–30). $13\frac{1}{2}$ inches long.

Godden of Worthing

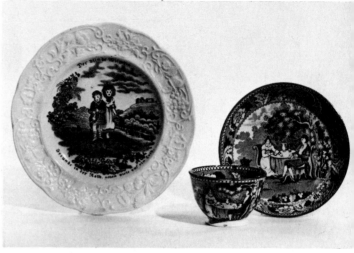

525. William Smith & Co's Stockton pottery, bearing impressed marks "W S & Co's/Wedgwood/Ware" and "W S & Co's/Queen's Ware/ Stockton". The printed cup and saucer is of the 1825–30 period, the German market place c. 1850.

T. SNEYD, HANLEY, SOUTH WALES POTTERY c. 1839–58

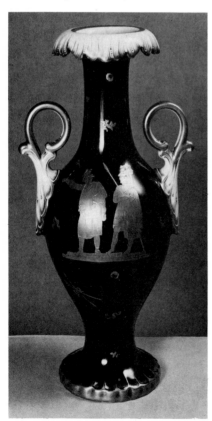

526. Blue ground porcelain vase by Thomas Sneyd of Hanley. Rate record 1846–7 only. Figures, etc., in gold. Impressed name mark: $12\frac{7}{8}$ inches high.

Victoria & Albert Museum

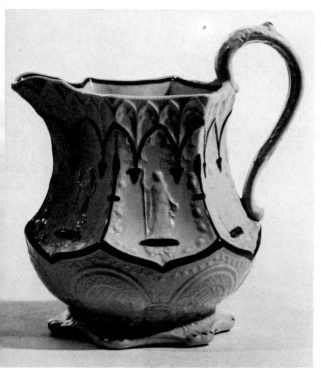

527. *"South Wales Pottery" impressed marked, moulded pink-coloured earthenware jug (c. 1839–58). A similar moulded jug had been made by Wedgwoods and occurs in the 1817 catalogue (see Plate 613). 5¼ inches high.*

Godden of Worthing

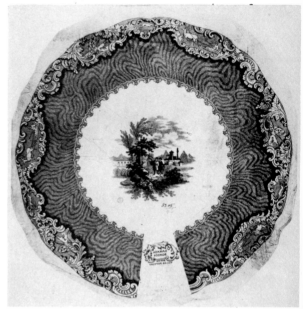

528. *Pull from "South Wales Pottery" copper plate. Note mark (in reverse on the pull) engraved on the copper plate with the main design. The mark is cut out and transferred to the base of article bearing the main print.*

Victoria & Albert Museum

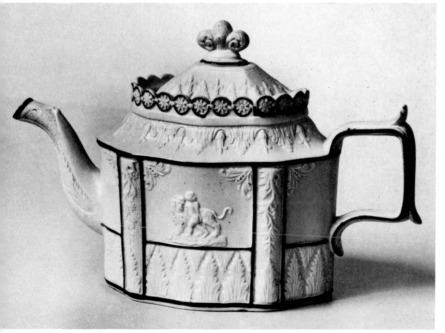

SOWTER AND CO

529. *Sowter & Co of Mex-borough teapot of the so-called Castleford stoneware type with sliding cover and blue line edging (see page xxiii). Impressed mark "S & oC" (c. 1795–1804).*

Castle Museum, Norwich

297

Spode

The Spode works were established in 1770 by the first Josiah Spode (1733–97). The early products were earthenware, often decorated with underglaze blue printed patterns; the forms were similar to those of most other manufacturers of the period, but the Spode specimens were always well potted and have a neat appearance. Some fine basalt wares were also made (see Plate 530). Most Spode earthenwares from about 1790 bear the name "Spode" impressed into the body or printed in blue.

The manufacture of porcelain was introduced in the 1790's and, like the earlier Spode earthen-wares, it was well potted, thin, and neat. It is highly translucent, and the glaze is well fitting and seldom crazes or discolours. Josiah Spode is credited with first using bone ash in his porcelain, and so introducing the world-famous English Bone China. As with other Spode wares, the designs and forms were neat, well made and proportioned, also attractively decorated. Tea and dessert services formed an important part of the factory's output from about 1795 onwards. About 1815 an improved porcelain body containing felspar was introduced, a fact recorded on printed marks of the period 1815–30. Prior to August 1822 Henry Daniel was responsible for most, if not all, enamel painting on Spode's porcelains. He subsequently established his own works at Stoke and traded as "Daniel & Son" and as "Henry & Richard Daniel" (see page 115).

An important new body—"Stone China" or "New Stone"—was introduced in 1805. Shaw, writing in 1829, states that this Spode body was really "Turner's Patent" body which was patented by William and John Turner in January 1800 (patent no. 2367). Josiah Spode, according to Shaw, purchased the right to manufacture the new ware and he naturally re-named it. Fine dinner and dessert services were made in this compact, durable body. The potting is thinner and crisper than the later Mason's Ironstone services. Most patterns owe their origin to Chinese porcelains (see Plate 535). These patterns were usually outlined by means of transfer printing which was then coloured in by hand.

Apart from the porcelains and the Stone China body mentioned above many Spode services and other objects were produced in the ordinary light cream-coloured earthenware of the period. The general high standard demanded by Spode is well seen in the blue printed earthenware, as well as in the finest porcelains.

Josiah Spode the second died in 1827. His son, also Josiah, succeeded him, but only survived his father by two years. The business was continued by the executors and William Taylor Copeland until 1 March 1833, when Copeland purchased the concern. He took into partnership Thomas Garrett (Spode's principal traveller), and the Copeland and Garrett partnership continued from 1833 to the middle of 1847 (see page 109). A. Hayden's *Spode and His Successors* (1924) contains much information on the Spode family and its wares. Leonard Whiter's *Spode a History of the Family, Factory and Wares from 1733 to 1833* (Barrie & Jenkins, London, 1970, revised edition 1978) must surely rank as the last word on this important factory and its superb and varied productions.

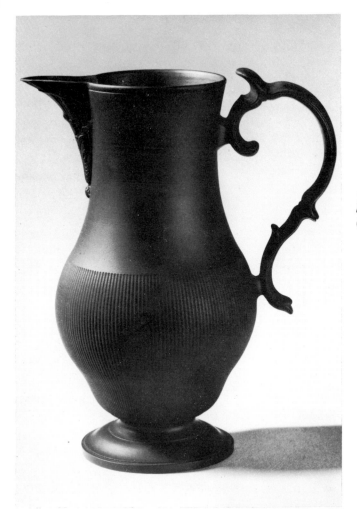

530. *An early and rare impressed marked "Spode" basalt jug of elegant form and fine workmanship (c. 1785–95). $8\frac{1}{4}$ inches high.*

531. *Very rare early impressed marked "Spode" porcelain covered sugar basin, cover and stand. Simple floral sprays in blue enamel (c. 1790–5).*

Worthing Museum

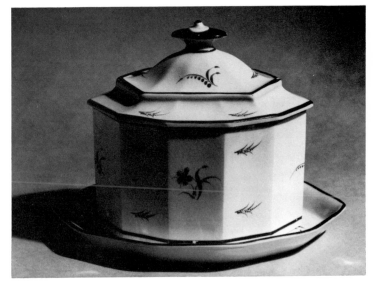

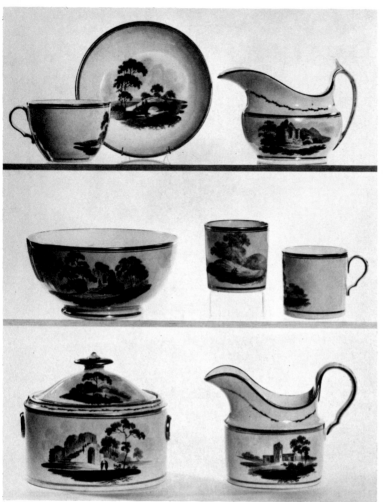

532. Early Spode porcelain part tea service, finely painted with landscape in monochrome. Early Spode porcelains were seldom marked. This set bears only the pattern no. 382, which matches the original factory pattern book (see below). The design is drawn on 1794 water-marked paper. These teaware shapes, especially the handles, should be noted as being typical Spode forms of the 1795–1805 period. The upper creamer is later (c. 1810).

Godden of Worthing

533. Page from Spode pattern book of the 1790's, showing pattern no. 382 which appears on the teaset above.

W. T. Copeland & Sons Ltd

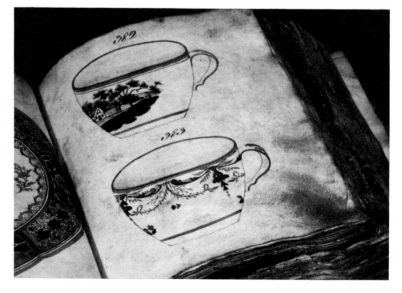

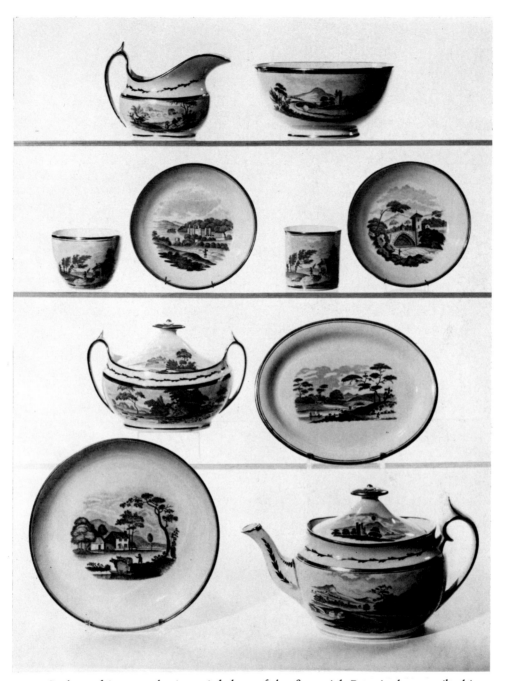

534. *Spode porcelain teaset, showing typical shapes of the 1800 period. Bat printed scenes, gilt edging. Pattern no. 557. Spode porcelain before* c. *1810 often have only a pattern number rather than the written name "Spode". Teapot 6¼ inches high.*

Godden of Worthing

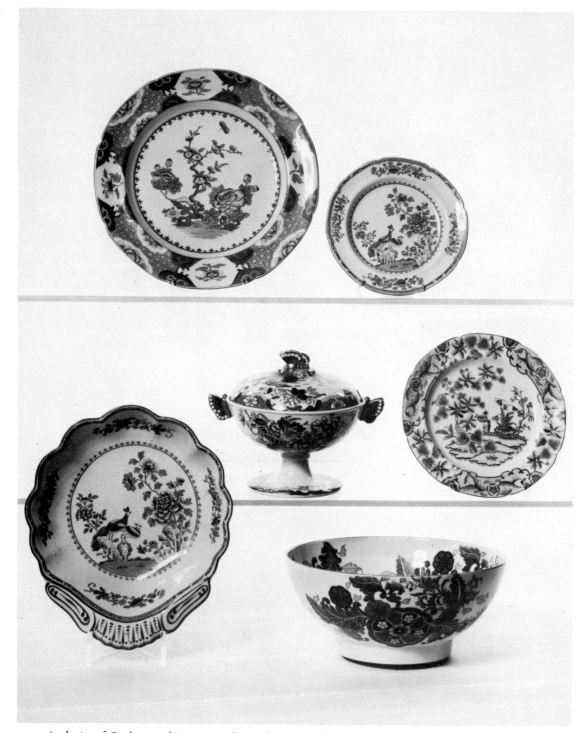

535. *A selection of Spode stone china wares with typical patterns of the 1805–15 period. Impressed or printed "New Stone" and "Stone China" marks with name Spode. Handled dish (pattern no. 2118) 9½ inches long. Many fine dinner services were made in this durable body (see page xxiii).*

Godden of Worthing

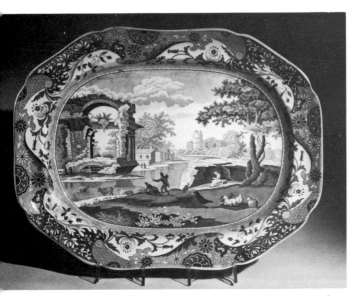

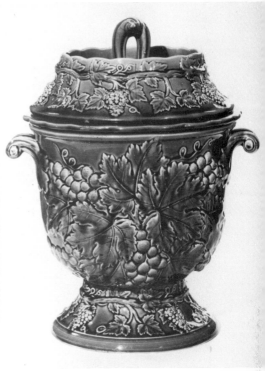

536. Large impressed marked "Spode" earthenware platter, decorated with fine quality underglaze print. This platter is part of a large dinner service. Many finely designed useful wares were produced in underglaze blue printed earthenware, at relatively low cost, for the home and export markets.

537. Spode (impressed marked) ice pail in moulded earthenware with green glaze which serves to accentuate the pattern (c. 1815–25). 12¾ inches high. Several firms made similar designs.

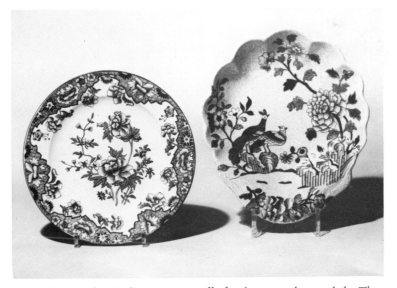

538. Two popular Spode patterns, normally found on an earthenware body. The plate is pattern no. 3184 (c. 1815), and the dish no. 4079 (c. 1820). Impressed mark "Spode".

Godden of Worthing

303

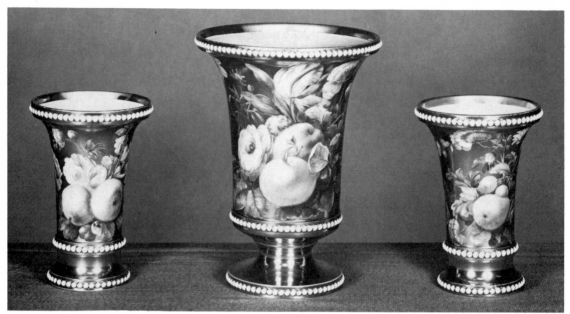

539. *A set of Spode porcelain spill vases, painted with fruit and flowers on a gold ground. Painted mark "Spode" with pattern no. 711 (c. 1810).*

Delomosne & Son

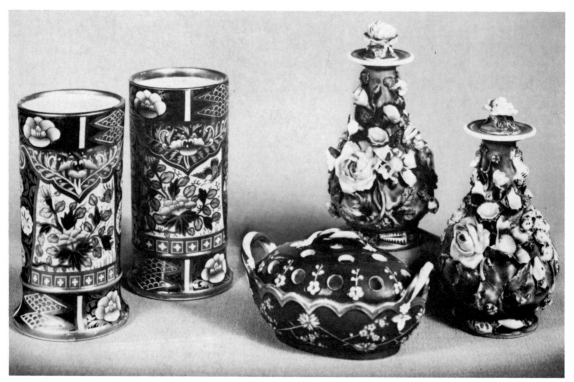

540. *Spode porcelains, with painted "Spode" mark. The spill vases are decorated with a class of pattern known as "Japan". The Derby and Worcester factories used similar colourful Japan patterns (c. 1810). Spill vases 4 inches high.*

Delomosne & Son

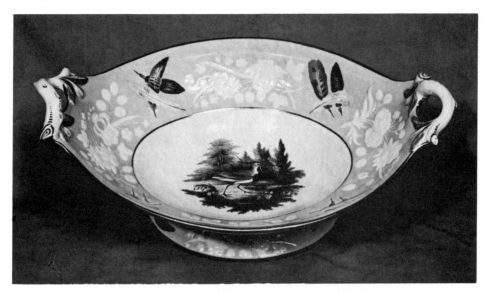

541. *Spode porcelain centrepiece. Painted mark "Spode 1979". The raised floral motifs occur with various painted motifs or without further decoration (c. 1805). 14¾ inches long. Fine dessert services and other objects were decorated with this popular pattern.*

Copeland Works Museum

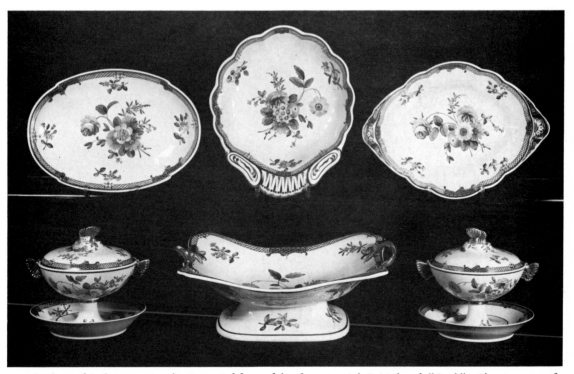

542. *Spode porcelain dessert service, showing typical forms of the 1805–15 period. Painted mark "Spode" with pattern no. 2783 (c. 1810). Centrepiece 11½ inches long.*

Delomosne & Son

305

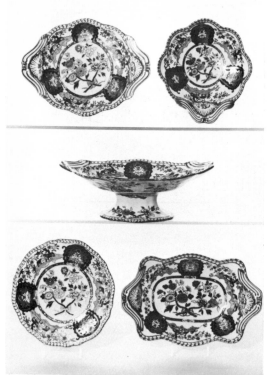

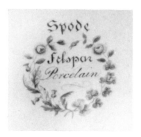

543. a. Standard "Spode Felspar Porcelain" mark (no. 3657) found on fine quality porcelains of the 1815–27 period.

543. Spode "Felspar" porcelain dessert service, showing typical forms of the 1815–20 period. Printed "Spode Felspar" mark (no. 3657) and impressed circle mark, no. 3649. Centre dish 13¾ inches long.

Godden of Worthing

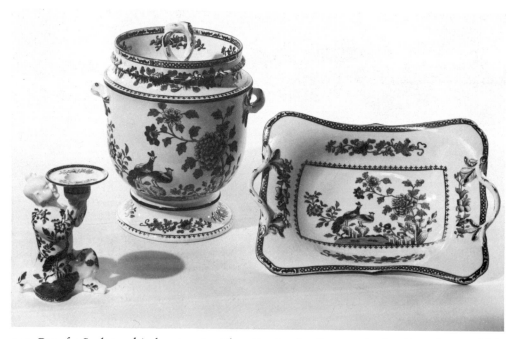

544. Part of a Spode porcelain dessert service. The pattern is coloured over a printed outline, and is copied from a Chinese original. The "Indian Clown" candle-holder (one of a pair) is very rare. Pattern no. 2083. Painted and printed "Spode" marks (c. 1805–15). Fruit cooler 11 inches high.

Godden of Worthing

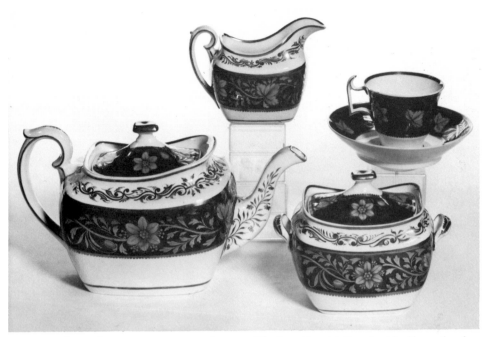

545. *Spode porcelain teaset, pattern no. 3569. Printed "Felspar Porcelain" mark with addresses (mark no. 3658) (c. 1820–5). Teapot 5½ inches high.*

Godden of Worthing

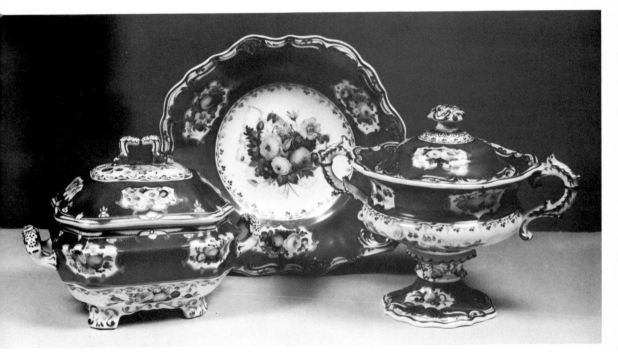

546. *Part of a Spode "Felspar" porcelain dessert and dinner service, decorated with very finely painted panels of fruit and flowers. Pale blue borders. Painted Spode mark in script. Pattern no. 4964 (c. 1820). Sauce tureen 6¾ inches high.*

Victoria & Albert Museum

307

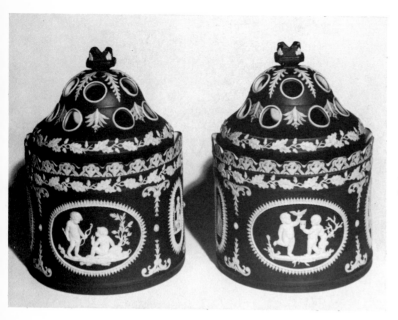

547. *"Steel"* (*impressed marked*) *blue and white jasperware crocus pots and covers. All bulb pots are now rare, but would seem to have been very popular and were made by several firms* (c. 1790–1824). *6½ inches high.*

D. M. & P. Manheim

STEVENSON, COBRIDGE *c.* 1816–30

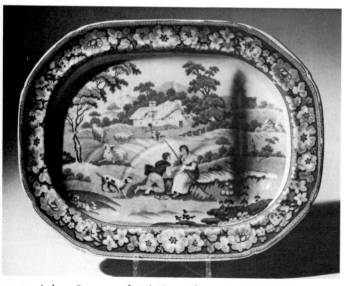

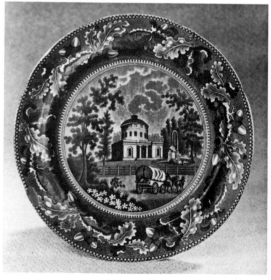

548. *Andrew Stevenson of Cobridge. A fine quality blue printed earthenware meat dish (the shadow is caused by the gravy well). Impressed mark no. 3700—the name "Stevenson" over the outline of a sailing ship* (c. 1816–30). *12½ inches long.*

549. *Stevenson & Williams ("R S W" printed mark) earthenware plate with underglaze blue print, showing the waterworks at Philadelphia, U.S.A. Messrs Stevenson & Williams of Cobridge are mentioned in a deed dated 1825.*

City Museum & Art Gallery, Stoke-on-Trent

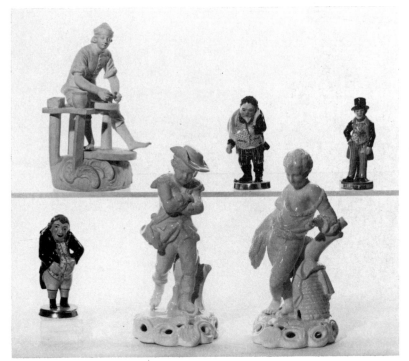

550. *Stevenson & Hancock Derby figure made at the King Street Works. "S & H" Derby mark no. 1267 (c. 1865–95).*

Godden of Worthing

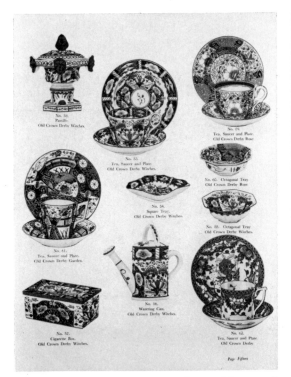

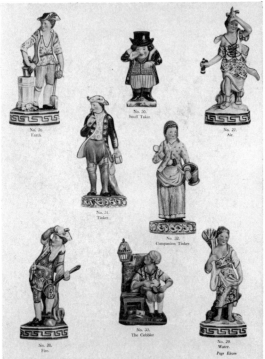

551–2. *Derby "Japan" pattern porcelains and decorative figures made at Stevenson & Hancock's Works at King Street, Derby. Most patterns and models were taken from Derby originals of the 1780–1830 period. Mark no. 1267. Reproduced from an original catalogue.*

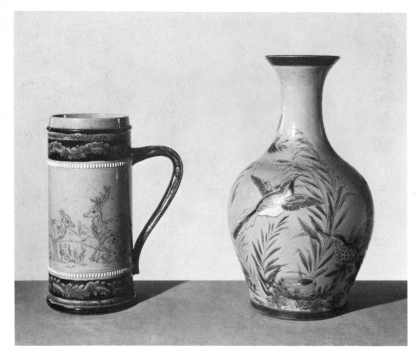

553. Tankard and vase in stoneware. Impressed marks "J Stiff & Sons. Lambeth" (c. 1880). Vase $11\frac{3}{4}$ inches high.

Victoria & Albert Museum

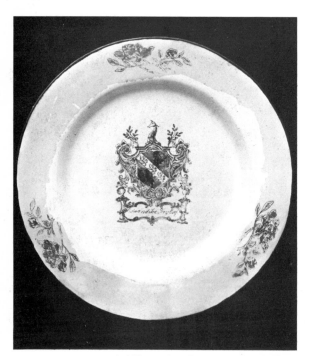

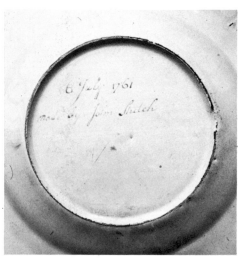

554 & a. Limerick delftware (tin glazed earthenware) plate decorated with coloured-over transfer printed motifs. Signed by John Stritch and dated 1761 (see detail). In the following year Stritch and C. Bridson were awarded a premium "for erecting a manufactory of earthenware in imitation of delft or white ware".

National Museum of Ireland

Sunderland Pottery

Several potteries in the Sunderland district produced utilitarian and decorative earthenwares in the eighteenth and nineteenth centuries. A class of "Splash" lustre with characteristic irregular splash designs on a pale pink lustry ground are associated with this group of potters, but most specimens are unmarked. Reproductions are made today. Many specimens are decorated with printed designs depicting the local Wearmouth Bridge and some printed designs incorporate the name of the manufacturer in or near the print.

Some typical marked specimens of Sunderland Pottery are illustrated in Plates 555–8. The Director of the local Museum & Art Gallery, Mr J. T. Shaw, has written a booklet, *The Potteries of Sunderland and District*, which gives a good account of the various local potters and their wares.

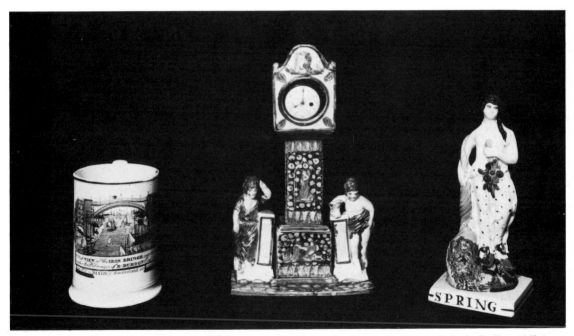

555. *Mug printed with view of the Wearmouth Bridge. Printed mark, "Dixon & Co. Sunderland. 1813". Modelled frog inside the mug. Rare watch-stand with pink lustre decoration. Impressed mark, "Dixon Austin & Co" (c. 1820–6). 10 inches high. Figure of Spring, one of a set of four seasons. Impressed mark, "Dixon Austin & Co". Similar figures are found with lustre decoration (c. 1820–6).*

Sunderland Museum

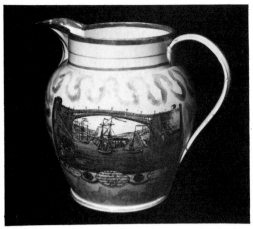

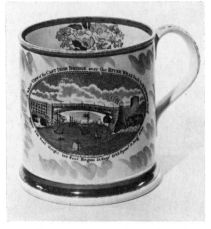

556. *A typical Sunderland earthenware jug with lustre rim, etc., and printed subject—the Wearmouth Bridge. Mark "J Phillips. Hylton Pottery" incorporated in the print (c. 1807–12). 8½ inches high.*

Sunderland Museum

557. *Sunderland lustre and printed mug by "Scott & Sons, Southwick", signed under main print. The date—1796—on these bridge prints should not be taken for the date of manufacture. "Scott & Sons" mark used c. 1829–41. 5¼ inches high.*

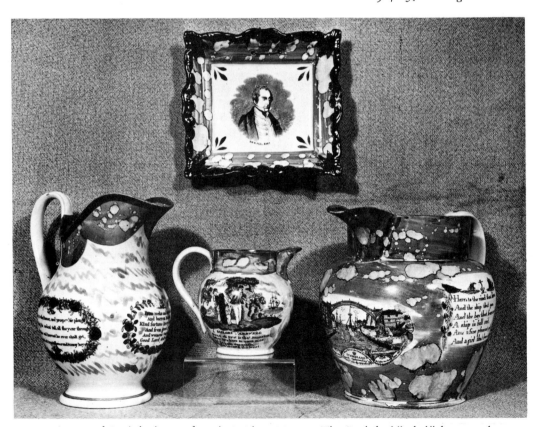

558. *A group of Sunderland wares from the Brighton Museum. The Sunderland "splash" lustre can be seen clearly (c. 1820–80). The plaque is marked "Dixon Phillips & Co" impressed.*

Brighton Museum & Art Gallery

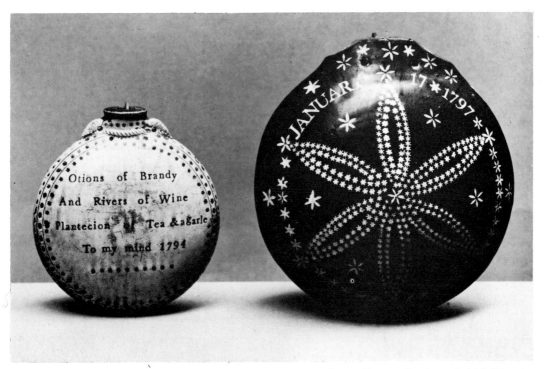

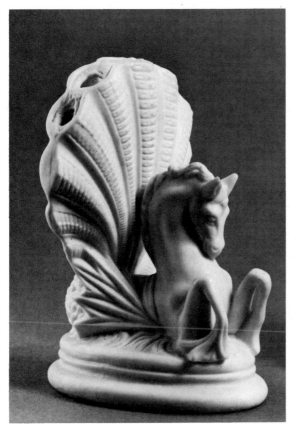

559. Sussex Pottery, showing typical inlaid inscriptions and decorative motifs. Pottery of this type was
mainly made at Chailey and Dicker. Dated 1794 and
1797. Signed examples by John Siggery of Herst-
monceux bear dates up to, at least, 1836.

Victoria & Albert Museum

D. SUTHERLAND AND SONS, LONGTON

560. Parian flower holder, with impressed initial
mark—"S & S" of D. Sutherland & Sons of
Longton (c. 1865–75). $6\frac{1}{4}$ inches high.

Swansea Pottery and Porcelain

Pottery was made at Swansea (Glamorganshire, Wales) from about 1764 at the Cambrian Pottery. The early wares were unmarked. Many changes in ownership of the pottery took place and the situation is further complicated by the establishment of other potteries in or near Swansea. E. M. Nance's monumental book, *The Pottery and Porcelain of Swansea and Nantgarw* (1942), gives a wealth of information with numerous illustrations of typical Swansea earthenwares. Some fine creamwares were made and painted with flowers (often named on the reverse of the article); such wares may bear the impressed mark S W A N S E A or C A M B R I A N. Various types of earthenware were made at Swansea for over one hundred years up to about 1870. Other potteries were situated near Swansea (see Ynismedw, page 318).

Lewis Weston Dillwyn of Swansea was asked to visit the small porcelain works at Nantgarw in 1814, as the proprietors, William Billingsley and Samuel Walker, were seeking financial help. Dillwyn was obviously impressed by the fine Nantgarw porcelain for he invited Billingsley and Walker to continue their work at his pottery at Swansea (see page 245). They remained there, producing a wonderfully translucent warm feeling porcelain until 1817 when they returned to Nantgarw. In the same year Dillwyn temporarily retired, leaving the works to T. & J. Bevington, who seem to have produced little porcelain. The manufacture of most Swansea porcelain therefore falls within the period 1813–17, but undecorated blanks were sold and decorated up to at least 1826. Overglaze painted marks have been faked; the standard mark is the name S W A N S E A printed or stencilled in red. The most reliable marks are those impressed S W A N S E A, with or without crossed tridents.

The white Swansea porcelain was in great demand by the leading London decorators who painted it in a pretentious style, quite different from the mainly floral patterns favoured for the factory's local customers. Typical examples of all styles are illustrated in W. D. John's *Swansea Porcelain* (1958) and in Nance's *The Pottery and Porcelain of Swansea and Nantgarw* (1942).

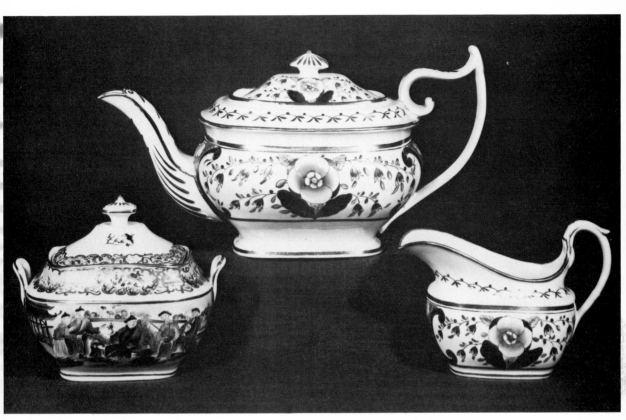

561. *Swansea (printed marked) teawares. The teapot and creamer are pattern no. 436, the covered sugar pattern no. 164. This colourful pattern is based on a printed outline, coloured over by hand (c. 1814–22).*

Messrs J. & E. Vandekar

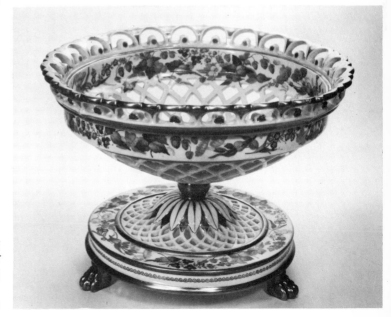

562. *Swansea porcelain fruit stand of fine quality and typical form. Wild flowers painted in the manner of David Evans. "Swansea" printed mark in red (c. 1814–22). 7 inches high.*

Sotheby & Co

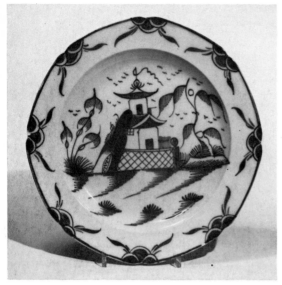

563. "Swansea" (impressed marked) earthenware plate, decorated in underglaze blue. One of several simple mock Chinese patterns (c. 1797–1810). $9\frac{3}{4}$ inches diameter.

Mr & Mrs J. F. Breeze Collection

564. Marked "Dillwyn & Co. Swansea" earthenware plate, painted in purple lustre. Similar plates were made at Sunderland; these have eighty-two pierced panels in the border, against sixty-four on Swansea, Spode and Herculaneum (Liverpool) examples (c. 1800–10). $7\frac{3}{4}$ inches diameter.

Mr & Mrs J. F. Breeze Collection

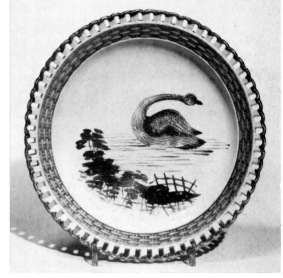

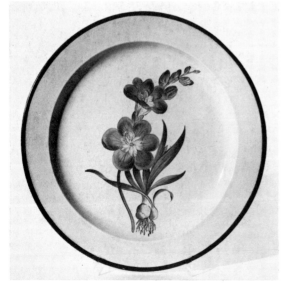

565. Swansea creamware botanical plate. Impressed marks "Swansea" and spade-shaped device (mark no. 3761). Name of flower written on back (c. 1800–10). $9\frac{1}{4}$ inches diameter.

Godden of Worthing

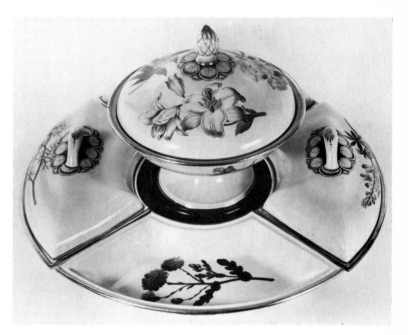

566. *Swansea creamware complete supper or sandwich set (normally on a mahogany carrying tray), painted with named botanical specimens in the style of Thomas Pardoe. Impressed mark "Swansea" (c. 1800–10). Centrepiece 9 inches high.*

Sotheby & Co

Other supper sets are oval rather than circular, all are rarely found undamaged.

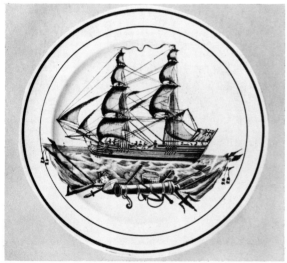

567. (Above) *Swansea earthenware plate, decorated with black printed pattern. Impressed mark "Dillwyn" (c. 1830–6).*

Godden of Worthing

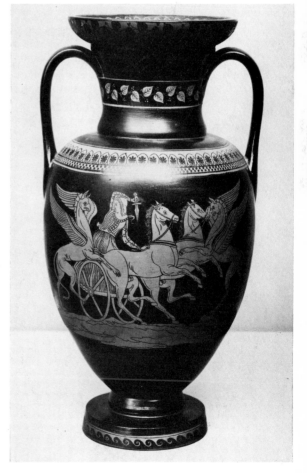

568. (Right) *"Dillwyn's Etruscan ware" (printed mark) earthenware vase. Many fine Etruscan patterned wares were made at the Swansea Pottery during the 1847–50 period. 14⅜ inches high.*

Victoria & Albert Museum

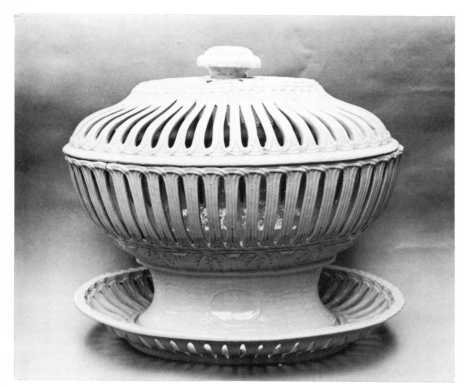

569. Buff coloured earthenware covered basket and stand with rare impressed mark "Ynismedw/Pottery/ Swansea Vale" (c. 1850–9) 10½ inches high.

Royal Institute of South Wales, Swansea

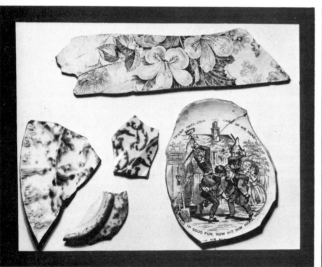

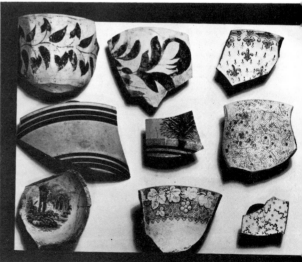

570–1. Fragments from the site of the little known Ynismedw factory near Swansea, recently excavated by Mr and Mrs Derek Harper. These fragments and matching finished specimens bear the following initial or name marks: Y M P; Y P; Ynismedw Pottery, Swansea Vale (all impressed) or printed marks incorporating the initials L & M or the name Williams (c. 1850–70).

Harper Collection

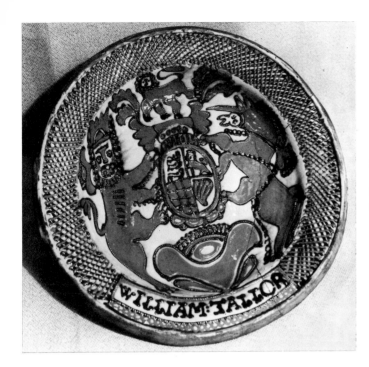
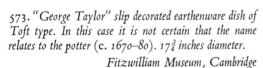

572. Staffordshire slipware dish by William Tallor. Similar examples are inscribed William Talor; one is dated 1700. 17 inches diameter.

Willett Collection, Brighton Museum

GEORGE TAYLOR, LATE SEVENTEENTH–EARLY EIGHTEENTH CENTURY

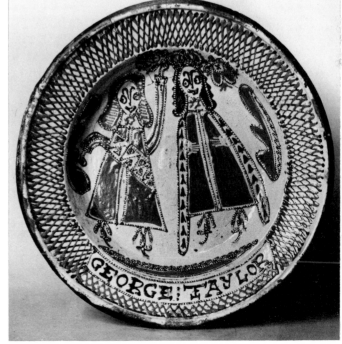

573. "George Taylor" slip decorated earthenware dish of Toft type. In this case it is not certain that the name relates to the potter (c. 1670–80). 17¾ inches diameter.

Fitzwilliam Museum, Cambridge

The Modeller Tebo

Bow, Bristol, Plymouth, and Worcester porcelains will be found marked with the impressed or moulded "To" or initial "T" marks or, very rarely, "IT".

These marks have been attributed to an eighteenth-century modeller or repairer (a skilled workman who assembles the finished figure or group from the many different moulded sections) called Tebo, perhaps an anglicized version of the name Thibauld. He worked for several different factories, including Wedgwood (c. 1774). Several letters in the Wedgwood archives mention Mr Tebo and one indicates that he was of French origin.

The "To", "T", or "IT" will be found on Bow porcelains of the 1750–60 period; Worcester porcelains c. 1760–9; Plymouth porcelains c. 1769–70; and Bristol porcelains of the 1770–3 period. The marks also occur on baskets bearing the printed Caughley "c" mark c. 1775–85. The moulded initial "T" also occurs on early Chamberlain-Worcester porcelains of the late 1780s or early 1790s, and here at least the initial can be linked with a modeller, John Toulouse. It is quite possible that all the above mentioned so-called Tebo marks really relate to Toulouse.

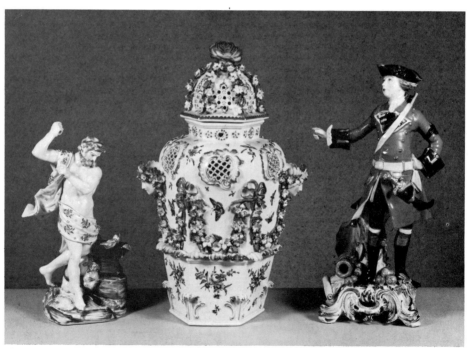

574. *Bristol hard-paste figure of Fire from the four elements. (Purchased by Lady Schreiber at Metz, in 1874.) A letter from Champion of the Bristol factory relates to the modelling of these figures and is dated "Feb 1772". Worcester porcelain vase (of a type also made at Bristol) (c. 1770). 16½ inches high. Bow figure of General Wolfe on typical Bow rocco base (c. 1760). 13⅞ inches high.*
Schreiber Collection, Victoria & Albert Museum

575. *Important impressed marked "Tittensor" earthenware group (c. 1815). 8 inches high.*

W. F. Greenwood & Sons Ltd

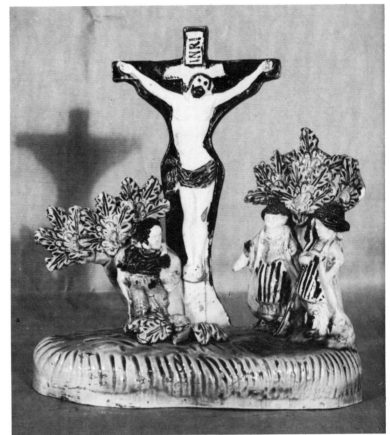

576. *Typical impressed marked "Tittensor" earthenware figures, decorated with semi-translucent coloured glazes. Marked examples are rare. Centre figures 6 inches high. For further information on the Tittensors see* Apollo *magazine, May 1943 and December 1950.*

Sotheby & Co

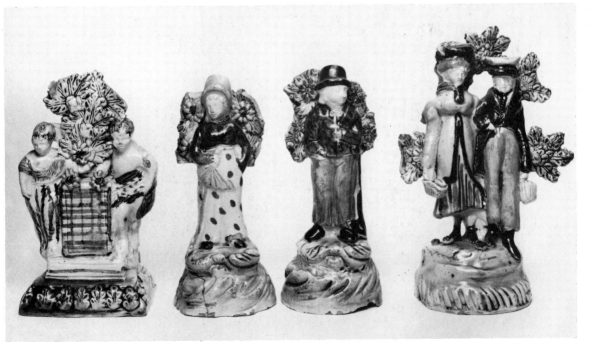

The Toft Family

The name "Toft" appears on the surface of several seventeenth- and eighteenth-century earthenware dishes, etc., decorated with white or tinted slip, which represents a traditional form of decorating earthenware and may be compared to icing a cake.

The name of Thomas Toft (died 1689) is most often seen, but James Toft (dated examples 1695 and 1705) and Ralph Toft (dated examples 1676, 1677, 1683) have also been recorded. Typical examples of Toft slip decorated earthenwares can be seen at the Victoria & Albert and the British Museums in London and at several provincial ones, including the Hanley Museum at Stoke-on-Trent (see Plates 519, 577–9). Other names or initials occur on similar Staffordshire slip decorated earthenware (see Plates 274, 370, 464, 516–17, 572–3). All specimens are rare and are often damaged.

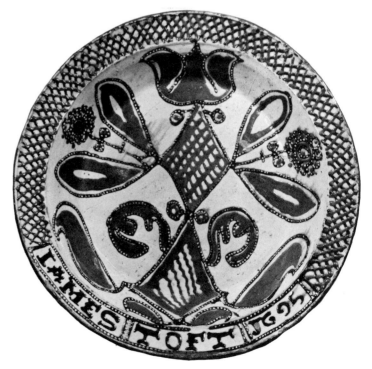

577. *A slip decorated earthenware dish by James Toft. Dated 1695, with formal floral pattern, the criss-cross border is typical.*

Royal Canadian Museum, Toronto

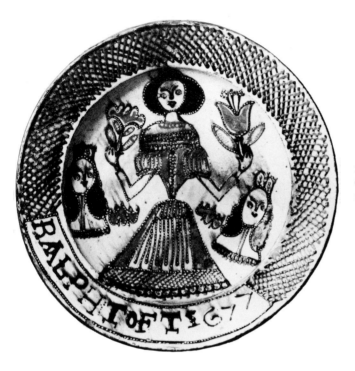

578. *"Ralph Toft" slip decorated earthenware circular dish, dated 1677. Similar dishes are recorded with different dates. 18 inches diameter.*

Fitzwilliam Museum, Cambridge

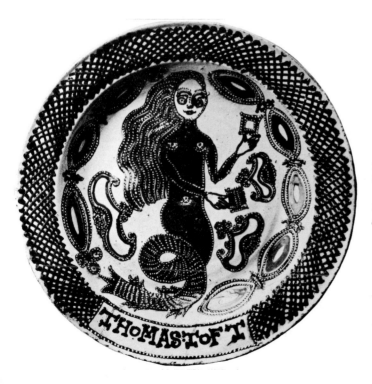

579. *A typical slip decorated earthenware circular dish bearing the "signature" of Thomas Toft of Hanley. Dated examples range between 1671 and 1689. 17¼ inches diameter.*

Victoria & Albert Museum

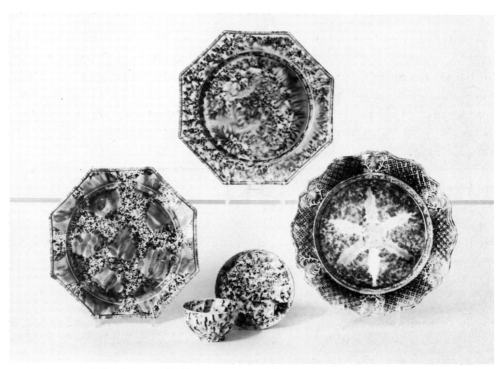

580. *"Tortoiseshell" glazed Staffordshire earthenwares of a type made by many potters from c. 1750 to c. 1785. Specimens are never marked. The mottled glazes are usually of green, brown and blue tints.*

Godden of Worthing

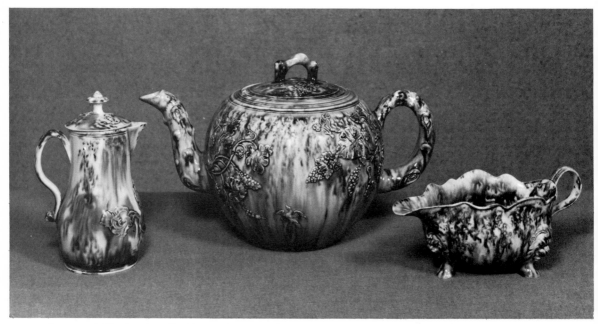

581. *"Tortoiseshell" glazed Staffordshire earthenwares of Astbury or Whieldon type. The forms, with raised leaf motifs, are typical of the 1750–60 period. Such wares are unmarked. Tea (or punch) pot 7¼ inches high.*

Victoria & Albert Museum

John Turner was born in 1738; he established his famous Pottery at Lane End in the Staffordshire Potteries in or before 1762, after being apprenticed to Daniel Bird and later in partnership with William Banks. Recent research suggests that John Turner may have commenced potting (salt-glazed earthenware) on his own account as early as 1759—his earliest wares are usually unmarked and impressed marked "Turner" earthenwares normally date from about 1775 onwards. Some very good Wedgwood-type jasper wares were made with white reliefs; the light blue jasper ground is very smooth to the touch and is of a slaty tint. He also made good black basalt wares, often with a slight silvery or grey tint. Good quality creamwares, too, were produced; some marked porcelain is recorded but this is very rare.

From c. 1781 to August 1792 John Turner (and after his death in December 1787 his sons William and John) and Andrew Abbott had a retail shop in London and in 1784 were appointed Potters to the Prince of Wales. An advertisement issued in January 1785 is interesting as it lists the wares made or, to be exact, sold by this firm in 1785:

Turner and Abbott, Potters to his Royal Highness the Prince of Wales, and Manufacturers of Queen's, and all other sorts of Staffordshire Ware, No. 82, Fleet Street have the honor to acquaint the Nobility and Public in general, that since they have established a Manufactory in London, for enamelling their goods, they are enabled, and will engage to finish a service of Ware to any Pattern, in the course of three or four days after the order is given, either with Crests, Cyphers or Borders. They also flatter themselves that the great variety of table services, desert setts, dejeunes, and other things which they have lately finished, and are now ready for sale, far exceeds that of any other house in the kingdom. Any single piece, or part of a service may be had separately, or broken services made up to any pattern. They likewise manufacture a very general assortment of Egyptian Black, and Bamboo, or Cane Colour Tea-Pots, some elegantly mounted with silver spouts and chains, and Mugs and Jugs, with silver rims and covers; also Mortars and Pestles of so hard a composition, that the strongest acids cannot penetrate them.

The "Mugs and Jugs with silver rims and covers" represent the best known type of Turner ware; they are of a creamy-white, hard compact stoneware body, attractively decorated with relief motifs—hunting scenes, drinking subjects, etc. (see Plate 582). Other potters made similar pieces, but these are not as neatly worked as the marked Turner specimens. The contemporary silver rims often bear hall-marks and year stamp, so that the period of the example can be ascertained. S. Shaw, writing in 1829 (*History of the Staffordshire Potteries*), noted: "About 1780 he discovered a vein of fine clay on the land at Green Dock. From this he obtained all his supplies for manufacturing his beautiful and excellent Stone Ware of a cane colour, which he formed into very beautiful Jugs with ornamental designs, and the most tasteful articles of domestic use. . . ."

After John Turner's death in December 1787 the Pottery was continued by his sons, John and William until November 1804 when John Turner withdrew from the partnership. They continued the staple lines of their father—creamwares, relief patterned stoneware jugs, etc., but business declined and they became heavily in debt. In January 1800 they patented a new type of hard, durable opaque earthenware, the forerunner of Ironstone china. This new body was used for dessert services and other useful wares, always neatly potted and often decorated with colourful "Japan" patterns (see Plate 588). The body bears the painted mark "Turner's Patent"; examples are rare. It is recorded that Josiah Spode purchased the patent rights about 1805 and renamed the body "Stone China". Much fine Spode stone china was produced in dinner and dessert services (see

Plate 535). In July 1806 the Turner brothers went bankrupt, and although William Turner continued potting until 1829, the true period of Turner wares ceased in 1806.

Most Turner wares are marked "TURNER" or "TURNER & CO" (this mark was probably used *c.* 1780–6 and 1803–6). The mark "TURNER & ABBOTT" is recorded (*c.* 1783–7) but it is very rare. All Turner wares are of good quality and represent a neglected field for discriminating collectors. It is interesting to see that Turner & Abbott's London address—82 Fleet Street—later occurs in the mark of J. Mist (see Plate 425) and is given on Davenport's bill for the 1835 Dinner service shown in Colour Plate V.

A recent very well illustrated reference book is *Master Potters of the Industrial Revolution, The Turners of Lane End* by Bevis Hillier (1965).

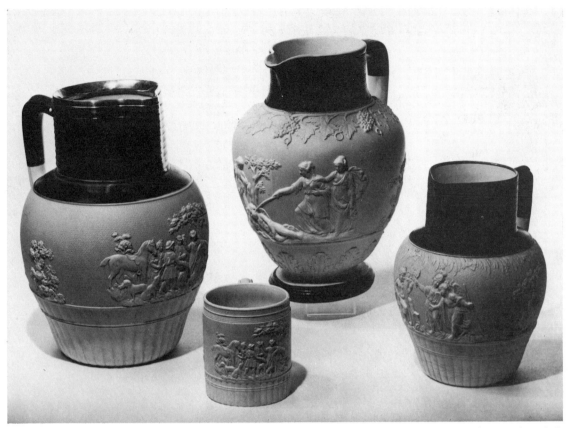

582. Turner (impressed marked) stoneware jugs with typical applied relief motifs (c. 1775–90). Centre jug 10¼ inches high. John Turner potted at Lane End from c. 1762. Other potters made similar stonewares but not of such fine quality as Turner's examples.

Godden of Worthing

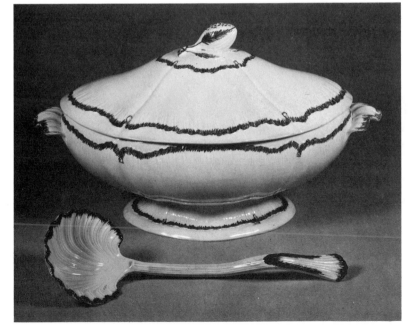

583. "Turner" impressed marked creamware tureen and ladle. Decorated with simple blue border (c. 1775–90). 9½ inches high.

Victoria & Albert Museum

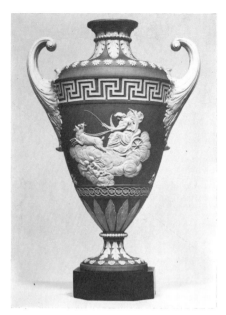

584. *Turner (impressed marked) blue jasper vase with white reliefs in the Wedgwood manner. Turner jasper is always of the finest quality* (c. 1790). *12½ inches high.*

British Museum

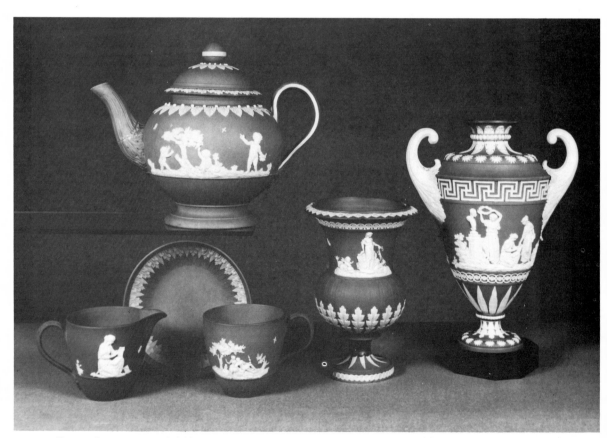

585. *"Turner" impressed marked blue jasper wares with white relief motifs in the Wedgwood manner. All pieces show fine workmanship* (c. 1780–1800). *Vase 5¾ inches high.*

Victoria & Albert Museum

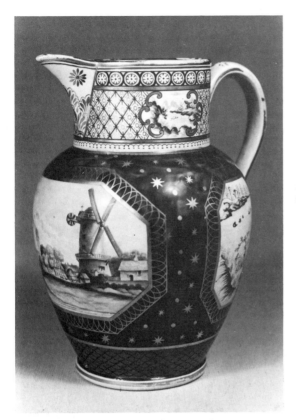

586. *"Turner Patent" earthenware jug of the finest quality, with rich blue ground (c. 1800–5). $8\frac{1}{8}$ inches high.*
Museum & Art Gallery, Stoke-on-Trent

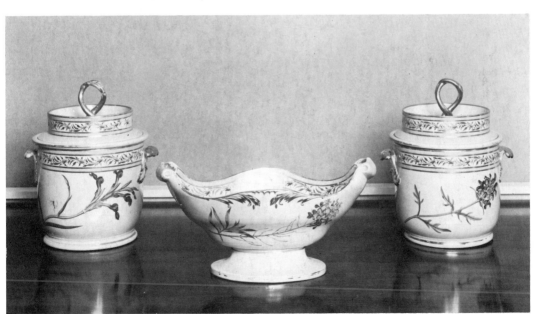

587. *A fruit cooler and centrepiece from a dessert service in "Turner's Patent" stone china-type body, patented in January 1800. This large service is finely gilt and has yellow bands in the borders. The botanical studies are a favourite form of ceramic decoration of the 1800–20 period (c. 1800–5).*
Ayer & Co (Antiques) Ltd

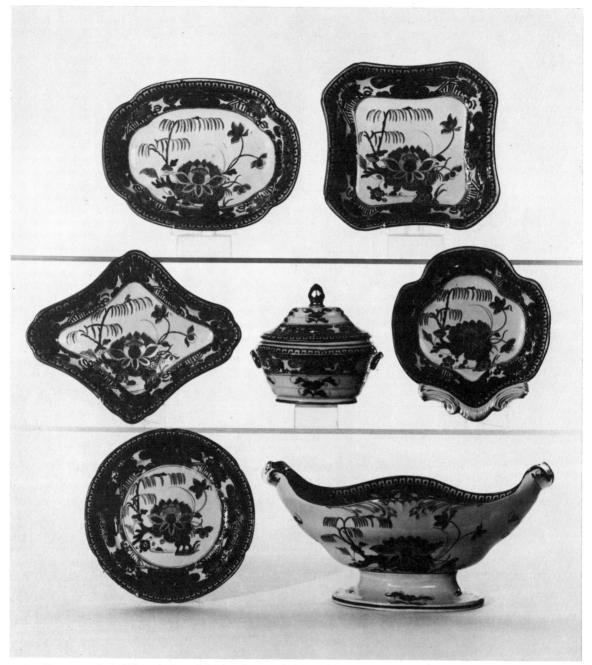

588. *Dessert service in "Turner's Patent" hard earthenware body introduced in 1800. Painted "Turner's Patent" mark. Centre-piece* 13¾ *inches long. The pattern and dessert ware forms are typical of this ware.*

Godden of Worthing

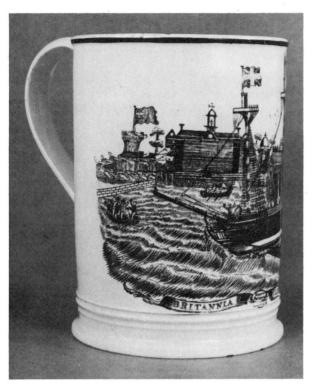

589. *Very rare creamware mug transfer printed in black with a view of Sunderland. Marked on print "Union Pottery". Very little is known of this pottery, apart from an advertisement of 1802. 5½ inches high.*

Willett Collection, Brighton Museum

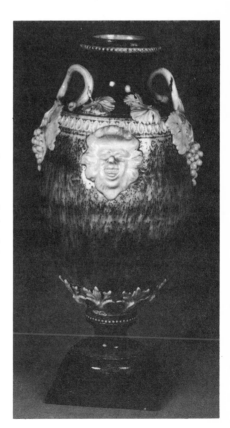

590. *"Voyez & Hales fecit" impressed marked creamware vase, decorated with mottled glaze (c. 1770). 9⅘ inches high.*

British Museum

Jean (John) Voyez was a modeller, best known for his "Fair Hebe" jugs (see Plate 18). For further information on Voyez see Transactions of the English Ceramic Circle, *vol. 5, part 1, and new 15th edition of Chaffer's* Marks and Monograms *(1965).*

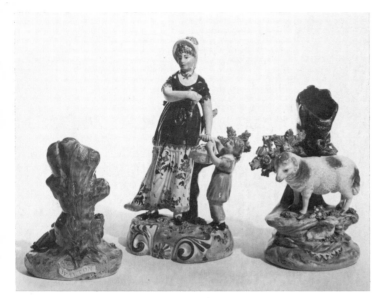

591. *Walton marked figures (c. 1820–5). One reversed to show normal form of name mark on a scroll at the back of the figure. Centre figure 9 inches high.*

Godden of Worthing

592. *Walton earthenware figures, marked with the name on a moulded scroll at the back of the bases. John Walton potted at Burslem, and these examples are typical of the 1815–25 period. "Flight into Egypt" group 7¼ inches high.*

Victoria & Albert Museum

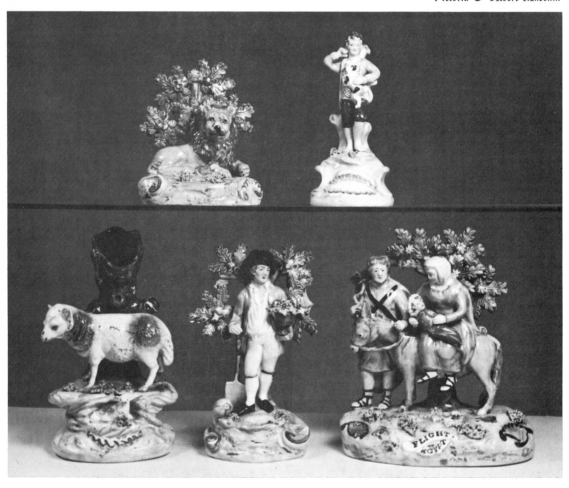

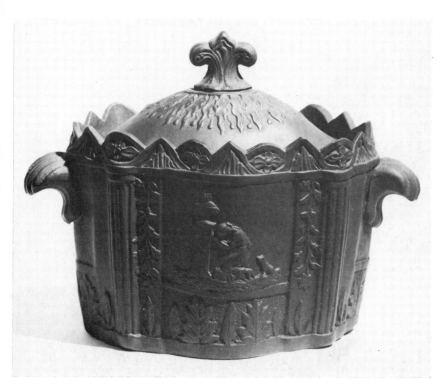

593. *"Warburton" (impressed marked) moulded basalt covered sugar. John Warburton potted at Cobridge between 1802 and 1823. Marked examples are extremely rare.* 5¾ *inches long.*

Godden of Worthing

WARBURTON, NEWCASTLE UPON TYNE *c.* 1750–95

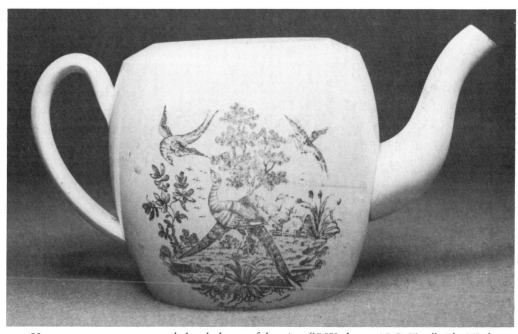

594. *Very rare creamware teapot, marked at the bottom of the print—"J Warburton. N.C. Tyne". John Warburton worked the Carr's Hill Pottery at Newcastle upon Tyne from* c. 1750 *to* c. 1795. *Cover missing.* 4¼ *inches high.*

Willett Collection, Brighton Museum

333

Wedgwood & Co

Many good eighteenth- and nineteenth-century creamwares (and other types of pottery) bear the name "Wedgwood & Co" impressed or printed. These were *not* made by the main Wedgwood firm.

The eighteenth-century "Wedgwood & Co" wares were made by Ralph Wedgwood of Burslem and Knottingley, Yorkshire. Little is known of this Burslem potter, apart from the fact that Josiah Wedgwood noted in April 1793: "I believe too that Ralph Wedgwood is tottering he has parted with many of his men." It may well be that his wares were too good and expensive for the normal trade of his day, for the marked examples are of very good quality, both in decoration and in the potting. He probably continued potting on a reduced scale at Burslem until 1796.

Ralph Wedgwood subsequently (late 1796) went to the Knottingley (Ferrybridge) Pottery in Yorkshire and joined the firm of William Tomlinson & Co. The partners then found it prudent to drop their own names and mark their products with the short title "Wedgwood & Co". The creamwares, Castleford-type stonewares, and basalt wares are of above average quality. It is often difficult to decide if marked pieces were made by Ralph Wedgwood at Burslem (*c.* 1790-5) or subsequently at Knottingley. The only dated examples bearing the "Wedgood & Co" impressed mark are the harvest jug and beaker shown in Plate 596. Ralph Wedgwood left the partnership *c.* 1800-1, and the remaining partners reverted to the old title "Tomlinson & Co", so that the period of use of the "Wedgwood & Co" mark is *c.* 1790-1801.

In the nineteenth century Messrs Podmore, Walker & Co (1834-59) of Tunstall used the title "Wedgwood & Co" as a mark, as did their successors Wedgwood & Co (Ltd) from 1860 to 1965. The marked wares of both these firms are often taken for the products of Josiah Wedgwood & Sons by those who do not know that the latter firm never added "& Co" to their name— WEDGWOOD. In order to avoid confusion the title Wedgwood & Co Ltd was changed, in 1965, to Enoch Wedgwood (Tunstall) Ltd.

Other misleading Wedgwood-type marks were used by John Wedg Wood of Burslem and Tunstall between 1841 and 1860. His marks often show the initial "J" and a slight space between the two words "Wedg" and "Wood", although the purchaser was doubtless intended to read it as Wedgwood and presume it was made by the famous firm of that name.

William Smith & Co of the Stafford Pottery, Stockton-on-Tees also employed misleading Wedgwood marks, including the names "Wedgewood" (note the middle "e"), Vedgwood, Wedgwood Ware, Queen's Ware. These Stafford Pottery wares are inferior in quality to the true Wedgwood examples. They also made children's motto plates and rather coarsely printed wares (see Plate 525).

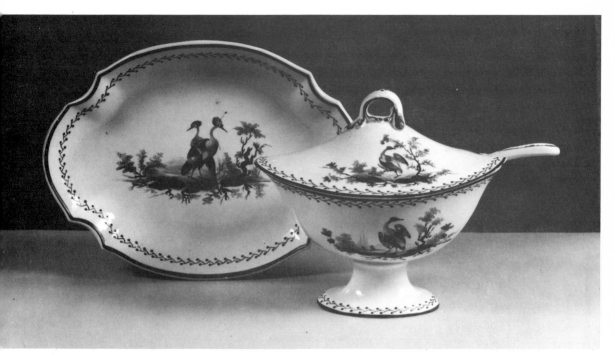

595. *"Wedgwood & Co" (impressed marked) creamware tureen and stand, painted in bright enamel colours in an attractive manner (c. 1790–1800). 6¼ inches high.*

Victoria & Albert Museum

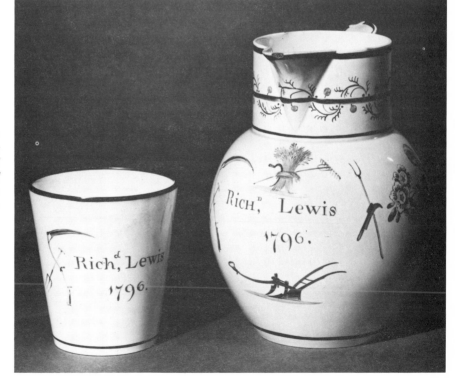

96. *"Wedgwood & Co" (impressed marked) creamware harvest jug and beaker of fine quality (dated 796). Made by Ralph Wedgwood at Burslem or at his Ferrybridge Pottery in Yorkshire. Jug 6½ inches high.*

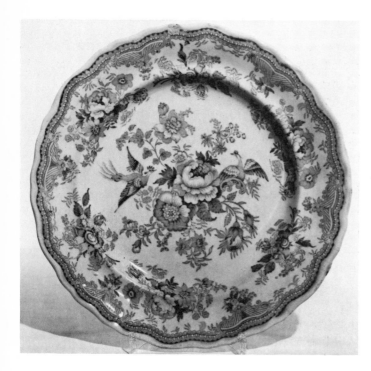

597. *"Asiatic Pheasants" pattern plate, bearing impressed and printed marks—"Wedgwood & Co". This form of mark relates to Wedgwood & Co of the Unicorn Works, Tunstall, not to Josiah Wedgwood & Sons (c. 1860–70).*

J. WEDG WOOD, BURSLEM AND TUNSTALL 1841–60

598. *"J Wedg. Wood" (printed mark, no. 4276b, also WW impressed) earthenware plate, printed in sepia (c. 1841–50). The wares and marks of John Wedg(e) Wood are often mistaken for those of Josiah Wedgwood & Sons. This was probably intended. See page 334.*

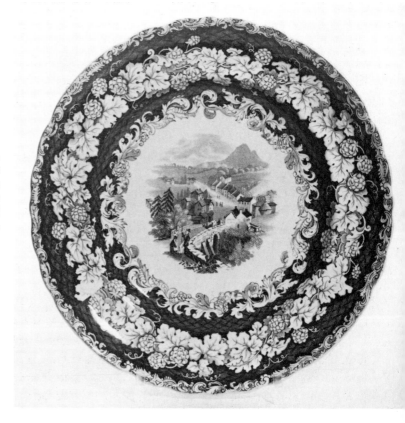

Josiah Wedgwood was born at Burslem in 1730. At an early age he was sent to work in the Churchyard Pottery which had passed, on his father's death, to the eldest son, Thomas. He was apprenticed there until 1749 and remained with his brother until *c.* 1752, when he went to Thomas Alders of Stoke. In 1754 he joined Thomas Whieldon of Fenton Low. At this period Josiah Wedgwood carried out many experiments in an effort to improve the standard bodies and glazes then in general use. In 1759 he was successful in producing a fine green semi-translucent glaze. Having undergone a thorough apprenticeship, he had practical experience of pottery management, had shown an inquiring mind, and was now ready to start up on his own.

In May 1759 he took this important step and laid the foundation of a firm that has done more to spread the knowledge and enhance the reputation of British ceramic art than any other manu-facturer. Prior to 1770 the articles were, in the main, of a useful nature to meet the everyday needs of the housewife; the early wares are seldom marked and are difficult to distinguish with certainty. Moulded earthenwares of leaf form, cauliflower-shaped teapots, creamers, etc., were an early innovation and the fine semi-translucent green glaze served to accentuate the moulded design.

In contrast to these utilitarian wares (finely potted and well designed as they were) Josiah Wedgwood soon felt the need (and challenge) to produce ornamental wares, vases, library busts, and so forth. These ornamental objects were produced from June 1769 at the new Etruria works, the utilitarian wares being still made at the Burslem factory. Elegantly shaped classical vases are included in the firm's Shape Book of 1770 and these early wares may be found in earthenware veined in imitation of marble, agate, porphyry, granite, and onyx or in the matt black "basalt" body (some basalt wares were painted with classical figure subjects—a bill of June 1771 lists—"1 large Etruscan vase painted, £31 10 –". Most of this painted decoration on early Wedgwood was added in London) or in blue and other coloured jasper bodies with the traditional white relief motifs. It should be noted that the gold on the relief festoons, handles, etc, of the early variegated vases was not durable and it has, in most cases, worn off, exposing the cream-coloured earthenware beneath the original gilding (see Plate 600).

The body that did Josiah Wedgwood more lasting good and won him world-wide repute was not so much the famous coloured jasper body, but the more everyday cream-coloured earthenware known as Creamware or Queen's ware. This could be neatly potted and was relatively easy and therefore inexpensive to produce. It lent itself to simple, tastefully painted border motifs that could again be carried out cheaply, or it could be decorated with printed patterns. It was light in weight —an important consideration that greatly helped Wedgwood's export trade, as both freight charges and import dues were cut to a minimum. From the customer's point of view, the new refined creamware was popular, as it was attractive in form and decoration as well as being reasonably durable—the glaze was sound, brilliant and clear, and the price low on account of the already indicated manufacturing advantages that the ware afforded. Josiah Wedgwood made huge dinner services (Plate 607), dessert and tea services, and a host of special objects (jelly moulds, spoons, etc.). It is difficult to think of any household item that was not made by Wedgwood in creamware.

Queen Charlotte ordered a teaset in 1765—so pleased was she with it that she allowed her name to be associated with the body and the term "Queen's ware" was adopted. This new name occurs on surviving accounts dated 1767 and may have been used before this date. The new Wedgwood wares were exported to the Continent in vast amounts and caused widespread concern to the manufacturers there. Its many advantages over the soft-bodied faience and Delft-type wares were so noticeable that many Continental potters were put out of business or forced to try to copy the new English wares. Not only did the Continental potters need to emulate Wedgwood's creamware body, so did nearly every English potter and it soon became the staple earthenware body of the country (see page xv). No other potters, however, consistently rivalled Josiah Wedgwood in the purity of their forms, in the quality of the body and glaze, or in the attractiveness of the ornamentation. Several, however, did undercut him in price by lowering their standards of body and workmanship. Donald Towner's excellent reference book *English Cream Coloured Earthenware* (1957) contains detailed information and good illustrations of creamwares made by the better known makers. Other examples are illustrated in Plates 59, 63, 191–2, 306, 317, 334, 336, 339, 434, 515, 634 of this illustrated encyclopaedia. Most examples of Wedgwood's creamware bear the simple impressed mark WEDGWOOD; pieces marked WEDGWOOD & CO or WEDGEWOOD (with a middle "e") were not made by this firm (see pages 334–6).

In 1769 Josiah Wedgwood and Thomas Bentley formed their celebrated partnership. This partnership had been discussed as early as 1767, but the Wedgwood & Bentley mark was probably not used before 1769. Bentley ably managed the fashionable London showrooms and decorating establishment. Their combined good taste and judgment of market trends did much to enhance the name of Wedgwood's pottery. The numerous letters that were exchanged between the two partners have thrown light on many ceramic problems and on matters of everyday life and fashion in the eighteenth century. Several are quoted in early reference books such as the *Life of Josiah Wedgwood* by E. Meteyard (2 vols., 1865–6) and *A Group of Englishmen* also by E. Meteyard (1871) and *The Selected Letters of Josiah Wedgwood*, edited by Ann Finer and George Savage (1965).

It will be observed that the "Wedgwood & Bentley" mark only appears on ornamental wares, not on purely useful objects such as plates. Wedgwood suggested in 1770: "May not useful ware be comprehended under his simple definition of such vessels as are made use of at meals". It will be further observed that marked "Wedgwood & Bentley" objects are of superb quality; many examples were sold through the London shop to the nobility and were regarded as prestige pieces. This is not to say that the contemporary utilitarian "Wedgwood" wares were of inferior quality—it is simply that the "Wedgwood & Bentley" pieces seem to have had special care bestowed upon them. Thomas Bentley died in 1780 (an event that has been written of as "the greatest misfortune in Wedgwood's life") and the partnership therefore came to an end. Marked examples of this period are today highly valued, both for their rarity and for their quality. All wares marked "Wedgwood & Bentley" (the initials "W. & B." were sometimes impressed on very small objects) were made between 1769 and 1780. In November 1772 Wedgwood wrote: "We are going upon a plan to mark the whole if practicable", a remark which suggests that all pieces had not previously been marked.

The ornamental matt jasper body which could be tinted to various colours, or used in the white, was a natural development of the black basalt body (introduced *c.* 1767). The jasper body was introduced to the market in 1775 after countless experiments. The official Wedgwood booklet, *The Story of Wedgwood*, describes it as "an unglazed, vitreous fine stoneware or semi-porcelain. It has been made in several shades of blue, green, lilac, yellow, maroon, black or white and sometimes one piece combines three or more of these colours. . . ." This is the body that calls to mind the name "Wedgwood" wherever it is seen, with its traditional white relief motifs on a coloured ground. The jasper body has been produced continuously from 1775 to the present day and it seems likely to continue until man tires of gracious living. The early examples are of very fine grain and feel silky to the touch. Vases, portrait, and other plaques and medallions, teawares and a host of interesting items were made in this decorative body. The vast range of portrait and other medallions offer fine scope for the collector with limited space (see Plates 604-5). Finely tooled reliefs with undercutting mark the earlier examples.

The jasper may be solid—that is, tinted throughout the body, or "dipped"; in the latter case the main body is white with a tinted surface caused by dipping it in tinted jasper slip, a system first used in 1777. In this case the inner layer can be exposed by turning away part of the upper tinted layer. It should be mentioned that many manufacturers, other than Wedgwood, produced jasper wares (see Plates 8, 9, 436, 547, 585, 632).

An important new decorative style of lustre was introduced during the 1805-10 period. This all-over splashed pink lustre decoration, with grey, brown, or yellowish marbled effects, often called "Moonlight lustre", is well illustrated in Plate 615. The shell forms of the service are traditional Wedgwood shapes found with various styles of decoration over a long period. This rare type of splashed pink lustre was made for a short period and its production was probably limited to the period 1805-15. The impressed standard mark "WEDGWOOD" is often very difficult to find on specimens of this type as the lustre tends to fill and hide the impressions. It should be noted that the plain all-over silver or gold lustre is rarely found on marked Wedgwood earthenwares. Further specimens of Wedgwood lustre are illustrated in W. D. John and J. Simcox's joint work *Early Wedgwood Lustre Wares* (1963).

Several different bodies were in use during the early years of the nineteenth century; some were of the so-called "dry body" type, others have a slight smear of glaze. Most staple shapes could be purchased in several different bodies and tints (see the page reproduced from the pattern books, Plate 613).

Trade was not good during the early years of the nineteenth century and in an effort to take a greater share of the available business, the second Josiah Wedgwood introduced the manufacture of porcelain (as made by Minton, Spode, the Derby works, and the Worcester factories, to name only the most important) by mid 1812. This was an answer to demands from the London shop. Byerley, the manager, wrote in 1811: "Every day we are asked for China Tea Ware—our sales of it would be immense if we had any—Earthenware Teaware is quite out of fashion. . . ." The Wedgwood bone china is quite characteristic; once handled it cannot be mistaken. The glaze is a soft, mellow, close-fitting one that appears to have tin or a similar ingredient to make it seem opaque. The opaqueness, however, is only imagined and is probably due more to the pure white body of the porcelain.

The porcelain shapes are pure and graceful and the decorative painted or printed patterns restrained (see Plates 616-17). The porcelain body was not a great success from a commercial point of view, and it is recorded that in 1814 Wedgwood had thoughts of abandoning its manufacture. This may have been due to the relatively high price of the fine quality hand-painted Wedgwood porcelains; a letter dated 1816 reports back to the factory that "No. 701 teaset £4/4/– I find is too high, if it could be reduced it might go off—they get all Landscapes up now, printed, and render them at 4/10 for 6 cups and saucers, not gilt. . . ." The production of porcelain gradually diminished from 1816 to the final cessation in 1822, ten years after its introduction. All early Wedgwood bone china is therefore rare. It normally bears the simple printed mark "WEDGWOOD".

The production of translucent porcelain was recommenced in 1878 and it continues to this day. Various forms of the Portland vase mark have been used on it (see the companion *Encyclopaedia of British Pottery and Porcelain Marks* (1964).

In an effort to rival the durable Ironstone china, popularized by the Mason firm, Wedgwoods made a "Stone China" from *c.* 1827 to 1861, but production was limited and specimens are rarely found. They normally bear a self-explanatory printed mark—"WEDGWOOD'S STONE CHINA". Good services and other objects were also made in the "Pearl" earthenware body from *c.* 1820 to 1868. Wares made in this body normally have the word "PEARL" impressed or incorporated in the printed mark. The initial "P" also occurs impressed on this body. The Pearl body had been introduced about 1780, but no distinguishing mark was then employed.

During the nineteenth century the earlier wares, creamware, black basalt, and coloured jaspers, were continued and many of the old forms and popular relief motifs were still produced. As the century progressed new objects were added to the long list of Wedgwood lines, often indicating their late date by the form and general appearance, although the traditional white relief motifs remain much the same as the eighteenth-century examples. Biscuit barrels with electro-plated silver mounts and cheese dishes are cases in point. Many late nineteenth-century objects would pass for those of an earlier period were it not for the three impressed letters in the body of most wares from 1860 onwards. The key to this dating system is given in the companion encyclopaedia of marks.

Like other manufacturers Messrs Wedgwoods produced wares in two typical Victorian bodies— Majolica, with its green or tinted semi-translucent glazes in 1860 and the white matt Parian body (called "Carrara" by Wedgwoods) in 1848. Some ornate groups in this Parian body are very fine.

Of all the Victorian innovations, the most costly and popular with collectors are those cream-wares bearing the charming and free painting of Emile Lessore (see Colour Plate XV). Lessore was trained in Paris, working for several decorating establishments and also for the French National Sèvres factory. In 1858 he came to England and, after a few months at Mintons, joined Wedgwoods staff—"free to name my own conditions, to choose my own workmen, my own materials. Mr. Wedgwood reposed confidence in me. I did not abuse it. I have drawn and coloured 4,000 pieces in two years . . . my heart is full of joy. I am my own master, and my benefactors are satisfied with me. . . ."

Emile Lessore's charming mellow ceramic paintings in a cheerful, light, free manner were included in several international exhibitions, and were warmly received and gained much publicity, mainly on account of his new, free style of ceramic painting, so different from the normal, rather laboured, miniature style. But the English climate and Staffordshire atmosphere—"the black smoke of the furnaces, which never ceases day or night, Sundays excepted"—did not suit Lessore or his children and by 1867 he had returned to his native France. Such was his fame and value to Wedgwoods that the blanks were shipped over to France to be decorated by Lessore, and returned to England for firing and resale—an arrangement probably unique in the history of pottery.

Lessore died in 1876. Mortlock's, the London retailers, purchased all his remaining work and held an exhibition of two hundred and seventy pieces—the prices ranging from one hundred and fifty guineas for a large plaque to ten shillings for small card trays. Most of Lessore's work was signed (or initialled) on the face of the object; the first "s" is an old-fashioned long "s", giving the signature resembling "Lefsore". Because of the popularity of Lessore's style of painting, several other artists sought to emulate it. At Wedgwoods, Henry Brownsword painted in a similar manner. Other members of Lessore's family, Therese Lessore and Louise Powell (granddaughter of Emile), also painted for Wedgwoods at a later date; their work is rare and attractive. Several contemporary Victorian reviews of Lessore's art are incorporated in an article printed in *The Studio*, July 1960.

The study of Victorian Wedgwood is one that could be most rewarding for collectors unable to pay the high prices of eighteenth-century wares, or other "collectable" types, such as three-colour jasper (in which two or more colours are used in addition to white, see Plate 618). Various novelties, both in form and style of decoration, were produced, sometimes for brief periods, as experiments. Some of these are featured in an article in *Country Life* of 13 October 1960.

With regard to twentieth-century Wedgwood, the paintings of Alfred and Louise Powell have been neglected by collectors, but the "Fairyland" lustres designed by Miss Makeig-Jones have lately attracted attention. The standard work on these designs is *Wedgwood Fairyland Lustre* by Una des Fontaines (1975).

Some ninety per cent of all Wedgwood is marked in a clear and straightforward manner. The staple marks, with their periods of use, are given in the companion *Encyclopaedia of British Pottery and Porcelain Marks* (1964) with the signature or device of the foremost artists. The addition of the word ENGLAND denotes a date after 1891, MADE IN ENGLAND denotes a twentieth-century date.

No general book can hope to deal fully with so vast a story as the history of Wedgwood, and the reader is recommended to study as many of the following selected reference books as he can. The early ones should not be neglected as they contain much interesting information with which modern stream-lined books cannot compete.

The Life of Josiah Wedgwood, E. Meteyard, 2 vols., 1865–6

The Wedgwoods, being a life of Josiah Wedgwood, J. Jewitt, 1865

A Group of Englishmen, E. Meteyard, 1871

Wedgwood and His Works, E. Meteyard, 1873

Memorials of Wedgwood, E. Meteyard, 1874

Handbook of Wedgwood Ware, E. Meteyard, 1875

Wedgwood's Letters to Bentley, Lady Farrer, 3 vols., 1902–7, reprinted 1962

Josiah Wedgwood, Master Potter, A. Church, 1903

Josiah Wedgwood and His Pottery, W. Burton, 1922

Wedgwood Ware, W. B. Honey, 1947

Wedgwood, a living tradition, J. M. Graham and H. C. Wedgwood, 1948

Wedgwood, W. Mankowitz, 1953

Proceedings of the English Wedgwood Society, 1956 onwards

Wedgwood and Artists, H. M. Buten, 1960

The Story of Wedgwood, A. Kelly, 1962

Early Wedgwood Lustre Wares, W. D. John and J. Simcox, 1963

The Selected Letters of Josiah Wedgwood, A. Finer and G. Savage, 1965

Decorative Wedgwood in Architecture and Furniture, A. Kelly, 1965

Wedgwood Ware, A. Kelly, 1970

Wedgwood Jasper, R. Reilly, 1972

Wedgwood, the portrait medallions, R. Reilly and G. Savage, 1973

In addition to these specialist books, most general reference books include a good general account of Wedgwoods' varied products.

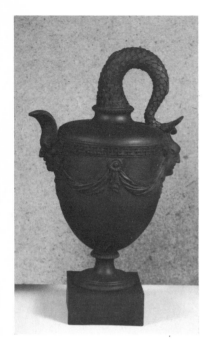

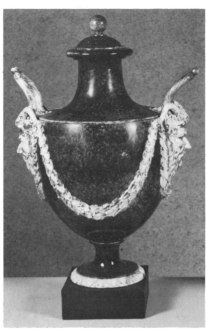

599. (Far left) *"Wedgwood &*
Bentley. Etruria" impressed marked
basalt vase of unusual form (c.
1771–80). 12⅝ inches high. Vases
made in sections joined by a bolt and
screw post-date April 1771.

Victoria & Albert Museum

600. *"Wedgwood & Bentley.*
Etruria" impressed marked vase.
Marbled ground with gilt swags and
handles. Mounted on basalt base
(c. 1771–80). 14 inches high.

Victoria & Albert Museum

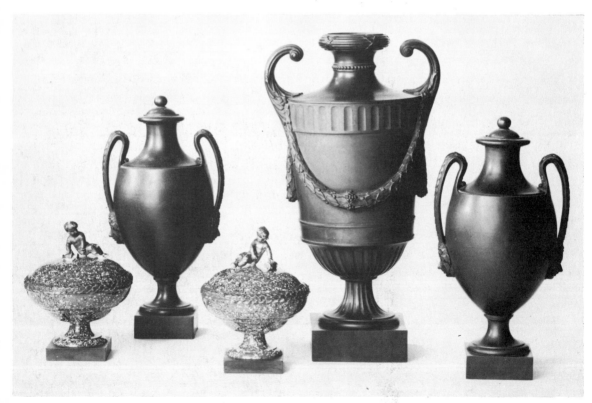

601. *Wedgwood & Bentley (impressed marks in circular form) basalt and imitation stone vases (c. 1771–80). Centre vase*
13½ inches high. The low "marbled" vases on basalt plinths are extremely rare.

Godden of Worthing

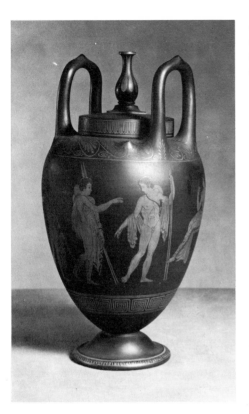

602. *Wedgwood basalt vase, decorated with encaustic paintings of Etruscan figure subject, similar painting occurs on the first vases made at Wedgwood's Etruria Works in 1769. In most cases this decoration was added in London (c. 1769–75). $13\frac{7}{8}$ inches high.*

Victoria & Albert Museum

603. *"Wedgwood" (impressed marked) creamwares printed by Sadler & Green at Liverpool. Other potters also had their wares printed at Liverpool in a similar manner. A fine dinner service has these "Liverpool Bird" prints but no factory marks (c. 1772–5). In April 1772 Wedgwood wrote,"We are sending a quantity of table ware to Liverpool to be printed in black, the bird pattern, and intend to gild some of it on the edges" as the covered jug here illustrated.*

Schreiber Collection, Victoria & Albert Museum

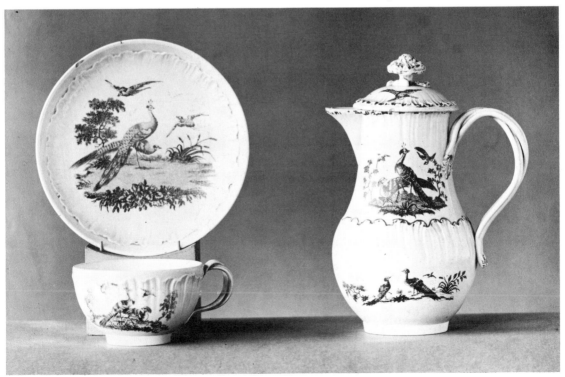

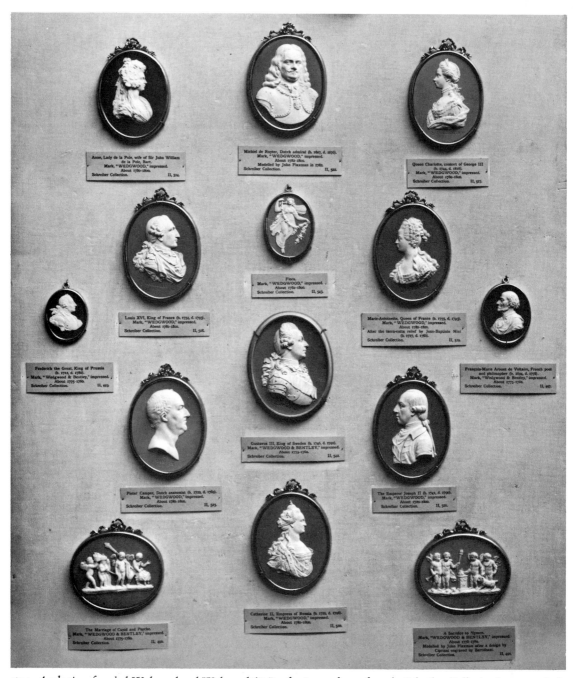

604. *A selection of marked Wedgwood, and Wedgwood & Bentley jasper plaques from the Schreiber Collection (c. 1775–1800).*
Victoria & Albert Museum

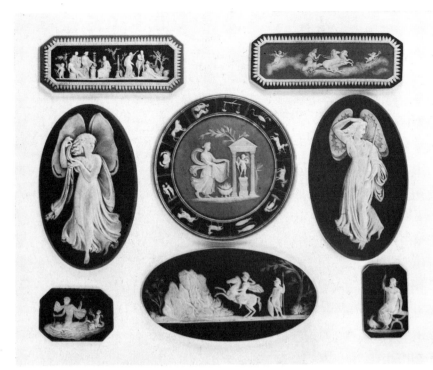

605. *Impressed marked "Wedgwood" jasper plaques of small size. The top two and the centre plaque are in the rare three-colour technique, others blue jasper ground.*

Sotheby & Co

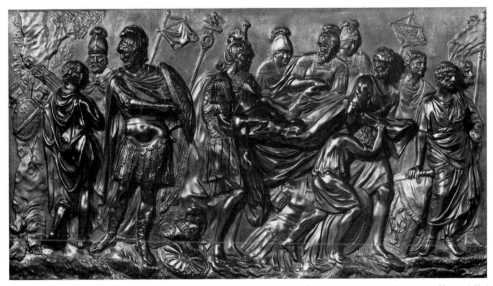

606. *A fine Wedgwood impressed marked basalt plaque—"Death of a Roman Warrior". Originally modelled in 1782 but reissued over many years; examples with "England" impressed are subsequent to 1891. 20 inches long.*

Godden of Worthing

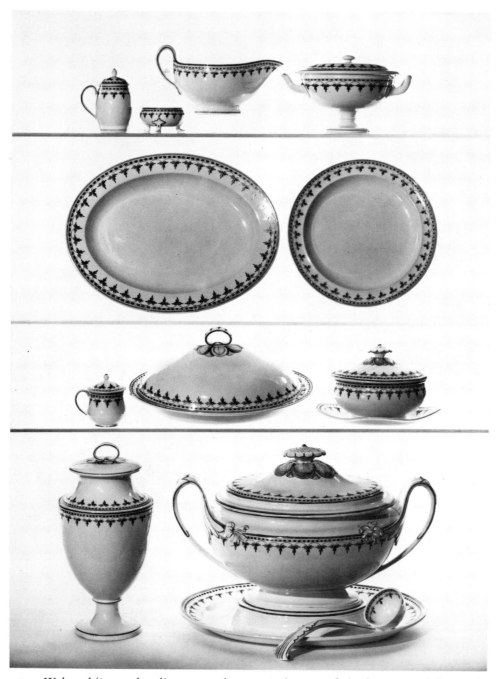

607. *Wedgwood (impressed mark) creamware dinner service (c. 1790–1800), showing typical shapes and simple border design. Tureen 11¾ inches high.*

Godden of Worthing

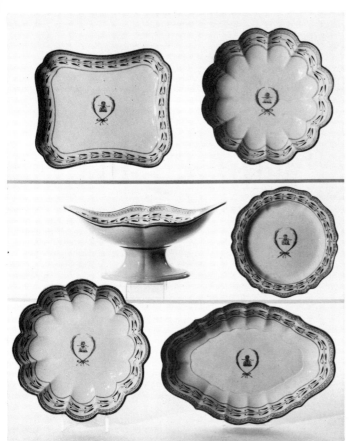

608. Impressed marked "Wedgwood" creamware dessert service of the 1790 period. Note simple enamelled border motifs, characteristic of Wedgwood creamwares. Comport 12 inches long.

Godden of Worthing

609. Impressed marked "Wedgwood" part teaset in the caneware body. Hackwood's infants in relief. Slight blue enamel borders. Many attractive objects were made in caneware with painted motifs (c. 1795–1805). Teapot $5\frac{1}{4}$ inches high.

Sotheby & Co

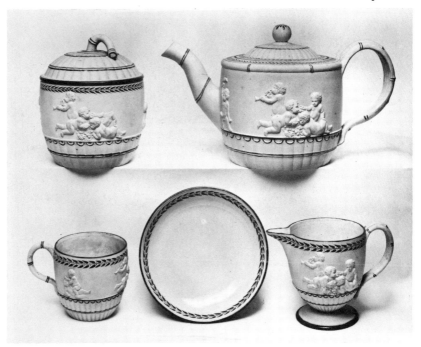

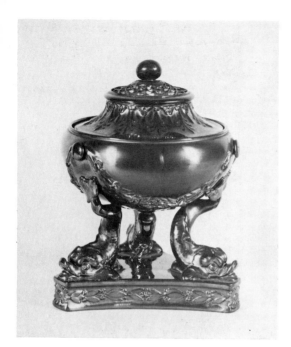

610. *Wedgwood "copper" lustred incense-burner. Rare mark—"Josiah Wedgwood. Feb. 2. 1805". Other ornaments of this form also bear this rare dated mark. 5¾ inches high.*

Victoria & Albert Museum

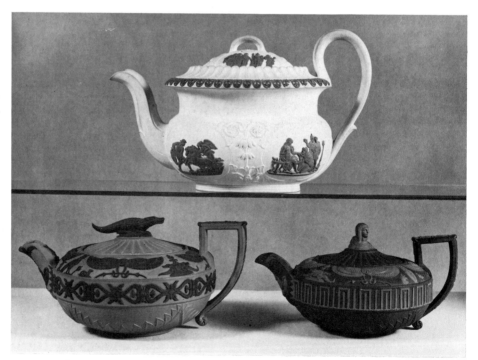

611. *Wedgwood (impressed marked) teapots of fine quality. The top example of cane-coloured "dry" body with red "Rosso Antico" reliefs. The lower examples with their Egyptian motifs occur in various colour combinations and date from c. 1805. Matching creamers, covered sugars and bowls were made (c. 1805–15). Top pot 5¾ inches high.*

Victoria & Albert Museum

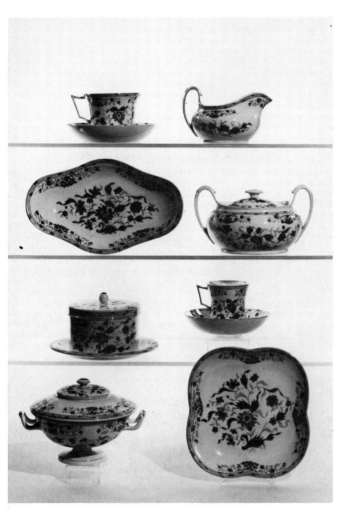

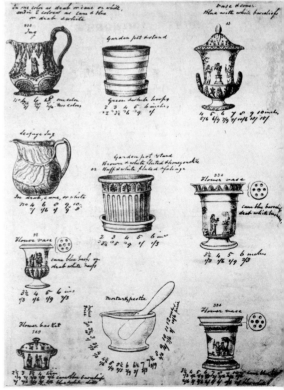

612. *Wedgwood (impressed marked) earthenware breakfast service, showing forms of the 1805–15 period. Pattern no. 26, decorated in underglaze blue, and overglaze enamels and gold. Square dish 7½ inches diameter.*

Godden of Worthing

613. *Jugs, vases, etc., from Wedgwood's 1817 catalogue. As can be seen, all designs were made in various sizes, or in different colours and effects. The 1817 prices are given in shillings and pence.*

Josiah Wedgwood & Sons Ltd

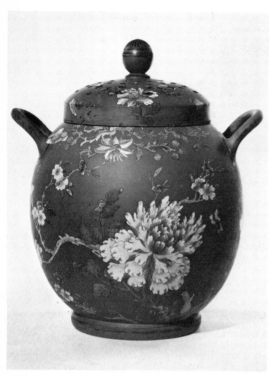

614. *Wedgwood terracotta coloured potpourri vase with perforated cover, and close-fitting inner cover. Enamelled in the Chinese taste (c. 1810). 11 inches high.*

Godden of Worthing

615. *A very rare and complete Wedgwood creamware dessert service decorated with "moonlight" lustre of mottled pink colour. Impressed "Wedgwood" marks (c. 1810). These shell forms occur with various styles of decoration.*

Delomosne & Son

"Moonlight" lustre is discussed by W. D. John, and J. Simcox in Early Wedgwood Lustre Wares (1963).

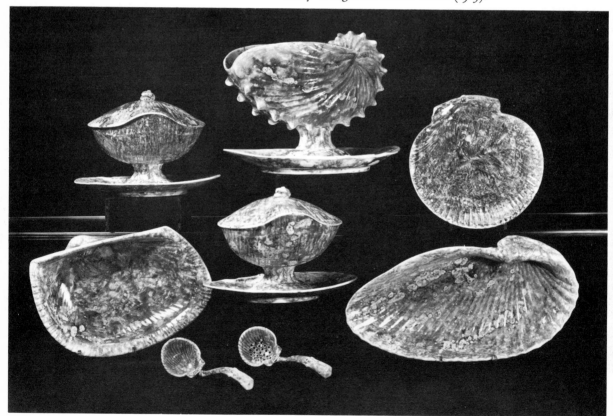

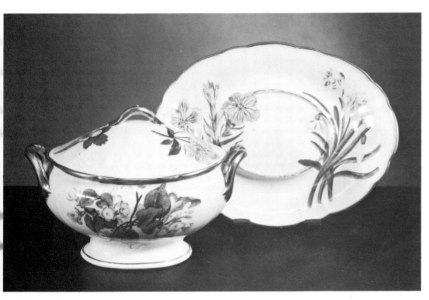

616. *Wedgwood porcelain sauce tureen, cover and stand, painted with botanical studies. Printed "Wedgwood" mark in red (c. 1812–22).*

Lucile Pillow Collection, Beaverbrook Art Gallery, Fredericton, Canada

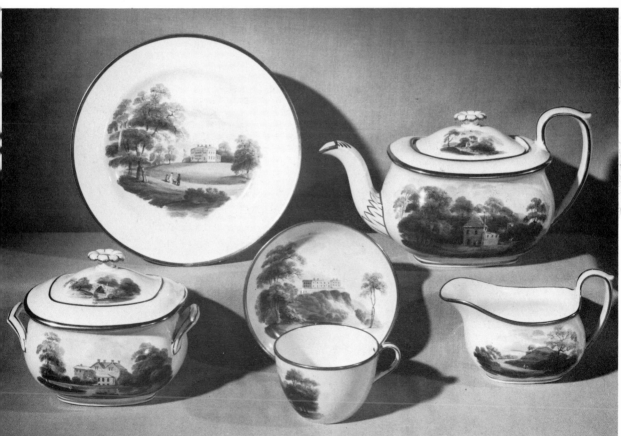

617. *Wedgwood bone china part teaset of fine quality, painted with named views. Printed "Wedgwood" mark (c. 1815). Teapot 5 inches high.*

Josiah Wedgwood & Sons Ltd

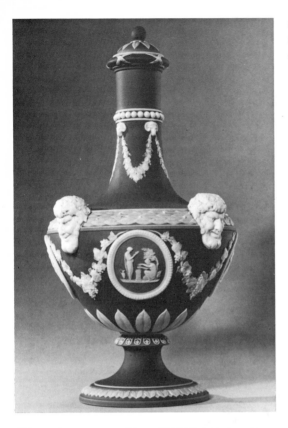

618. *A three-colour jasper vase of 1110 shape, introduced c. 1830. This form of vase was made in several colour combinations. Impressed year letter for 1867. 10¼ inches high.*

Godden of Worthing

619. *Impressed marked "Wedgwood" coffee cup and saucer in three colours—light blue, green and white, jasper. Mid nineteenth century.*

Godden of Worthing

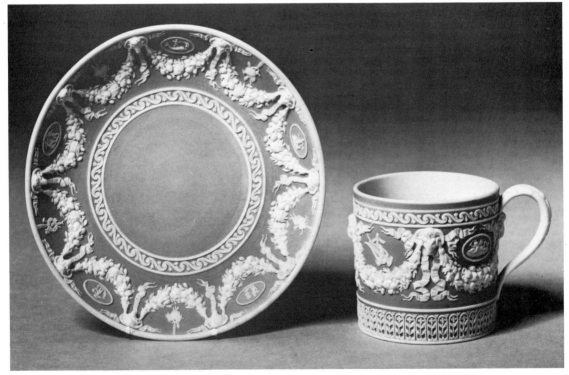

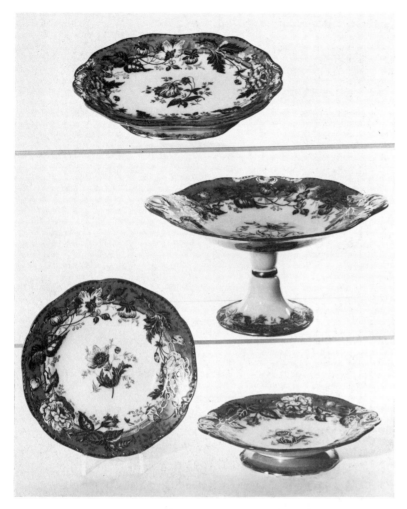

620. *Wedgwood pearlware dessert service of the 1840–68 period, showing typical early Victorian forms. Impressed mark "Wedgwood/ Pearl". Printed pattern "Horticultural". Comport 6½ inches high.*

Godden of Worthing

621. *Wedgwood (impressed marked) library busts in the basalt body. (Left) "Moore", modelled by E. W. Wyon, year mark for 1871. (Right) "R Stevenson", modelled by Wyon and "published 1858". 13¾ inches high. Wedgwoods made many fine basalt busts from the Wedgwood & Bentley period onwards.*

Godden of Worthing

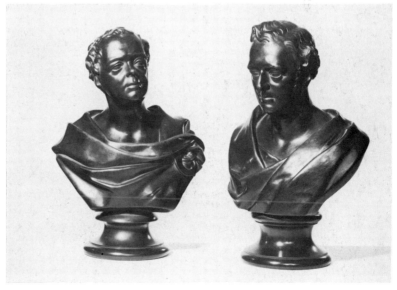

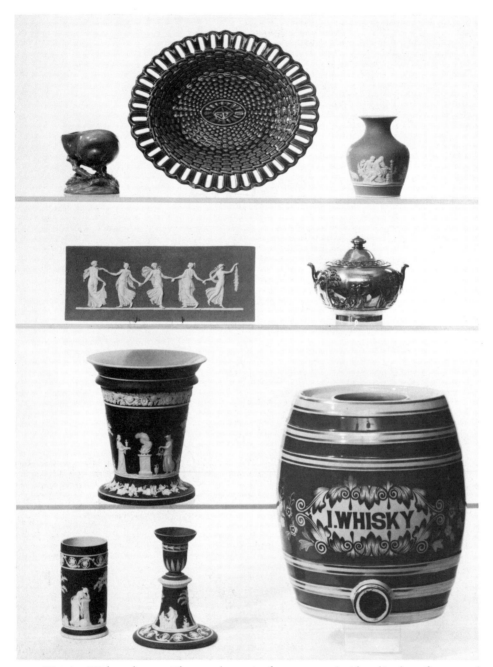

622. *Victorian Wedgwood wares. The covered sugar is of a type covered with a thin sheet of copper and silver plated. Whisky barrel (also made by other potters)* 10½ *inches high. All examples with impressed "Wedgwood" mark, plaque and jardinière also with "England" and therefore subsequent to 1891.*

Godden of Worthing

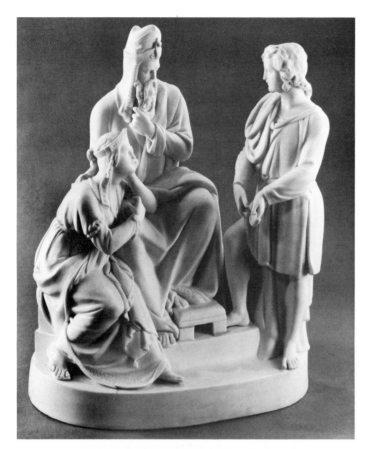

623. *Wedgwood Parian group, "Joseph before Pharaoh", modelled by William Beattie in 1856. $19\frac{1}{2}$ inches high. Mark "Wedgwood" impressed. Messrs Wedgwood called their Parian body "Carrara".*

Godden of Worthing

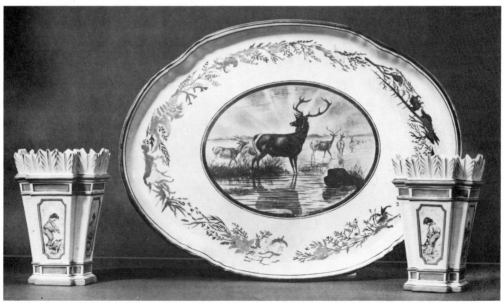

624. *Wedgwood (impressed marked) creamware, decorated by a photographic process. Signed and dated—H Hope Crealocke. 1876. Several other designs by Colonel Hope Crealocke were produced in the 1870's. The vases are painted by H. Brownsword (c. 1873). 6 inches high.*

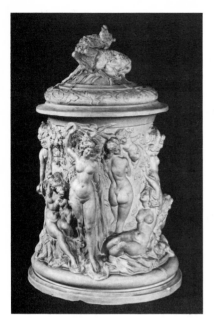

625. *Wills Bros terracotta covered jar with ornate relief decoration. Shown at the 1862 Exhibition. Inscribed "Wills Bros. Scpts, London. Published as the Act directs, 1858". 10½ inches high.*

Victoria & Albert Museum

D. WILSON, HANLEY *c.* 1801–18

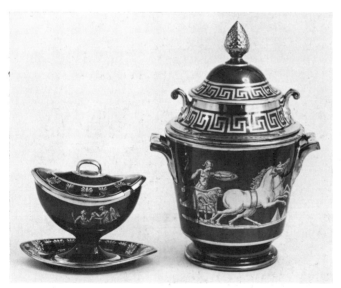

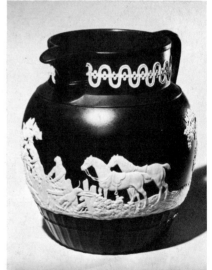

626. *"Wilson" (impressed marked) earthenware part dessert service, decorated with gilt classical figures, etc., over a rich chocolate ground (c. 1805–15). Ice pail 13¼ inches high.*

Godden of Worthing

627. *"Wilson" (impressed marked) earthenware jug, with applied white reliefs on a chocolate ground (c. 1805–17). 7½ inches high. David Wilson of Hanley worked from 1801 to 1817.*

Godden of Worthing

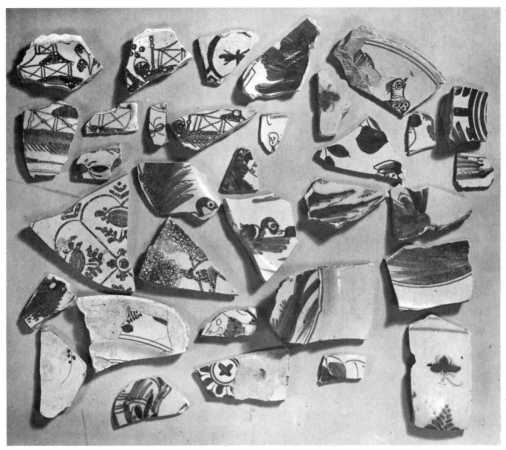

628. *Wincanton delft-type earthenware fragments found on the site of this Somerset factory. Most specimens are unmarked (c. 1735–50).*

Victoria & Albert Museum

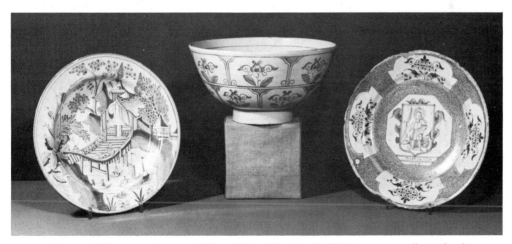

629. *Wincanton delft-type earthenwares (left to right): Plate inscribed "Wincanton, 1739". 9 inches diameter. Bowl inscribed "Wincanton, 1738". 8¾ inches diameter. Plate inscribed "Wincanton, 1738". 8¾ inches diameter.*

Fitzwilliam Museum, Cambridge

357

Enoch Wood

Enoch Wood was born in January 1759; he was apprenticed to Humphrey Palmer and reputedly also worked at Wedgwoods before starting on his own account at Burslem about 1784. The 1792 dated dinner service in the creamware body, illustrated in Plate 634, is very important as it shows the excellence of his productions in this type of ware. Enoch Wood is not known for dinner services (or even for creamwares), although his trade card lists "table-services enamel'd with arms, crests or other ornaments; Egyptian black Teapots, Vases, Busts, Figures, Seals &c. Colour'd ware in all its Branches".

Wood was a talented modeller and several fine relief pattern plaques bearing his signature or impressed mark are recorded; the word "Sculpsit" occurs after his name on several items which he modelled. Fine portrait busts were also a feature of his work. The plaques are often in the Wedgwood tradition—white reliefs on a blue jasper ground.

About 1790 Enoch Wood took as a partner James Caldwell, and some wares of high quality of the 1790–1818 period bear the impressed mark "Wood & Caldwell". Such wares include figures and busts. From 1818 to 1846 the style was "Enoch Wood & Sons" (many impressed and printed name or initial marks occur). Fine underglaze blue printed patterns were made by this firm, the blue being dark and rich; many special designs were produced for the American market. A contemporary account states that Enoch Wood & Sons was the largest exporter of earthenwares to America.

For further information on Enoch Wood the reader is referred to *The Wood Family of Burslem*, F. Falkner (1912), which also contains information on the talented figure modellers and manufacturers Ralph Wood, three generations of which produced fine figures and groups in the eighteenth century, see Plates 639–43.

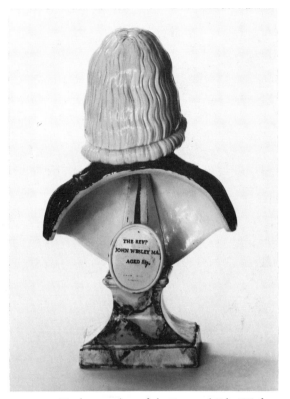 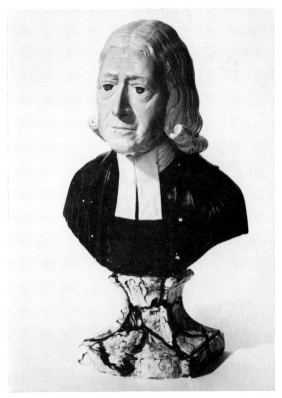

630 & a. *Earthenware bust of the Reverend John Wesley, modelled and signed "E Wood, Sculp. Burslem". 11½ inches high. This bust was copied at later dates by many potters (c. 1785).*

Godden of Worthing

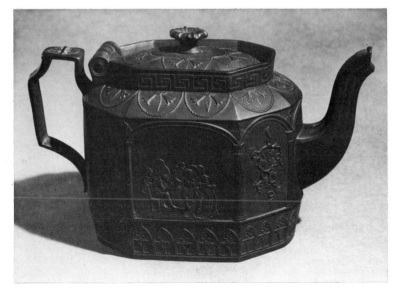

631. *Moulded basalt (Egyptian black) teapot of the 1785–95 period. Impressed initial "W" under handle. This may relate to Enoch Wood of Burslem; his trade card mentions "Egyptian black tea-pots". The initial could also relate to other manufacturers.*

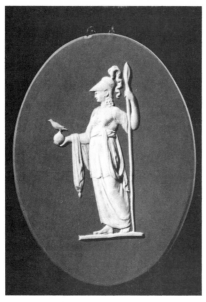

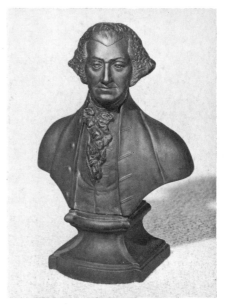

632. *Enoch Wood (impressed marked) blue and white jasper plaque of Minerva in the Wedgwood style (c. 1790–1800). 5¼ × 4 inches.*

Godden of Worthing

633. *Enoch Wood basalt bust of George Washington. Impressed mark—Enoch Wood Sculpst. 1818. 8 inches high.*

Museum & Art Gallery, Stoke-on-Trent

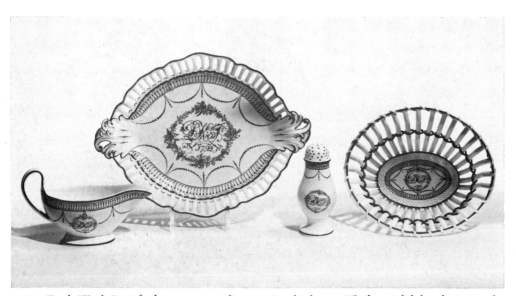

634. *Enoch Wood. Part of a large creamware dinner service, dated 1792. The largest dish has the impressed mark "E Wood", and a few other pieces have the impressed initial "W". Most of Enoch Wood's early creamwares are unmarked and specimens are attributed to other potters. Sauce boat 7 inches long.*

Trevor Antiques, Brighton

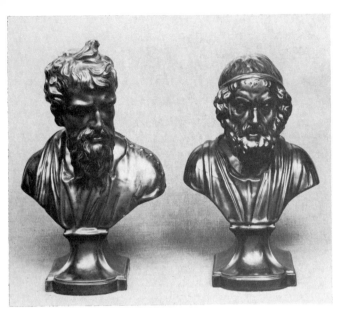

635. *Wood & Caldwell (impressed marked) earthenware busts of Plato and Homer. Decorated with bronzed effect (c. 1790–1818). 12½ and 11½ inches high.*

D. M. & P. Manheim

636. *"Wood & Caldwell" impressed marked earthenware figures, two with unusual bronze effect. Several very fine figures were made by this partnership between Enoch Wood and James Caldwell from 1790 to 1818. Wood continued as Enoch Wood & Sons. Neptune candle-holder 9¼ inches high.*

Victoria & Albert Museum

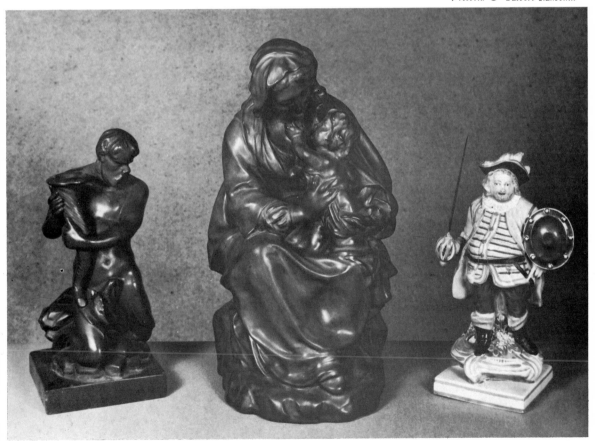

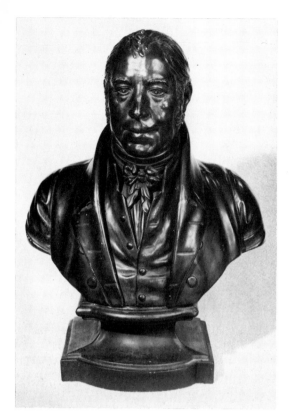

637. *Enoch Wood, master potter of Burslem, an important earthenware bust (23 inches high) signed by Enoch Wood and dated 1821.*

City Museum & Art Gallery, Stoke-on-Trent

638. (Right) *Blue transfer printed earthenware bowl by "Enoch Wood & Sons", depicting the "Entrance to the Erie Canal into the Hudson"; this is one of many American views produced by this firm at Burslem between 1818 and 1846.*

Ellouise Baker Larsen Collection, Smithsonian Institution, U.S.A.

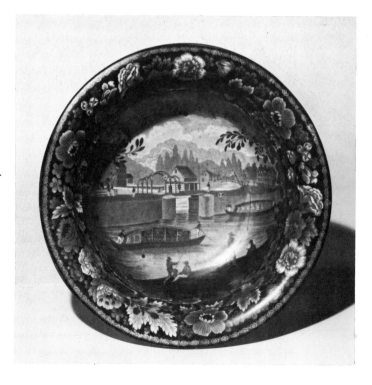

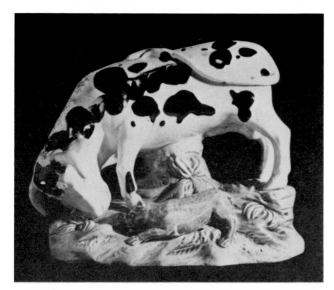

639. R. Wood (impressed marked) pottery group of a bull and dog, decorated with semi-translucent glazes (c. 1770). 6¾ inches long.

D. M. & P. Manheim

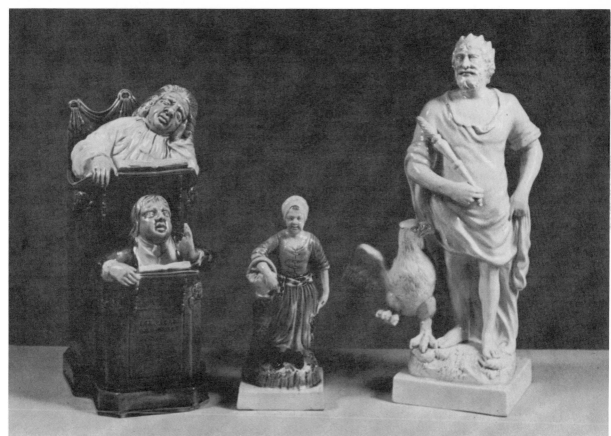

640. Ralph Wood earthenware figures (impressed marks "Ra Wood/Burslem" Vicar and Moses and on Jupiter. "R. Wood", Dutch peasant). Note the attractive semi-translucent coloured glazes on the two coloured figures. After c. 1790 the colours were opaque (c. 1770–80). Jupiter 10¼ inches high.

Victoria & Albert Museum

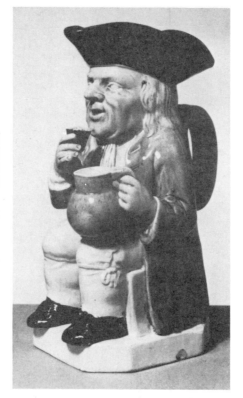

641. *"Ra Wood. Burslem" (impressed marked) earthenware Toby jug, decorated with typical semi-translucent coloured glazes. Most Toby jugs are unmarked (c. 1770–5). 9¾ inches high.*

Victoria & Albert Museum

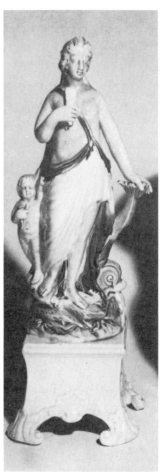

642. *"Ralph Wood. Burslem" (impressed marked) earthenware figure of c. 1770. 10¾ inches high. Note the semi-translucent coloured glazes used on Staffordshire figures, etc., before c. 1790.*

D. M. & P. Manheim

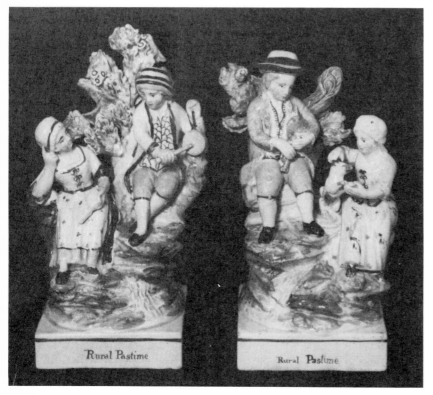

643. *Rural Pastime groups in enamelled earthenware. Impressed mark "Ra Wood. Burslem" (c. 1790). 8¾ inches high.*

D. M. & P. Manheim

The Partnership Deeds of the first Worcester Porcelain Company, originally titled the "Worcester Tonquin Manufacture", are dated 4 June 1751. It would appear from these articles that Dr John Wall and William Davis had already "invented" (or acquired) the knowledge necessary to manufacture porcelain on a commercial scale and that further, in June 1751, they already employed workmen and possessed working materials; the 18th, 19th, and 20th articles make this plain:

That all the materials and utensils that the inventors (John Wall and William Davis) are now possessed of and which are proper to carry on the work be purchased for the use of the subscribers. . . .

That the workmen and boys now employed by the inventors be deemed to have entered into the service of the subscribers in general in the said Manufacture from the eleventh day of May last.

That for the encouragement of Robert Podmore and John Lyes workmen who have for some time been employed by the inventors in the said Manufacture . . .

It is possible that Dr John Wall and William Davis had carried on lengthy experiments at Worcester before reaching the stage when they could present their "invention" to local business people for their financial support in June 1751. It is, however, more likely that they acquired the knowledge, trained workmen, and working materials from an already established porcelain works. It is probable that the factory concerned was that carried on by Benjamin Lund (and William Miller) of Bristol to whom a licence to mine soap-rock was granted in 1748 (this was purchased by Richard Holdship of the Worcester Company in 1752). The Bristol soft-paste porcelain of the late 1740's and early 1750's is remarkably similar in the type of body (containing soap-rock) and in style of decoration to the earliest Worcester porcelains. The same type of painter's signs also occurs on both porcelains and the relief mark "BRISTOL" on some sauce boats (see Plate 80) may be compared with the name "WIGORNIA" (the Roman name for Worcester) on the unique cream boat illustrated in Plate 644.

There is documentary proof that the Worcester partners, early in 1752,

on considering the state and condition of the said Bristol Manufactory had resolved it would be in their interest either to procure a Union of the said Worcester and Bristol Porcelain companies or to purchase of the said William Miller and Benjamin Lund their works or Manufactory at Bristol and the process thereof and to discontinue the same there and carry on by the said company at Worcester a Manufactory of Earthenware of both China and Dresden and that the said Richard Holdship at their request had accordingly purchased of the said William Miller and Benjamin Lund their stock, utensils and effects and the process of the said Bristol Manufactory. . . .

(quoted in H. Rissik Marshall's *Coloured Worcester Porcelain of the First Period* (1954).

This is confirmed by an announcement in the *Bristol Intelligencer* of 24 July 1752 to the effect that the Bristol porcelain manufactory was "now united with the Worcester Porcelain Company where for the future the whole Business will be carried on". The first apprentice to the Worcester works was taken on in August 1752 and on 20 September 1752 the first sale of Worcester porcelain was held "with a great variety of ware and at a reasonable price". Benjamin Lund was certainly in Worcester in February 1753 when he was described as "china maker".

It is possible that the elaborate partnership deeds of the Worcester Company signed in June 1751 were drawn up purely with the intention of acquiring the Bristol stock, utensils and materials, and that in 1751 Dr Wall and William Davis had not "invented" or produced porcelain themselves.

The workmen mentioned as being in their employment "for some time" may well have been Bristol workmen. This theory is supported in part by an advertisement in the *British Intelligencer* of 20 July 1751 which includes the following notice: "For the future no Ware will be sold at the Place where it is manufactured; nor will any Person be admitted to enter there without Leave of the Proprietors". It can be construed from this that the secrecy was imposed because negotiations were then being carried on to sell the concern to the newly formed Worcester Company. It must also be remembered that the first recorded sale of Worcester porcelain was held in September 1752, not in 1751.

It has always been thought that porcelain was first produced at Worcester in 1751 (not 1752 as now put forward as a possibility). This traditional 1751 date has always been taken for granted as the Articles of Partnership and the Lease of the Works are dated 1751, but these could have been drawn up and signed in anticipation of the purchase and transfer of the Bristol works. Mention must be made of a tureen dated on the base 1751 (or 1754), but if the indistinct date is in fact 1751 there is no proof that it was made in 1751; it could have been made in 1752, dated to commemorate the formation of the company in the previous year.

Be this as it may, porcelain was being made at Worcester in 1752 (if not in 1751) and it is very similar to soft-paste Bristol porcelain of the period *c.* 1749–52. It is similar in its neat potting, charming raised motifs, best seen on sauce or cream boats, and its neat and attractive underglaze blue painting—nearly always of Chinese figures in landscape or other designs with strong Chinese influence. The enamel painting is again neat and restrained. Ground colours were not used at this period and gilding was seldom employed. If marks occur on Worcester porcelains of the early 1750's they are in the form of painter's signs; these vary greatly and also occur on other porcelains of the period. The identification of early Worcester porcelain is based on known forms and/or patterns (see Plates 645–652), on the neat potting and close uncrazed glaze on a compact soap-rock porcelain—this can be readily recognized only by handling as often as possible authentic specimens. The Worcester paste is greenish when viewed by transmitted light.

By far the greatest proportion of early Worcester porcelain was painted with motifs in underglaze blue (that is, painted on the once fired but unglazed body); this was subsequently glazed. These charming "blue and white pieces" are illustrated in Dr B. Watney's *English Blue and White Porcelain* (1963) and in S. W. Fisher's earlier work (1947) of the same title. Other typical examples are illustrated in Plate 646. A large selection may be seen in the Dyson Perrins Museum at the Royal Worcester Works and in the Victoria & Albert Museum's collection.

By the latter half of the 1750's the now recognized factory marks—a crescent or a square Chinese fret mark (of which many different variations were employed)—were in general use, but many specimens were unmarked or bear one of the rarer marks, a "W" or the Dresden-type crossed swords. The body is rather thicker in the potting and gilding was often employed as were ground colours. The usual ground colour was underglaze blue; a popular variation of this was painted (or wiped out) into a fish scale design known as "Scale Blue" (see Plate 649, Colour Plate XVI). The blue pigment was also blown on, giving a granular effect known as "powder blue"; this occurs in a dark tint and in a lighter greyish blue. The scale blue is highly favoured with most collectors. The scale design also occurs with other overglaze colours—yellow, red, pink, or purple, but these are very rare.

All ground colours are decorative and rare and consequently highly valued. Yellow is one of the most sought after. A pale, warm yellow occurs on quite early pieces (*c.* 1755–60) while harder yellows are found on later wares of the 1770s. It must always be remembered that these desirable ground colours have often been added to enrich ordinary patterns; such work was carried out in the nineteenth century, and specimens can be found today in the oldest and most respected collections. Harsh opaque colours should be treated with great suspicion, especially if the body or glaze shows black specks. Other rare ground colours include sky blue, pink, purple, and the apple green. The gilding would not take on this last colour, so the gilt borders, etc., are always slightly away from the edge of the ground colour. Many of the "blue and white" pieces after about 1765 were produced by printing from engraved copperplates, the inked design being transferred from the copperplates to the unglazed porcelain by means of thin tissue-like paper. Pieces decorated by this method usually bear a cross-hatched or filled-in crescent as opposed to the outlined or open crescent mark found on other pieces. A very popular form of printing pre-dates the underglaze blue variety; this is overglaze and is generally in a black pigment (purple also occurs). There is great range and beauty in these black printed pieces, some of the best specimens of which bear the signature or initials of Robert Hancock, the master engraver, see Plate 645. Several of these printed patterns are washed over with enamels and slightly gilt. Few pieces bearing overglaze prints are marked—if a mark does appear it is often the crossed swords with or without numerals between the hilts. Cyril Cook's *The Life and Work of Robert Hancock* (1948) and the 1955 supplement are indispensable reference books for the collector of Worcester overglaze printed wares.

Most enamelled patterns are floral in character; some were based on Chinese and Japanese flower designs, others copy Dresden floral patterns, others again were painted with naturalistic English flowers or floral groups. A large and decorative group of Worcester porcelains were painted with exotic birds in landscape. Figure or animal subjects are very rare. Some charming paintings of Chinese style figures are associated with Chelsea artists who decorated Worcester porcelain after the closure of the Chelsea factory. Spirited animal painting, often depicting fable scenes, was done by O'Neale. Many attractive and unusual patterns were painted by outside decorators in London, of these the best known is James Giles of Kentish Town, who issued several advertisements to "procure and paint for any person Worcester porcelain to any or in any pattern". Colourful paintings of fruit, often with some cut open, are often attributed to Giles's workshop and also some of the colourful paintings of exotic birds in landscapes.

While the vast majority of early Worcester porcelains were confined to useful wares (tea services, dessert services, tankards, jugs, etc.) and vases, other objects were made, but these are very rare and are normally unmarked; such rarities include figures, cauliflower tureens, cornucopia, dove tureens (only one is recorded), partridge tureens, and shell centrepieces. A very large selection of patterns and forms are illustrated in H. Rissik Marshall's *Coloured Worcester Porcelain of the First Period* (1954). The following books by Henry Sandon are all but indispensable: *The Illustrated Guide to Worcester Porcelain* (1969); *Royal Worcester Porcelain* (3rd edition, 1978) and *Flight & Barr Worcester Porcelain* (1978). Large collections may be seen at the Worcester Works Museum and at the Victoria & Albert Museum in London.

In 1783 the "Dr. Wall" or "First Period" came to an end and in September 1783 the former London agent, Thomas Flight, purchased the concern for his sons, the price being three thousand pounds. New simple patterns were introduced; tasteful borders or floral springs and fluted forms were much favoured. The former blue crescent mark was continued, but was generally painted smaller than had been the case in the Dr Wall period. After a visit by George III and Queen Charlotte to the works in 1788 a crown was added to the crescent mark and the word "Royal" to the firm's title. The impressed mark "FLIGHT" also occurs as does several written marks incorporating the name.

One of the Flights (John) died in 1791, and in 1792 his brother Joseph took Martin Barr into partnership. The former marks were discontinued and the names "Flight & Barr" or the initials "F. & B." were used. The incised initial "B" with or without a small cross also occurs on pieces made between 1792 and 1807. In 1807 Martin Barr's son was taken into partnership under the style "Barr, Flight & Barr". Marks of this period include these names or the initials "B.F.B.". Martin Barr Senr. died in November 1813 and the style of the firm became "Flight, Barr & Barr", repeated in the many printed marks employed. The standard impressed mark was "F.B.B." under a crown. In 1840 the two firms of Flight, Barr & Barr and Messrs Chamberlains were combined and continued as "Chamberlain & Co" (see page 57). Messrs Chamberlain was succeeded by Kerr & Binns in 1852 and the present "Royal Worcester" Company was formed in 1862.

The quality of Worcester porcelains of the Barr, Flight & Barr and Flight, Barr & Barr period are of the highest standard, both in potting, in general design, and in the painted decoration. The management employed the then novel step of paying the artists by time instead of by the piece. The piece rate of course encouraged the painters to rush their work, whereas the time rate enabled them to lavish all their skill on the porcelain and the Barrs, on their twice daily inspection, frequently encouraged the painters to consider their work as jewellery and to take "all possible pains". Information on many of the artists of the period is included in my *British Pottery and Porcelain, 1780–1850* (1963) and in the new revised 15th edition of Chaffer's *Marks and Monograms* (1965). Typical specimens of the period are illustrated in Plates 660–3. Good representative displays can be seen at the Victoria & Albert Museum or at the Dyson Perrins Museum at the Worcester works.

Readers must be warned of reproductions of "Dr. Wall" or "First Period" Worcester of the more expensive kinds. Many of these have now acquired their own ageing as they were made over sixty years ago; some were made on the Continent and are of the hard, cold porcelain made there. Colourful scale-blue patterns with exotic bird panels were largely featured and the old marks were often copied. Another class of reproduction was made in England, by Booths of Tunstall; a crescent-like mark was often used, but these wares are of opaque earthenware rather than translucent porcelain. The most dangerous class of reproduction consists of the pieces that were "enhanced" by added decoration, ground colours, etc., in the nineteenth century for the original porcelain body was used; the decorators enriched a poorly decorated or blue and white specimen with all the correct characteristics of paste, glaze, etc., and, of course, the shape is correct. Experience only will teach the new collector to detect these pieces which, in general, appear "stiff" in the painting with rather bubbled opaque colours. Black spots appear on most refired examples; a black footrim should always be regarded with suspicion.

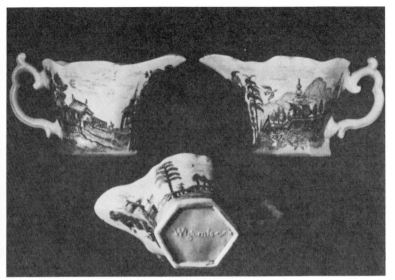

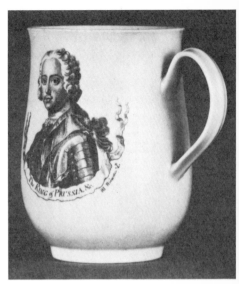

644. *Unique Worcester porcelain cream boat with moulded mark "Wigornia" (the Roman name for Worcester). Moulded and coloured over Chinese landscape pattern, other unmarked specimens are recorded (c. 1751). 2½ inches high.*

Present owner unknown.
Photo supplied by Tilley & Co

645. *Dr Wall, or first, period Worcester porcelain mug, decorated with black (jet) printed pattern, showing "R H", the initials of R. Hancock or of R. Holdship, the place-name "Worcester", and the anchor rebus of Holdship. In the ribbon above this mark is the further inscription "Hancock fecit. Worcester" (c. 1757). 5¼ inches high.*

Victoria & Albert Museum

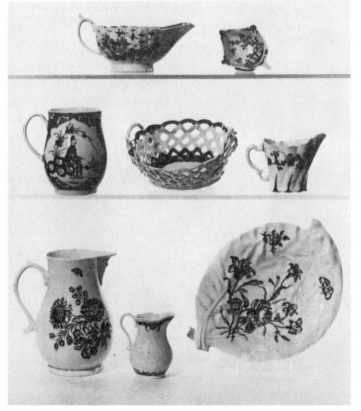

646. *First period Worcester porcelains, painted in underglaze blue (c. 1755–65). The small leaf dish has a painter's sign, the basket has a square mark, the other examples have an open crescent mark in underglaze blue. Large jug 6¾ inches high.*

Godden of Worthing

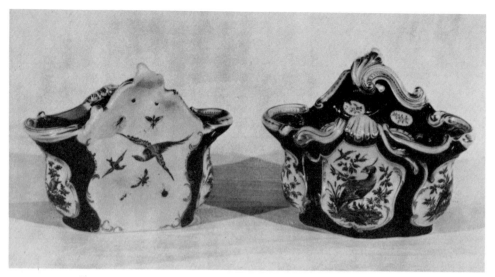

647. *Dr Wall period bulb pots with typical Worcester decoration—exotic birds in panels on a scale-blue ground. One is reversed to show typical bird and insect painting. Square mark in underglaze blue (see Plate 650a) (c. 1760).*

Godden of Worthing

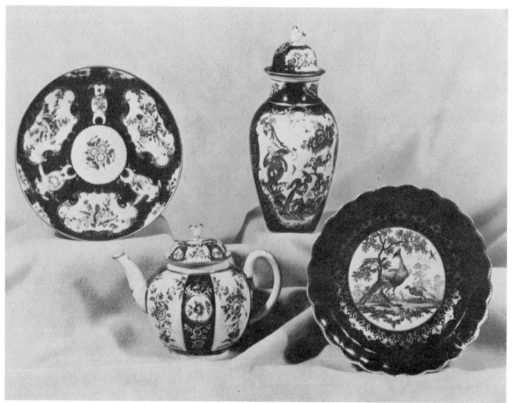

648. *Typical Worcester porcelains of the first, or Dr Wall, period, all marked with the square mark in underglaze blue (as mark no. 4315) (c. 1760–70).*

Worcester Works Museum

649. *Square marked Worcester porcelain vase (one of a pair) of the first period, showing typical exotic birds in panels, on a rich scale-blue ground (c. 1765–70). 16 inches high.*

Delomosne & Son

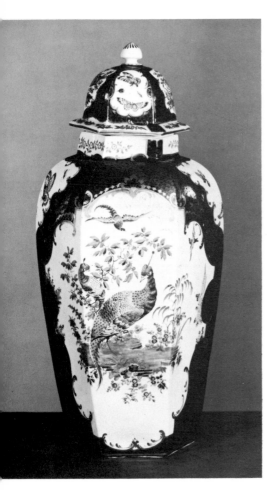

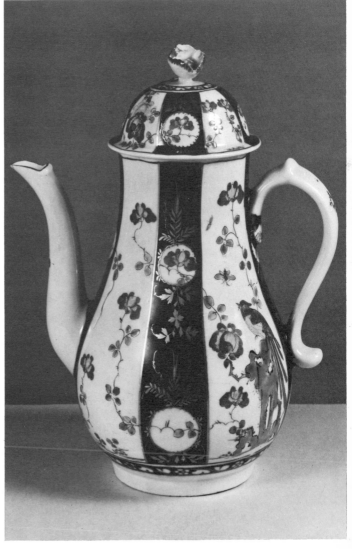

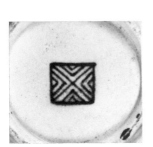

650. a. *Typical Worcester square mark in underglaze blue.*

650. *Square marked Worcester porcelain coffee pot of the first, or Dr Wall, period. This graceful shape is typical, also the use of underglaze blue panels and borders in conjunction with overglaze enamels (c. 1765–75). 9 inches high.*

Victoria & Albert Museum

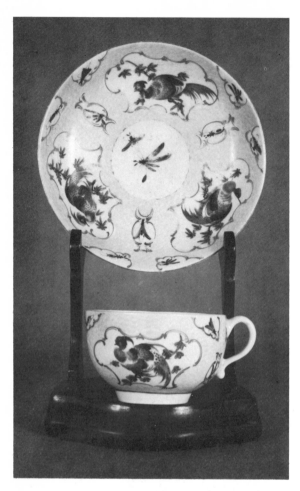

651. *Worcester porcelain cup and saucer with rare yellow scale ground. Crossed swords and "9" mark in underglaze blue (c. 1760–70).*

G. Stevens Collection, Brighton Museum

652. *A very rare pair of Dr Wall, or first, period Worcester porcelain plates. Crescent mark painted in underglaze blue (c. 1770).*

Delomosne & Son

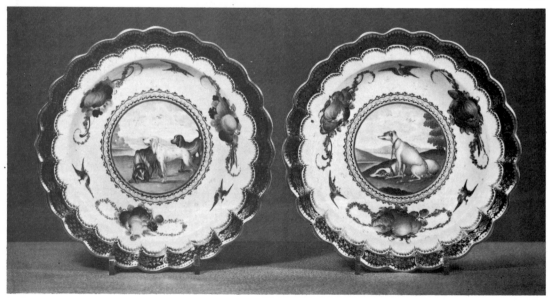

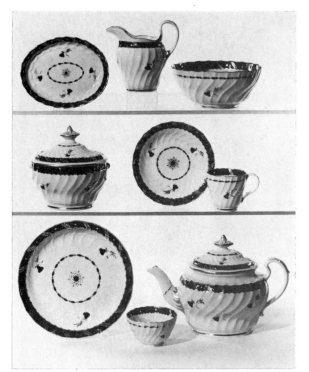

653. *Flight period Worcester teaset, showing typical fluted forms of the 1783–8 period, and restrained decoration in underglaze blue with gilt enrichments. Blue painted "Flight" and crescent mark. Teapot 6½ inches high.*

Godden of Worthing

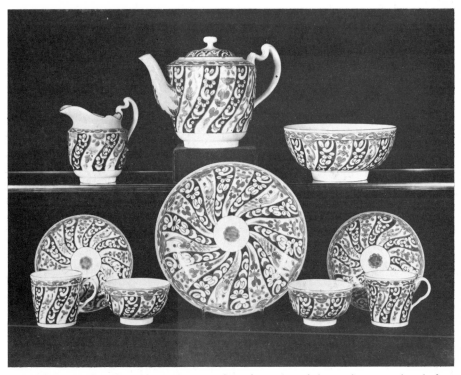

654. *Flight period (1783–92) Worcester porcelain of a traditional design—known as the wheel, or whorl, pattern. Mark "Flight" written in underglaze blue.*

Delomosne & Son

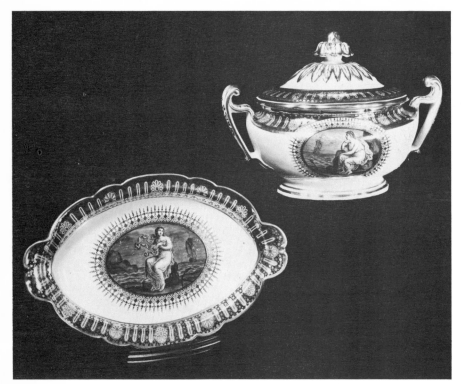

655. *Flight period Worcester tureen cover and under dish from a dinner service made in 1792 for the Duke of Clarence (later to become William IV). This service, often called the Hope service on account of the figure subjects depicting Hope, was painted by John Pennington. This form of tureen is confined to the Flight period (1783–92). Painted mark (in underglaze blue)—crown, the word "Flight" with a crescent below.*

Marshall Field & Co, Chicago

656. *Worcester porcelains of the 1785–1820 period. Barr, Flight & Barr cup and saucer, painted with panels of shells on a marbled ground. Written mark no. 4340 (c. 1807–13). Mask head jug, decorated in blue and gold. Blue "Flight" mark (c. 1783–92). Fine quality mug, written mark "Flight & Barr, Worcester" (under a crown) (c. 1792–1807). Covered vase of the finest quality, impressed mark "FBB" with crown, also written name and address mark (1813–30).*

Worcester Works Museum

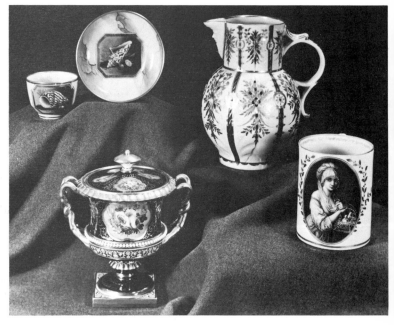

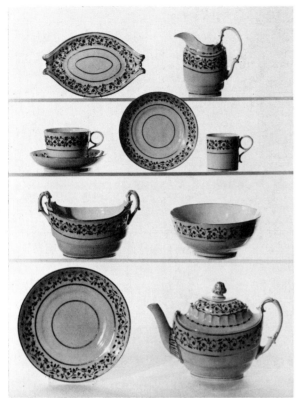

657. *Barr Worcester tea service, showing typical forms and restrained style of decoration. Incised marks "B" and "Bx" (c. 1792–1807). Teapot 6¾ inches high.*

Godden of Worthing

658. *Part of a Barr, Flight & Barr Worcester dessert service, bearing printed mark, no. 4341, and impressed initial mark, no. 4339. This colourful pattern called Bishop Sumner was produced by the main Worcester factory from c. 1780 to c. 1840, also by the Chamberlain factory at Worcester and at the Caughley and Coalport Works. These shapes are typical of the period. Ice pail and cover 11½ inches high.*

Godden of Worthing

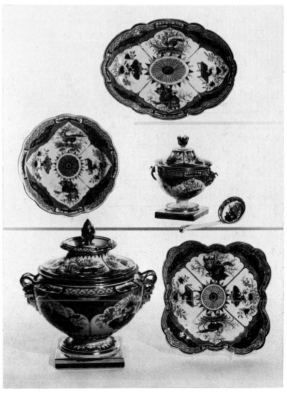

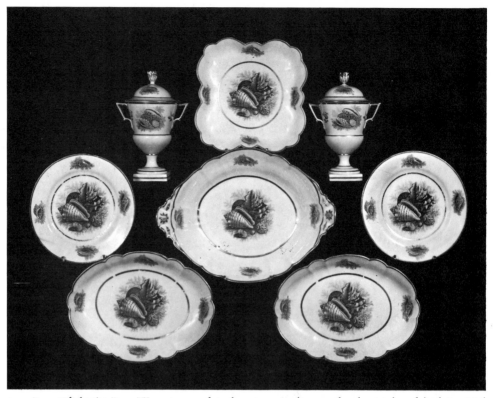

659. *Barr, Flight & Barr Worcester porcelain dessert service (impressed and printed marks), bat printed with shell motifs. The dish shapes are typical Worcester forms, but the vase shaped sauce tureens are very rare. Shell motifs, both printed and painted, occur on fine quality Worcester porcelains of this period (c. 1807–13).*
Delomosne & Son

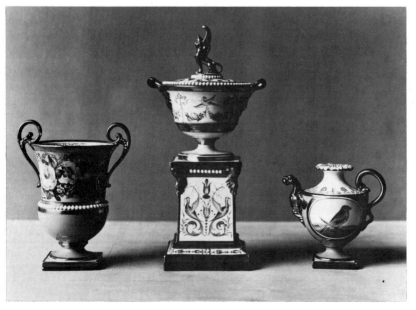

660. *Barr, Flight & Barr (written mark with address) potpourri vase with two covers, one pierced (1807–13). The two small open vases are Flight, Barr & Barr (c. 1813–20) and bear full written marks. All three examples show the fine quality of Worcester porcelains of this period. The simple square bases with gilt top edges are typical. Centre vase 8¾ inches high.*

Victoria & Albert Museum

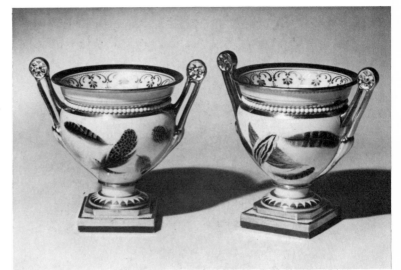

661. *Flight, Barr & Barr vases painted with feathers. This style of decoration is rare and examples are always of fine quality (c. 1813–20). Impressed initial mark no. 4343, also painted name and address mark. 5½ inches high.*

Godden of Worthing

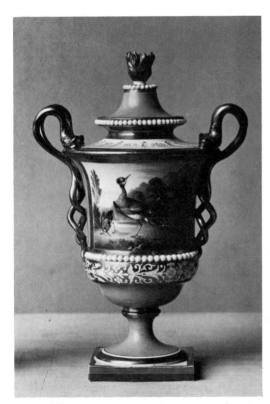

662. *Flight, Barr & Barr Worcester vase with written mark—"Flight Barr & Barr/Royal Porcelain Works/Worcester/London House/1 Coventry Street". Also standard impressed mark "FBB" with crown above (c. 1813–20). 9⅛ inches high.*

Victoria & Albert Museum

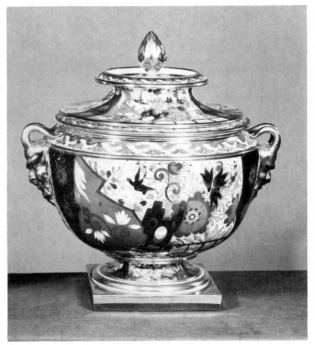

663. *Impressed marked "FBB" (under a crown) Worcester ice pail (one of a pair) decorated with typical, fine quality "Japan" pattern (c. 1813–20). 11 inches high.*

Delomosne & Son

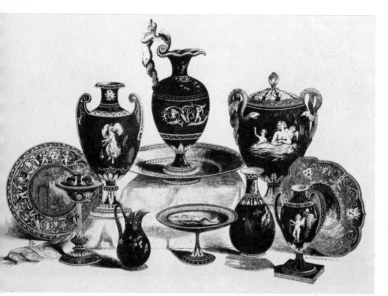

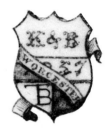

664. *Kerr & Binns' "Worcester Enamels", painted in the Limoges enamel style by Thomas Bott. Reproduced from the* Art Journal, *1857, such wares will bear the printed shield shaped mark no. 4346, shown above.*

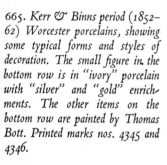

665. *Kerr & Binns period (1852–62) Worcester porcelains, showing some typical forms and styles of decoration. The small figure in the bottom row is in "ivory" porcelain with "silver" and "gold" enrichments. The other items on the bottom row are painted by Thomas Bott. Printed marks nos. 4345 and 4346.*

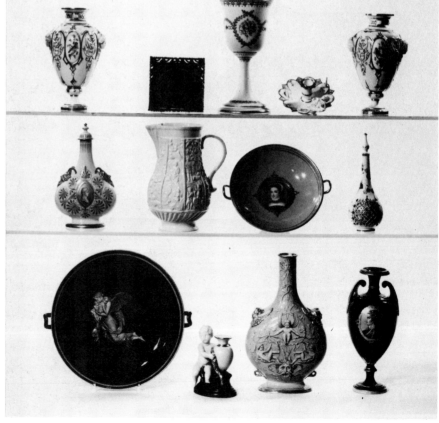

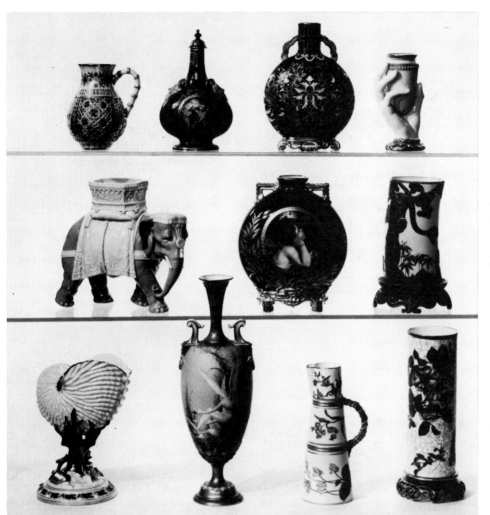

666. Royal Worcester porcelains, bearing standard printed marks nos. 4349, 4350 and 4354, often with code letters showing year of production (see companion Encyclopaedia of Marks). These vase shapes occur with other types of decoration. The swan painting is by C. H. Baldwyn; this vase is 13 inches high.

Godden of Worthing

667. Royal Worcester "Jewelled" porcelain of the finest quality. Part of a special service made for the Countess of Dudley in 1865. Painted heads by Thomas Callowhill, gilding and jewelling by Samuel Randford. Printed mark no. 4349.

Worcester Works Museum

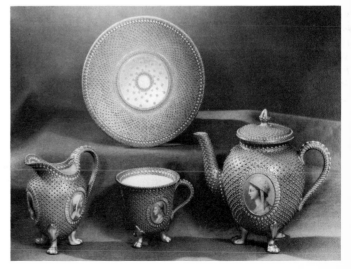

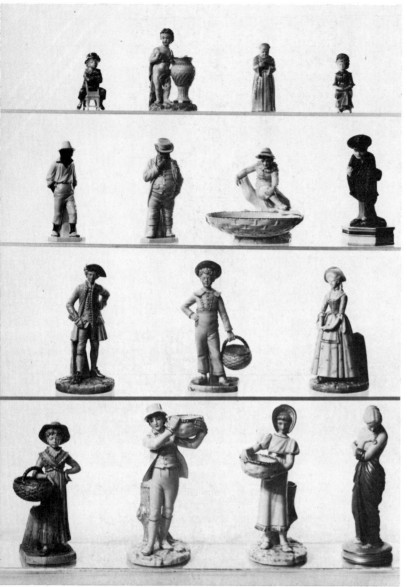

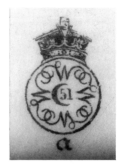

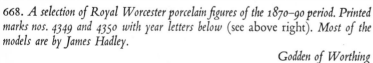

668. *A selection of Royal Worcester porcelain figures of the 1870–90 period. Printed marks nos. 4349 and 4350 with year letters below (see above right). Most of the models are by James Hadley.*

Godden of Worthing

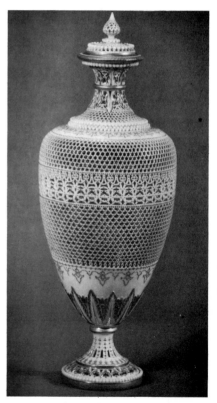

669. *Royal Worcester reticulated vase, worked by George Owen. The finest specimens in this delicate style bear Owen's signature as well as the printed mark no. 4354. Most examples date from the 1880's.*

Worcester Works Museum (Pottery Gazette copyright)

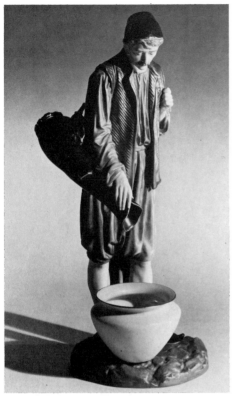

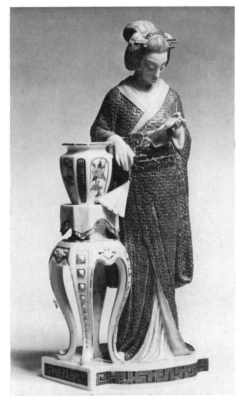

670. *Royal Worcester figure of a water-carrier, one of a pair modelled by James Hadley (c. 1883). This model shows the fine quality Royal Worcester tinted gold decoration, both matt and burnished. Printed mark no. 4350. 18 inches high.*

Godden of Worthing

671. *Royal Worcester figure (one of a pair) modelled by James Hadley, and shown at the 1873 Vienna Exhibition. Printed mark no. 4349. 15½ inches high.*

J. YATES, HANLEY *c.* 1784–1835

672. *Yates (impressed marked) basalt teapot (c. 1820–5), 6⅜ inches high. Marked examples by John Yates of Shelton are rare, although this potter worked from c. 1784 to c. 1828. Several other Yates are recorded.*

Victoria & Albert Museum

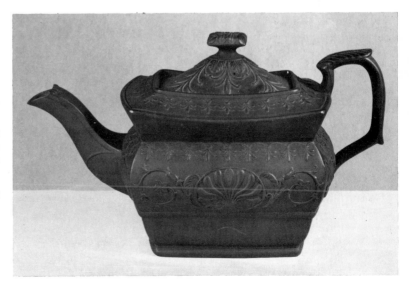

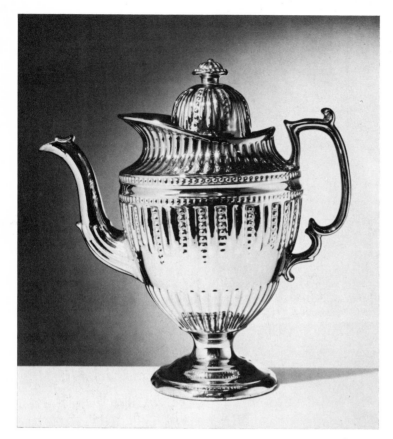

673. *Silver lustre tea or coffee pot. Rare impressed anchor mark, maker unknown (c. 1825). 5¾ inches high.*
Victoria & Albert Museum

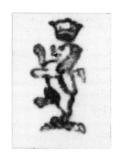

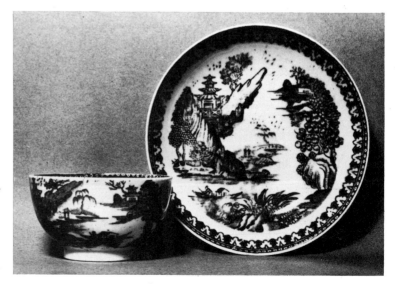

674. *New Hall-type blue printed porcelain teabowl and saucer, with the very rare crowned lion mark (c. 1790). Attribution open to some doubt.*

National Museum of Wales

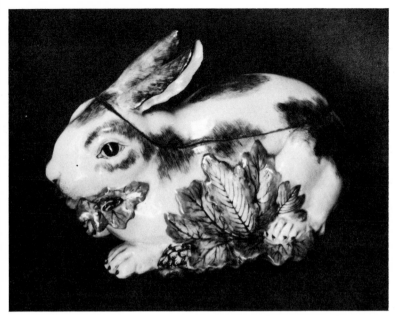

675. *Hard-paste copy of a Chelsea rabbit tureen. In this case the mark was not copied and this specimen bears the Samson cross mark, see mark book, page 730.* $8\frac{3}{4}$ *inches long.*

Sotheby's "Rogues" Gallery

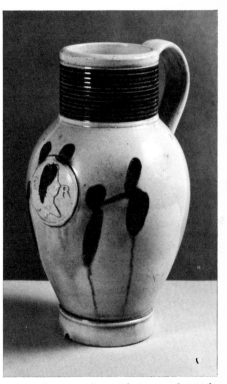

677. *Stoneware jug with impressed initial mark "W T & Co". I have been unable to trace an eighteenth-century English firm with these initials before William Tomlinson & Co of the Knottingley Pottery, Yorkshire,* c. 1792–6. $6\frac{1}{4}$ *inches high.*

Victoria & Albert Museum

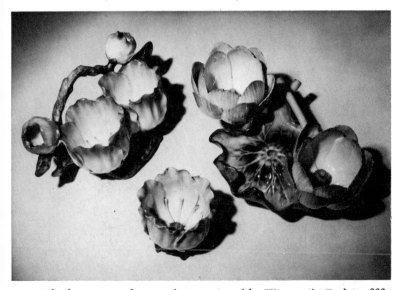

676. *Floral ornaments of various designs registered by Wittman & Roth in 1888. These specimens which bear the painted initials W & R with a number, are often attributed to English firms of an earlier period. Right hand example 11 inches long.*

Godden of Worthing

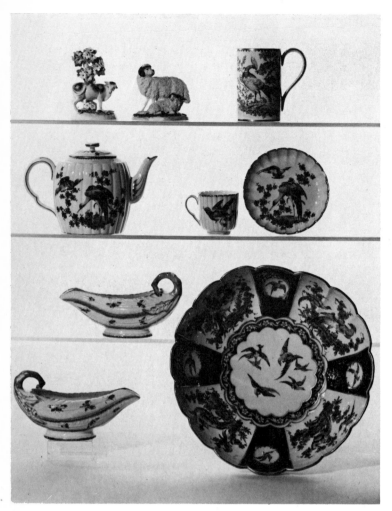

678. *Hard-paste Continental fakes of English porcelains. Specimens on the top two rows are marked with a large gold anchor. The leaf-pattern sauce boats (the originals are usually unmarked) have a very large red anchor mark. The circular Worcester-type dish is unmarked, but other reproductions of this type have a faked square mark, or crescent mark as used at Worcester. Some fake Worcester bears the gold anchor mark of Chelsea, as is the case with the teapot and cup and saucer (late nineteenth century). Dish $11\frac{3}{4}$ inches diameter.*

679. *Advertisement showing typical Worcester and Lowestoft reproductions produced in Paris in the early years of the present century, in hard paste, not soft paste (see page xviii).*

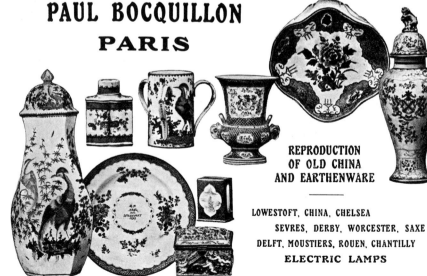

PAUL BOCQUILLON
PARIS

**REPRODUCTION
OF OLD CHINA
AND EARTHENWARE**

LOWESTOFT, CHINA, CHELSEA
SEVRES, DERBY, WORCESTER, SAXE
DELFT, MOUSTIERS, ROUEN, CHANTILLY
ELECTRIC LAMPS

Selected Bibliography

This list includes only general ceramic reference books—specialized works are listed in the appropriate outline histories of the main firms or in the historical introduction. The general books are listed below in date order:

History of the Staffordshire Potteries, S. Shaw, 1829

The Ceramic Art of Great Britain, L. Jewitt, 1878, revised 1883

The Art of the Old English Potter, M. L. Solon, 1883

A History and Description of English Porcelain, W. Burton, 1902

Catalogue of the Collection of English Pottery . . . in the British Museum, R. L. Hobson, 1903

English Earthenware and Stoneware, W. Burton, 1904

Staffordshire Pots and Potters, G. W. & F. A. Rhead, 1906

The 1st century of English Porcelain, W. M. Binns, 1906

English Earthenware, A. H. Church, 1911

The A.B.C. of English Saltglaze Stoneware, J. F. Blacker, 1922

Scottish Pottery, J. A. Fleming, 1923

Guide to Collectors of Pottery and Porcelain, F. Litchfield, 1925

English Porcelain Figures of the 18th century, W. King, 1925

English Porcelain Circles Transactions, 1928–31, continued as *English Ceramic Circles Transactions*, 1931–

Catalogue of the Schreiber Collection, V. & A., vols.I and II, 1929

English Blue and White Porcelain of the 18th century, S. W. Fisher, 1947

English Pottery Figures, 1660–1860, R. G. Haggar, 1947

Medieval English Pottery, B. Rackham, 1948

English Delftware, F. H. Garner, 1948

English Country Pottery, R. G. Haggar, 1950

Old English Lustre Pottery, W. D. John, 1951

Nineteenth Century English Pottery and Porcelain, G. Bemrose, 1952

Eighteenth Century English Porcelain, G. Savage, 1952

Staffordshire Chimney Ornaments, R. G. Haggar, 1955

English Porcelain and Bone China, 1743–1850, B. & T. Hughes, 1955

A Picture History of English Pottery, G. Lewis, 1956

The Concise Encyclopaedia of English Pottery and Porcelain, R. G. Haggar and W. Mankowitz, 1957

English Cream-Coloured Earthenware, D. Towner, 1957

Victorian Pottery and Porcelain, G. B. Hughes, 1959

Victorian Porcelain, G. A. Godden, 1961

Victorian Pottery, H. Wakefield, 1962

English Pottery and Porcelain, W. B. Honey, 5th edition, 1962

English Blue and White Porcelain, Dr B. Watney, 1963

British Pottery and Porcelain, 1780–1850, G. A. Godden, 1963

Encyclopaedia of British Pottery and Porcelain Marks, G. A. Godden, 1964

British Porcelain, 1745–1850, edited by R. J. Charleston, 1965

Marks and Monograms . . ., W. Chaffer's 15th edition, vol. II revised by G. A. Godden, 1965

English Ceramics, S. Fisher, 1966

Eighteenth Century English Porcelain Figures, P. Bradshaw, 1981

Staffordshire Pottery, A. Oliver, 1982